Solid Organ Transplantation

A Handbook For
Primary Health Care Providers

Sandra Ann Cupples, DNSc., RN, is the Heart Transplant Coordinator at The Washington Hospital Center, Washington, DC. She received her BSN degree from Duquesne University, Pittsburgh, PA, her MSN from Boston University, and her doctorate from The Catholic University of America, Washington, DC. Dr. Cupples is an Associate Editor of *Progress in Transplantation* and has authored numerous articles about transplantation, including several studies that have examined quality of life issues associated with the pretransplant period. She has been invited to speak at national and international conferences on transplantation. As a Commander in the United States Navy Reserve Nurse Corps, Dr. Cupples serves as the Associate Director for Cardiovascular and Critical Care Services at the National Naval Medical Center, Bethesda, MD.

Linda Ohler, MSN, RN, CCTC, FAAN. At the time this book was written, Ms. Ohler was nurse manager of the Organ and Tissue Transplant Research Unit at the National Institutes of Health in Bethesda, Maryland. Before joining NIH, Linda was a heart and lung transplant coordinator at Temple University in Philadelphia and at Inova Fairfax Hospital in Falls Church, Virginia. Since 1994, Linda has served as Editor for *Progress in Transplantation* (formerly the *Journal of Transplant Coordination*). She has spoken on transplant-related issues throughout the United States, in Japan, Italy, Russia, Hungary, India and Canada. Ms. Ohler has served as a Co-Investigator in several multicenter transplant research studies. She received her BSN from Marymount University in Arlington, Virginia and her MSN from The Catholic University of America in Washington, DC.

Solid Organ Transplantation

A Handbook For
Primary Health Care Providers

Sandra A. Cupples, DNSc, RN
Linda Ohler, MSN, RN, CCTC, FAAN
Editors

 Springer Publishing Company

Springer Publishing Company, Inc.
536 Broadway
New York, NY 10012-3955

Acquisitions Editor: Ruth Chasek
Production Editor: Jeanne W. Libby
Cover design by Joanne E. Honigman

01 02 03 04 05 / 5 4 3 2 1

Library of Congress Cataloging-in-Publication Data

Solid organ transplantation : a handbook for primary health care providers / Sandra A. Cupples, Linda Ohler, editors.
  p. ; cm.
  Includes bibliographical references and index.
  ISBN 0-8261-1906-9
  1. Transplantation of organs, tissues, etc.—Handbooks, manuals, etc.   2. Primary care (Medicine)—Handbooks, manuals, etc.
  I. Cupples, Sandra A. (Sandra Ann)   II. Ohler, Linda.
  [DNLM: 1. Organ Transplantation.   2. Physicians, Family.
  3. Primary Health Care. WO 660 S6857 2002]
  RD120.7 .S654 2002
  617.9'5—dc21   2002070588

Printed in the United States of America by Maple-Vail Book Manufacturing Group

---

Every effort has been made to check the accuracy of the content of this book. However, medicine is always evolving and changing with new research findings and clinical practices. For this reason, readers are advised to check the most current product information provided by the manufacturers of each drug to verify recommended dose, method of administration, and contraindications. It is the responsibility of the treating physician, nurses, or other health care provider to determine the best treatment and dosages for each individual patient. Neither the Publisher nor the editors assumes any liability for any injury to persons or property arising from this publication.

Contents

Contributors

Vincent T. Armenti, MD, PhD, is a transplant surgeon and professor of surgery at Thomas Jefferson University. Dr. Armenti is principal investigator of the National Transplant Pregnancy Registry (NTPR).

Marilyn Rossman Bartucci, MSN, RN, CS, CCTC, received her Bachelor of Science degree in nursing from Marquette University and her Master of Science degree in nursing from Case Western Reserve University, Frances Payne Bolton School of Nursing. She has had 28 years of experience in the care of kidney and pancreas transplant recipients and is certified as a clinical transplant coordinator and clinical specialist. Ms. Bartucci is a clinical faculty member at Case Western Reserve University, Frances Payne Bolton School of Nursing and Kent State University College of Nursing. She currently is the Senior Medical Science Liaison for Fujisawa Healthcare, Inc.

Steven W. Boyce, MD, graduated from the University of Maryland Medical School and completed his residency at the University of California, San Francisco. He trained at UCLA in cardiothoracic surgery and later joined the Washington Hospital Center where he served as Director of Cardiac Transplantation and the Mechanical Circulatory Assist Device Programs. He is currently Assistant Clinical Professor of Surgery at Georgetown University.

Cyala Calhoun-Wilson, MSW, is a Clinical Transplant Social Worker at the Nazih Zuhdi Transplantation Institute, Oklahoma City, Oklahoma. She has her BA in Social Work, and MSW, both from the University of Oklahoma.

Lisa A. Coscia, BSN, RN, has worked with transplant recipients in various capacities for 10 years. She is currently a research coordinator for the National Transplant Pregnancy Registry and has coauthored several publications with the NTPR.

John M. Davison, MD, who has a particular interest in transplant recipients, is an obstetrician and gynecologist at the Royal Victoria Infirmary in Newcastle upon Tyne, England. Dr. Davison has published numerous articles and chapters on pregnancy after transplantation and has helped to develop a pregnancy registry in the United Kingdom. He has also collaborated with the NTPR.

Barbara S. DiMercurio, RN, is the Chief, Nurse Consultant for the Immune Tolerance Network, National Institutes of Health, Division of Allergy, Immunology and Transplantation. At the time this chapter was written, Ms. DiMercurio was a Research Nurse/Transplant Coordinator for the Renal and Islet Cell Transplant Program at the National Institutes of Health. She has worked in the field of solid organ transplantation for five years.

Mary Douglas, RN, MSN, CCTC, is the Senior Clinical Transplant Coordinator at the University of Wisconsin Hospital and Clinics. Ms. Douglas has served as a chairperson for Contemporary Forums' Advances in Transplantation for the past five years and has taught extensively on liver, kidney, and pancreas transplantation.

Isao Fukunishi, MD, PhD, is Director of Liaison Psychiatry at the Tokyo Institute of Psychiatry. He received his MD at Tokushima University School of Medicine, Tokushima, Japan, and his Ph.D. at Department of Neuropsychiatry, Kagawa Medical School, Kagawa, Japan, 1990.

William Garmoe, PhD, is a neuropsychologist who is the co-director of the Brain Injury Program and Coordinator of Neuropsychology Services at National Rehabilitation Hospital in Washington, D.C. His clinical work involves assessment and treatment of adults with brain injury, dementia, and other neurologic syndromes. He also is a consultant to the Washington Hospital Center cardiac transplant program. Dr. Garmoe performs research in the area of brain injury, and his publications include studies of self-awareness following traumatic brain injury, pharmacologic enhancement of cognition following brain dysfunction, and mild brain injury.

Daniele K. Gelone, PharmD, received her Doctor of Pharmacy from Temple University in 1999. She completed a pharmacy practice residency with an emphasis on long term/palliative care at Thomas Jefferson University Hospital in Philadelphia. Dr. Gelone is currently a Transplant and Immunology Pharmacotherapy Research Fellow at the University of Michigan. In 2002, Dr. Gelone was awarded the American College of Clinical Pharmacy Transplantation Research Fellowship.

David Harlan, MD, received his MD from Duke University. He currently serves as Chief of the Transplant and Autoimmunity Branch of the National Institute of Diabetes, Digestive, and Kidney Disease (NIDDK) at the National Institutes of Health. As an endocrinologist by training, with long-standing interest in the pathogenesis and treatment of Type 1 diabetes, Dr. Harlan is directing a research program exploring immune system function so as to better understand the cause of TIDM.

Jeanette Hasse, PhD, RN, LD, FADA, CSND, has worked in the critical care nutrition field for 17 years and has worked full-time with transplant patients since 1986. She has been involved in related research and development of nutrition care protocols. Jeanette has given many professional presentations and has several publications on nutrition and transplantation. Dr. Hasse is past Editor of *Support Line,* a publication of Dietitians in Nutrition Support. She is the recipient of the 1998 American Dietetic Association Foundation Award for Excellence in Clinical Nutrition and received the 1994 A.S.P.E.N. Dietitian Research Award. Jeanette received her BS degree in Nutrition at the University of Nebraska and received her MS and PhD degrees in Nutrition at Texas Women's University.

Leonard Henry, MD, is a Lt. Commander in the United States Navy and is Chief Resident in General Surgery at Bethesda Naval Hospital. Dr. Henry received his MD at the University of Michigan. His transplant rotation was at NIH with Dr. Allan Kirk.

Simon Horslen, MB, ChB, MRCP (UK), FRCPCH, is a Pediatric Hepatologist, Transplant Physician and Professor of Pediatrics at the University of Nebraska, Omaha. He is a graduate of Bristol University Medical School in England and did postgraduate training in general pediatrics, pediatric gastroenterology and hepatology in the United kingdom.

Donald E. Hricik, MD, is Professor of Medicine and Chief, Division of Nephrology at Case Western Reserve University and Medical Director, Transplantation Services, University Hospitals of Cleveland. Dr. Hricik's research interests are clinical outcomes after kidney and pancreas transplantation, complications of immunosuppression, and immune monitoring.

Allan D. Kirk, MD, PhD, is the Section Chief for Organ and Tissue Transplant Research in the Autoimmunity and Transplantation Branch of the National Institute of Diabetes, Digestive and Kidney Diseases (NIDDK), National Institutes of Health in Bethesda, Maryland. Dr. Kirk completed his MD at Duke University and his Residency and Fellowship at the University of Wisconsin as an abdominal transplant surgeon. He has published numerous articles on his research in tolerance, co-stimulation and transplantation.

Kathleen D. Lake, PharmD, BCPS, is the Director of Transplant Therapeutics at the University of Michigan Health Systems in Ann Arbor. She has worked in solid organ transplantation since 1985 and specializes in pharmacotherapy of transplant patients. Her research has focused on areas of drug interactions, immunosuppressant pharmacokinetics and dynamics. Dr. Lake's clinical focus has been in the management of posttransplant complications including hypertension, diabetes, hyperlipidemia, and osteoporosis. She has served as Editor of the Transplant Pharmacy Newsletter as well as Past-President and Fellow of the American College of Clinical Pharmacy. She is a graduate of the University of Minnesota.

Alan Langnas, DO, is a Professor of Surgery, Chief, Section of Transplantation and Director of Liver and Intestinal Transplantation Programs at the University of Nebraska.

Daniel R. Lucey, MD, MPH, FACP, is Chief of the Infectious Diseases Division, Washington Hospital Center, Washington, D.C. and Professor of Medicine, Uniformed Services University of the Health Sciences, Bethesda, MD. Dr. Lucey obtained his medical degree from Dartmouth Medical School and his master of public health degree from the Harvard School of Public Health. He completed his internal medicine residency at the University of California, San Francisco and his infectious disease fellowship at Harvard University Brigham & Womens' Hospital, Beth Israel Hospital, and the Dana Farber Cancer Institute.

Martha Markovitz, MSW, is a Clinical Pediatric Transplant Social Worker at the St. Louis Childrens Hospital at Washington University School of Medicine. She has a BA degree in Child Development from Connecticut College, and a MSW from the University of Pennsylvania.

Carolyn H. McGrory, MS, RN, is a research coordinator for the NTPR and has been a coauthor of numerous papers related to transplantation and pregnancy. Her particular areas of interest have included pancreas–kidney outcomes and research in systemic lupus erythematosus.

Michael J. Moritz, MD, a transplant surgeon, is the director of the Division of Transplantation Surgery and associate professor of surgery at Thomas Jefferson University. Dr. Moritz is a coinvestigator of the NTPR.

Steven Nathan, MD, has worked in the field of lung transplantation for over 13 years. Originally from South Africa, Dr. Nathan completed his university education there before coming to the United States. He did his Fellowship in Pulmonary, Critical Care and lung transplantation at Cedars-Sinai Medical Center in Los Angeles and is currently the medical director of lung transplantation at Inova Fairfax Hospital in Northern Virginia.

Wayne Paris, MSW, is a Clinical Transplant Social Worker at the Nazih Zuhdi Transplantation Institute, Oklahoma City, Oklahoma. He has a BA in History and Sociology from Northeastern Oklahoma State University, an MSW from the University of Oklahoma, and is currently a Doctoral Candidate at the University of Huddersfield, Huddersfield, Yorkshire, United Kingdom.

Lydia Z. Philips, BSN, RN, has been in the field of transplantation for 20 years. She has been a transplant coordinator in various organ groups and had roles in the field of management. She is now a full-time research coordinator at the NTPR.

John Pirsch, MD, is a Professor of Medicine and Surgery and Director of Medical Transplantation Service at the University of Wisconsin. Dr. Pirsch has published extensively on liver, kidney, and pancreas transplantation. His research includes work with polyoma virus, Cytomegalovirus as well as drug studies in immunosuppression.

Sotiris Stamou, MD, PhD, is a surgical resident at Georgetown University Hospital, Washington, DC. Dr. Stamou obtained his medical degree and Doctor of Philosophy degree from the University of Athens, Athens, Greece. His main interests are minimally invasive cardiac surgery and mechanisms of stroke after cardiac surgery. Dr. Stamou has authored numerous articles and has presented his research at national and international conferences.

Laurel Williams, RN, MSN, CCTC, is the Manager for Transplant Coordinators at the University of Nebraska's Liver and Intestinal Transplant Program. Laurel is a graduate of the University of Michigan and Wayne State University in Detroit. She is a past president of the North American Transplant Coordinators Organization (NATCO).

Linda Wright, MSW, is a Clinical Transplant Social Worker in the Multi Organ Transplant Programme at the University Health Network in Toronto and a student at the Joint Center for Bioethics at the University of Toronto, where she is studying for a Master of Health Sciences degree in Bioethics. She studied Sociology at the University of Liverpool, and later took a Master's degree in Social Work at McGill University, Montreal.

Foreword

Transplant experimentation began in the 18th century, perhaps long inspired by the ancient Greek myth of the Chimera, the creature composed of a seemingly incompatible lion, goat, and serpent, and by the legends of the early Christian era. Continued fascination combined with a relentless effort of multidisciplinary scientists led to the first successful kidney transplant in 1954. Since that time advances in surgical technique, tissue typing, immunology, and pharmacology have greatly contributed to the success of transplantation and to the continued attraction to this special area of medicine and surgery by physicians, nurses, scientists, social workers, psychologists, nutritionists, and many other health-related professionals.

Although some of the most significant advances were made in the early part of the last two decades, a number of innovative approaches to long-term survival have been developed during the last 5 to 10 years. These include specificity of immunosuppressive agents, immune modulation, widespread use of artificial devices to enhance candidacy, and finely tuned skills in managing comorbidities. The growing population of transplant recipients supports the success of these innovations.

In the last decade, although more than 200,000 solid organs have been transplanted, the number of patients waiting for transplantation far surpassed the number of available donors. Given this shortfall, the need for the best possible care of patients receiving these precious donor organs becomes even more apparent, as the demand for all solid organs continues to exceed supply.

Improved survival rates, coupled with the preference of managed care organizations for local care, has highlighted the need for health care providers, outside of transplant centers, to be knowledgeable about transplant care issues, and feel confident and comfortable caring for this select, but growing population of patients.

Experienced transplant clinicians realize that the most frequently encountered problems are not those originating from the primary transplanted organ, but rather primary care problems precipitated by the immunobiology of transplantation. Of course, each organ has its own set of attendant problems, but for the most part the majority of clinical work hours are devoted to problems related to long-term complications of transplantation and to co-morbidities.

The science and practice of transplantation medicine has expanded to the point that having a hospital-based team of well-informed experts is no longer sufficient. Community-based primary care physicians and nurse practitioners, as well as specialty practitioners, are needed to share the management and care of this select group of patients. Simultaneous with the realization that these practitioners are essential in transplantation, the management of these patients has become increasingly complex. Long-term management in the community is as critically important as acute care management in the intensive care unit. A thorough understanding of the delicate balance among immunosuppressive medications, their sequelae, and preexisting comorbidities, is essential.

In *Solid Organ Transplantation: A Handbook for Primary Health Care Providers,* Sandra Cupples and Linda Ohler skillfully integrate all of the important general, as well as organ-specific, issues indispensable for those health care providers who care for this fascinating group of patients. The editors have succeeded in putting together a comprehensive and scholarly book that theoretically presents the state of the art, while practically offering savvy clinical practice strategies. By reviewing core chapters on immunology, pharmacology, infection, neurocognitive factors, nutrition and psychosocial concerns, the reader is then prepared to benefit from the chapters related to organ-specific interests. The chapter on pregnancy and transplantation will be of interest to caregivers in all specialties, as this is a topic that has been infrequently addressed in the transplant literature.

This is a detailed, yet user-friendly reference book that will be well-received by its principal target audience—primary community healthcare providers and specialists—who will find it to be both an exceptional primer and important reference book. Additionally it will be useful to transplant physicians, clinical coordinators, nurse specialists, and staff nurses involved in all solid organ transplant programs. The individuals who may benefit the most, however, are the transplant recipients and their families.

Sharon M. Augustine, MS, RN, C-ANP
Nurse Practitioner
Cardiothoracic Transplant Program
University of Maryland
Baltimore, MD

William Baumgartner, MD
The Vincent L. Gott Professor
Cardiac Surgeon-in-Charge
Johns Hopkins University Hospital
Baltimore, MD

Preface

Solid Organ Transplantation: A Handbook for Primary Health Care Providers is intended for physicians and nurses in the community who care for transplant recipients on a primary care, home-care, emergency, or consultant basis. Many patients receive a transplant in hospitals far from their homes. Long-term, follow-up, and emergent care are often provided within the home and community settings. With that in mind, we decided to develop a reference guide for our community colleagues. To do this in a comprehensive yet user-friendly manner, in many cases, key information has been bulleted for quick reference. The book is also a useful review for those who are already working on transplant teams, or are preparing to do so.

The volume of single organ and multiorgan transplants performed annually in the United States increased by 44% between 1990 and 1999 (www.unos.org). The annual number of transplants in the United States has maintained a plateau of 20,000 to 22,000 for the past few years. With more than 80,000 candidates awaiting solid organ transplantation, the use of expanded criteria for cadaveric donors has become more prevalent. Living donor transplantation has doubled over the last decade and has proven to be an option for kidney, lung, and liver transplantation. Outcomes of living donors in kidney transplantation have been similar to those reported with human leukocyle antigen (HLA) matched cadaveric donors.

Transplantation has made many medical advances in the past 30 years. However, the morbidity from infection, rejection, and other complications continues to take its toll on long-term survival of grafts and patients. Care of transplant recipients can present many challenges to clinicians beginning with complex medication regimens to diagnosing potential complications such as rejection, infections, and malignancies. Each chapter is written in a way to extract the most salient issues that may confront health care providers. Although our book intends to provide readers with a guide to the various solid organ transplants, it also encompasses psychosocial, neurocognitive, pharmacological, and nutritional aspects of patient care that may face our colleagues in the community.

To demonstrate the multidisciplinary and collaborative nature of transplantation, each chapter on solid organ transplantation is written by a physician and a nurse who are experts in their field. This enabled us to provide readers with the most current information on clinical practice and patient care. Chapter 1 gives readers an overview of solid organ transplantation and includes a brief history of transplantation. Chapter 2 presents information on infectious complications. Infections are known to cause a high rate of morbidity and mortality in this patient population as a result of the immunosuppression used to prevent graft rejection. This chapter may prove to be the most frequently referenced.

Obesity, hyperlipidemia, osteoporosis, hypertension, and diabetes are addressed in Chapter 3. Because these complications often manifest themselves in the long-term follow-up phases after transplantation, they will be some of the most common problems presented to community health care providers. The chapter's author, Dr. Jeanette Hasse, provides readers with dietary interventions that may help to alleviate some of these complications. Immunosuppression therapy has become more complex with the increasing number of new drugs available to prevent rejection. In the early stages of transplantation, most centers used a triple therapy of cyclosporine, imuran, and prednisone. Although triple and monotherapy are being used to suppress rejection of transplanted organs, the regimens can vary greatly from center to center as well as from organ to organ. Drug interactions, drug-food interactions, and side effects pose a real challenge to clinicians and patients. Community providers are encouraged to consult with transplant centers with regard to drug interactions. Chapter 4, which covers pharmacotherapy issues, is an important and informative addition to this book.

Neurocognitive disorders are a relatively new area of investigation for this patient population. The purpose of chapter 5 is to increase the reader's awareness of complications that may lead to changes in behavior, concentration, or cognitive status.

Chapters 6 through 12 present readers with information on potential complications commonly reported in solid organ transplantation. Signs and symptoms of rejection vary with each organ. Thus, these chapters serve as a user-friendly guide to recognizing symptoms of rejection. In many cases, rejection may require a biopsy or specified laboratory tests to be definitively diagnosed. Close communication and collaboration with the transplant physicians and coordinators is important to maximize patient safety and outcome.

Transplant recipients may experience anxiety, depression, and other complex psychosocial problems. Chapter 13 addresses therapeutic interventions for some of the more commonly seen psychiatric problems reported after transplantation. Important issues related to helping patients return to work after transplantation are also presented. As younger patients return to an improved health status, they may want to consider having children. Chapter 14 on pregnancy after transplantation is a helpful guide to clinicians counseling recipients considering this option. Authors of this chapter provide information from the National Transplant Pregnancy Registry. Transplant recipients with a pregnancy or fathering a pregnancy should be included in this database. Again, close communication with the transplant center is important in monitoring rejection and immunosuppression dosing.

A brief checklist overview of transplant immunology is presented in the appendix. The most commonly requested immunology tests are described, and terms are defined.

We hope this book will serve as a guide for care and interventions with transplant recipients. We also hope it will serve to increase the important communication between transplant centers and community caregivers. Collaboration in the care of this complex patient population has great potential to improve transplant outcomes.

1

Overview of Solid Organ Transplantation

Sandra A. Cupples

Transplantation is an effective treatment modality for end-stage diseases of the kidney, pancreas, liver, heart, lung, and intestine. Thousands of neonates, children, and adults have benefited from these types of procedures. Transplantation is truly one of the most exciting medical success stories of the 20th century. This chapter provides an overview of various aspects of organ transplantation. It begins with a brief discussion of the concept of transplantation as evidenced in myths and legends. Folklore gave way to reality with Yu Yu Voronoy's pioneering renal transplantation surgery of the 1930s. This and other key transplantation milestones are reviewed, and current statistics regarding volume, survival rates, and the shortage of donor organs are presented. The responsibilities of the United Network for Organ Sharing (UNOS) are explained, and the roles of various transplant team members are discussed. Because the field of transplantation is rapidly changing, additional Internet-based sources of information are provided. The chapter concludes with a discussion of transplantation in the 21st century.

TRANSPLANTATION LEGENDS

There are many legends about transplantation. Perhaps the most famous is that of Saints Cosmos and Damien. These twin brothers and physicians

1

were martyred in A.D. 287. Many people made pilgrimages to their tombs in Syria to seek healing, including Emperor Justinian I. Miraculously cured of his affliction, Justinian constructed a basilica at the saints' gravesites. Subsequently, it became customary for the sick to pray at the basilica, then sleep in the church overnight, during which time supplicants hoped to be healed. In A.D. 348, the church sacristan happened to be suffering from a gangrenous leg. He appealed to Saints Cosmos and Damien and, hoping for a miracle, slept in the church overnight. According to legend, these saints appeared in the basilica, removed the sacristan's gangrenous leg, and replaced it with the leg of another individual who had died that very day. When the sacristan awoke, he discovered that his leg was cured. However, when he looked at his leg, he immediately knew it was not his, as the "transplanted" leg was that of a "donor" with dark skin (Loucks, 1998).

HISTORICAL PERSPECTIVE

Over 1500 years would elapse between the "Miracle of the Black Leg" and the first reported attempt at human solid organ transplantation—the Russian surgeon Voronoy's series of six pioneering but unsuccessful human cadaver renal transplantations in the 1930s (Morris, 1997; Voronoy, 1937). The first successful solid organ transplantation in humans occurred in 1954 when Joseph Murray and colleagues removed a kidney from one identical twin and implanted it in the other twin (Crumbley & Sade, 1991). The recipient survived for over 20 years (Starzl, 1990).

In the early 1960s, the introduction of two immunosuppressive agents, 6-mercaptopurine and azathioprine, facilitated the success of the first cadaveric kidney transplantation (Baumgartner, 1995). It wasn't until the discovery of cyclosporine in the mid-1970s and its introduction in 1983, however, that the number of solid organ transplantation procedures increased exponentially (UNOS, *Transplant milestones*, 2001). This new immunosuppressive drug dramatically increased survival rates and decreased morbidity among recipients of all solid organs. Consequently, solid organ transplantation has become an effective intervention for the treatment of adults and children afflicted with end-stage diseases of the kidney, liver, pancreas, heart, lung, and intestine. Table 1.1 lists the date of the first successful transplant for each of the solid organs (UNOS, *Transplant milestones in the United States and Canada*, 2001).

TABLE 1.1 Transplant Milestones in the United States and Canada

Organ	Date	Institution
Kidney*	1954	Brigham and Women's Hospital
Pancreas	1966	University of Minnesota
Liver*	1967	University of Colorado Health Sciences Center
Heart	1968	Stanford University Hospital
Heart—lung	1981	Stanford University Hospital
Lung—single	1983	Toronto General Hospital
Lung—double*	1986	Toronto General Hospital
Liver—living related	1989	University of Chicago Medical Center
Lung—living related	1990	Stanford University Medical Center

* Denotes first transplant of its kind in the world
Source: United Network for Organ Sharing. (2001). *Transplant milestones in the United States and Canada.*

UNITED NETWORK FOR ORGAN SHARING

Although many of the major medical problems associated with transplantation had been overcome, there still remained unresolved legal, ethical, economic, scientific, and social issues. Therefore, in October 1984 the U.S. Congress passed the National Organ Transplant Act (NOTA) and authorized the establishment of the Task Force on Organ Procurement and Transplantation. The task force recommended that a national Organ Procurement and Transplantation Network (OPTN) be established under NOTA. The United Network for Organ Sharing was awarded the OPTN and Scientific Registry contracts in 1986 and 1987, respectively. Although it is a private, nonprofit corporation, UNOS's policies are subject to review and approval by the U.S. Department of Health and Human Services.

PURPOSE OF UNOS

UNOS maintains the national, computerized waiting list of transplant candidates. Additionally, UNOS is charged with the responsibility of:

- Optimizing access to transplantation for all who can benefit from it
- Maximizing the number of organs donated, procured, and transplanted through policies and programs that improve quality, efficiency, efficacy, and survival
- Establishing standards for membership, access to the allocation of organs, organ acceptability, transplant program and organ procurement organization performance, and information collection and reporting
- Allocating organs equitably
- Functioning as a central resource for the collection, processing, storage, analysis, and reporting of data pertaining to donation and transplantation
- Collaborating with scientists and scientific/professional organizations to stimulate improvements in transplant technology
- Providing technological, analytical, and administrative services to members of the transplant community to improve effectiveness and efficiency
- Educating professionals and the public about donation and transplantation (U.S. Department of Health and Human Services, 1999, p. 374.

UNOS MEMBERSHIP

UNOS membership includes every transplant center, organ procurement organization, and tissue typing laboratory in the United States, as well as other professional health organizations and members of the public.

UNOS ORGAN ALLOCATION POLICY

UNOS donor organ allocation policies are based on objective factors such as acceptable preservation times, candidates' medical urgency, and immunological factors. Maximum preservation times for major organs are as follows:

Heart	4–6 hours
Lung	4–6 hours
Liver	24 hours
Pancreas	24 hours
Kidney	48–72 hours

Medical urgency is specific to the type of organ and is discussed in chapters 6 through 12. Immunological factors are of more importance for certain organs (e.g., kidneys) than others (e.g., livers). UNOS allocation policies are continuously reviewed by both the transplant community and the public. These policies are updated on the basis of advances in medical science (Bollinger, 1995).

TRANSPLANT VOLUME AND SURVIVAL RATES

As UNOS data indicate (Table 1.2), the total number of these organ transplants has increased yearly since 1988. Not only has the volume of solid organ transplantation increased, but survival rates have improved as well. Increased survival can be attributed to a number of factors including improvements in operative techniques, organ preservation techniques, tissue matching, immunosuppressive regimens, and rejection therapy. The most recent UNOS 1-, 3-, and 5-year graft and patient survival rates are summarized in Table 1.3. The survival of the longest living solid organ adult transplant recipients as of 1997 is depicted in Table 1.4.

TRANSPLANT CENTERS

As transplantation survival rates improved, the number of transplant centers increased accordingly. Today, there are 260 transplant centers in the United States (UNOS, *Number and type of UNOS members*, 2001). The number of organ transplant programs in the United States is listed in Table 1.5.

SHORTAGE OF DONOR ORGANS

Despite the increase in the number of transplant programs, there remains a dire shortage of donor organs. Every 14 minutes, a new patient is added to the waiting list (UNOS, *Online*, 2001). In March 2001, the number of patients on the UNOS waiting list surpassed the 75,000 mark (UNOS, *Patients on the UNOS national patient waiting list, 2001*). Within the span of a decade, the discrepancy between the number of transplant procedures performed and the number of individuals on the waiting list grew from 5,000 to over 50,000 (UNOS, *National organ transplant waiting list tops 75,000, 2001*). In 2000, 5,597 patients died while waiting for a donor organ—an average of 16 deaths per day. Between 1988 and 2000, a total

TABLE 1.2 U.S. Transplant Volume by Organ and Year

Organ*	1988	1989	1990	1991	1992	1993	1994	1995	1996	1997	1998	1999	2000	Total
Kidney	8,873	8,657	9,416	9,673	9,736	10,360	10,644	11,051	11,363	11,674	12,375	12,527	13,332	139,681
Pancreas	79	83	69	78	64	113	94	107	165	208	245	362	436	2,103
Kidney-Pancreas	170	334	459	452	493	661	748	917	860	851	971	932	910	8,758
Liver	1,713	2,200	2,690	2,953	3,062	3,440	3,651	3,924	4,072	4,176	4,502	4,707	4,950	46,040
Intestine	0	0	5	12	22	34	23	45	45	68	68	70	79	471
Heart	1,684	1,707	2,108	2,125	2,171	2,298	2,340	2,357	2,342	2,294	2,344	2,181	2,197	28,148
Lung	34	94	203	406	535	668	721	870	814	931	864	886	956	7,982
Heart/Lung	73	68	52	51	48	60	71	69	39	60	47	49	48	735
Total	12,626	13,143	15,002	15,750	16,131	17,634	18,292	19,340	19,700	20,262	21,416	21,714	22,908	233,918

* Includes Cadaveric and Living Donor Transplants

Source: UNOS. U.S. Transplants by Organ and Donor Type: January 1988–December 2000.

TABLE 1.3 Graft and Patient Survival Rates at 1, 3, and 5 Years

Organ/Donor Type		Number of Transplants 1997–1998	1-Year Survival (%)	Number of Transplants 1990–1998	3-Year Survival (%)	5-Year Survival (%)
Cadaveric donor kidney	Graft survival	13,235	89.4	56,352	76.3	64.7
	Patient survival	13,235	94.8	56,352	88.9	81.8
Living donor kidney	Graft survival	7,431	94.5	25,092	87.0	78.4
	Patient survival	7,431	97.6	25,092	94.6	91.0
Liver	Graft survival	7,196	81.4	26,652	71.5	66.1
	Patient survival	7,196	87.9	26,652	79.2	74.2
Pancreas	Graft survival	324	76.2	824	49.9	41.6
	Patient survival	324	93.4	824	88.7	84.2
Kidney/ pancreas	Kidney graft survival	1,709	91.8	6,148	80.4	70.7
	Pancreas graft survival	1,674	83.7	6,110	73.9	67.4
	Patient survival	1,716	94.4	6,156	88.0	82.7

continued

TABLE 1.3 (continued)

Organ/Donor Type		Number of Transplants 1997–1998	1-Year Survival (%)	Number of Transplants 1990–1998	3-Year Survival (%)	5-Year Survival (%)
Heart	Graft survival	4,316	85.1	19,269	76.0	68.5
	Patient survival	4,316	85.5	19,269	76.9	69.8
Lung	Graft survival	1,663	76.3	5,613	56.2	42.0
	Patient survival	1,663	77.0	5,613	58.1	44.2
Heart–lung	Graft survival	89	58.2	469	50.9	40.5
	Patient survival	89	60.0	469	51.4	41.7
Intestine	Graft survival	45	63.8	104	48.8	37.4
	Patient survival	45	78.9	104	62.0	49.6

Source: U.S. Department of Health and Human Services. (2000). *Annual Report of the U.S. Scientific Registry for Transplant Recipients and the Organ Procurement and Transplantation Network: Transplant Data, 1990–1999.*

TABLE 1.4 Longest Living Adult Solid Organ Transplant Recipients

Organ	Date of Transplant	Age at Transplant	Years of Continued Function
Kidney (living related donor)	1/31/63	38	34 years, 11 months
Kidney (cadaveric donor)	1/25/65	38	32 years, 11 months
Pancreas	12/3/80	25	17 years
Liver	1/22/70	3	27 years, 11 months
Heart	4/4/75	28	22 years, 8 months
Heart—lung	11/5/82	40	15 years, 1 month
Lung—single	9/6/88	59	9 years, 4 months
Lung—double	7/26/87	25	10 years, 5 months

Source: United Network for Organ Sharing. (2001). *Transplant patient survival in the U.S., longest living adult recipients.*

of 45,743 transplant candidates were removed from the national waiting list following their death (UNOS, Number of patients removed from the OPTN waiting list due to death, *2001*).

TRANSPLANT TEAM MEMBERS

Transplantation is a team process. In addition to the patient and family, a typical transplant team includes the following key members: physician, transplant surgeon, nurse coordinator, dietitian, social worker, pharmacist, and financial counselor. Although the roles of the medical members of the team are fairly straightforward, the responsibilities of the coordinator, pharmacist, social worker, dietitian, and financial counselor are more complex and are clarified here.

The *transplant coordinator* typically is a registered nurse who manages the care of the patient from the initial referral to the transplant team. This role is multifaceted and may vary from center to center. In general, however, in the pretransplant phase, the transplant coordinator obtains the patient's medical records from the referring physician, convenes the

TABLE 1.5   Number of Transplant Programs in the U. S.

Type of Program	Number
Kidney	245
Liver	122
Pancreas	137
Pancreas Islet Cell	32
Intestine	39
Heart	141
Heart-Lung	82
Lung	76
Total	884

Source: UNOS. Number and Type of Organ Transplant Programs.

initial evaluation conference, schedules the evaluation tests, compiles test results, and places the patient on the waiting list. In the posttransplant phase, the coordinator schedules biopsies and other routine follow-up tests, triages patient calls, obtains consults, and maintains patient records and UNOS databases. Large-volume transplant centers may have several coordinators assigned to specific types of organ transplantation, phases of transplantation (pretransplant vs posttransplant), or point of service (inpatient vs. outpatient). It is typically the transplant coordinator who is the initial point of contact for primary health care providers with questions or concerns about their pre- or posttransplant patients.

The *transplant social worker* often is the primary mental health care professional on the team, although many centers also have transplant psychiatrists and psychologists. A psychosocial assessment is an essential component of the transplant evaluation process. Patients are carefully screened in terms of their support systems, emotional stability, substance abuse history, compliance with previous medical therapy, and commitment to transplantation. In addition, the social worker assists patients and families in coping with transplant-related stressors, identifies community resources, locates affordable sources of posttransplant medications, and provides guidance regarding insurance issues, medical leave, and disability applications.

The *transplant dietitian* assists in the management of the patient's nutritional status pre- and posttransplant. Before the transplant, the dietitian may monitor specific lab values such as prealbumin levels and help under- or overweight patients to achieve a more optimal weight. Given that many transplant recipients experience problems with weight gain, diabetes, hypertension, and lipid metabolism, the dietitian also provides posttransplant patient education.

The *transplant pharmacist* helps the transplant physicians in managing the patient's immunosuppression therapy. In some centers, the pharmacist makes daily rounds with the transplant team and provides assistance with various aspects of the immunosuppression regimen, particularly with respect to the side effects of these drugs and their potential interactions with other medications. The transplant pharmacist may also be involved in patient education.

The *financial counselor* is primarily responsible for identifying the parameters of the patient's health insurance, particularly with respect to transplant benefits and prescription medication coverage. Conjointly, the social worker and financial counselor may help patients with applications for Medicare, Medicaid, Social Security, pharmacy assistance programs, and similar types of applications.

INFORMATION ON THE INTERNET

The Internet abounds with information for both transplant professionals and patients. The URL addresses of major transplantation-related Web sites are listed in Table 1.6. Of particular note, the American Share Foundation was developed as a central resource for links to over 1,000 transplantation Web sites.

More than 20 million Americans now use the Internet as a source of health care information (Eng et al., 1998). Although this technology affords patients access to over one billion documents on the World Wide Web (Lucky, 2000), health care providers have an obligation to help patients and family members evaluate Web-based information and remind them that

- Information obtained on the Internet is not a substitute for individualized medical advice.
- Infomation that is accurate and valid for one situation may be harmful in a different situation.
- Information does not have to be false to be harmful; correct information applied to the wrong situation can be dangerous (Health Summit Working Group, 2001).

TABLE 1.6 URL Addresses of Transplantation Web Sites

Organization	URL Address
United Network for Organ Sharing	http://www.unos.org
American Diabetes Association	http://www.diabetes.org
American Heart Association	http://amhrt.org
American Liver Foundation	http://gi.ucsf.edu/alf.html
American Share Foundation	http://www.asf.org
American Society of Transplantation	http://www.a-s-t.org
American Transplant Association	http://www.american-transplant.org
Centers for Disease Control and Prevention	http://www.cdc.gov
Division of Transplantation, Department of Health and Human Resources	http://www.hisa.dhhs.gov/osp/dot
National Institutes of Diabetes and Digestive and Kidney Diseases	http://www.niddk.nih.gov
National Kidney Foundation	http://www.nkf.org
Intestinal Transplant Registry	http://www.lhsc.on.ca/itr
Transplant Recipients International Organization	http://www.trioweb.org
Transweb	http://transweb.org

TRANSPLANTATION IN THE 21ST CENTURY

Given that the most critical issue in transplantation today is the shortage of donor organs, efforts in the 21st century will focus on strategies to mitigate this problem. Remarkable progress has already been made in the development of artificial organs. Future evolvement of this technology may include definitive organ replacements such as the totally implantable artificial heart (DiBardino, 1999), permanent left ventricular assist devices (Rodeheffer & McGregor, 1992), artificial pancreases, and miniature dialysis machines that provide 24-hour hemodialysis at home. Bioartificial hepatic assist devices are available in limited use. Liver support systems must maintain physiological support and enhance hemodynamic stability while either serving as a bridge to transplantation or providing opportunity for the patient's liver to recover or regenerate (Rosenthal, 2000). Both the bioartificial liver and the extracorporeal liver-assist device are in clinical trials (Sechser, Osorio, Freise, & Osorio, 2001).

Xenotransplantation offers the possibility of an unlimited source of organs from animals (Patterson & Patterson, 1997). However, several significant ethical concerns and immunological barriers to xenotransplantation must first be overcome. Gene therapy, molecular cloning, and enhanced or altered immunosuppression regimens may be useful in conquering the hyperacute rejection associated with xenotransplantation (Hardy & Marvin, 1999).

Future efforts will also be directed at the development of better immunosuppressive agents that have fewer side effects (Morris, 1997). Advances in immunosuppression regimens will likely include new combinations of calcineurin inhibitors, antimetabolites, anticytokines, and antibody therapies (Hardy & Marvin, 1999). Modern molecular techniques will yield important information about the mechanisms by which cells of the recipient enter the donor organ and cells of the donor organ peacefully coexist in the recipient (Bahnson, 1997; Calne, 1994).

REFERENCES

Bahnson, H. T. (1997). Transplantation of the heart: Reminiscences of the past and inklings of the future. *Annals of Thoracic Surgery, 64*, 1561–1563.

Baumgartner, W. A. (1995). Foreword. In M. T. Nolan & S. M. Augustine (Eds.), *Transplantation nursing: Acute and long-term management* (pp. vii–viii). Norwalk, CT: Appleton & Lange.

Bollinger, R. R. (1995). Organ sharing network. In L. Makowka & L. Sher (Eds.), *Handbook of organ transplantation* (pp. 65–87). Austin, TX: Landes.

Calne, R. (1994). The history and development of organ transplantation: Biology and rejection. *Bailliere's Clinical Gastroenterology, 8*(3), 389–397.

Crumbley, A. J., & Sade, R. M. (1991). The history of transplantation. *Journal of the South Carolina Medical Association, 87*(6), 361.

DiBardino, D. J. (1999). The history and development of cardiac transplantation. *Texas Heart Institute Journal, 26*(3), 198–205.

Eng, T. R., Maxfield, A., Patrick, K., Deering, M. J., Ratzan, S. C., & Gustafson, D. H. (1998). Access to health information and support: A public highway or a private road? *Journal of the American Medical Association, 280*(15), 1371–1375.

Hardy, M. A., & Marvin, M. R. (1999). Transplantation in the 21st century. *Transplantation Proceedings, 31*, 2929–2050.

Health Summit Working Group. *Criteria for assessing the quality of health information on the Internet: Policy paper.* Retrieved February 1, 2001, from the Health Summit Working Group Web Site: http://hitiweb.mitretek.org/hswg.

Loucks, E. B. (1998). The origin and future of transplantation surgery. *Journal of Investigative Surgery, 11*(2), iii–iv.

Lucky, R. (2000). The quickening of science communication. *Science, 289*(5477), 259–264.

Morris, P. J. (1997). Renal transplantation: A quarter century of achievement. *Seminars in Nephrology, 17*(3), 188–195.

Patterson, C., & Patterson, K. B. (1997). The history of heart transplantation. *American Journal of the Medical Sciences, 314*(3), 190–197.

Rodeheffer, R. J., & McGregor, C. G. A. (1992). The development of cardiac transplantation. *Mayo Clinic Proceedings, 67,* 480–484.

Rosenthal, P. (2000). Is there a future for liver-assist devices? *Current Gastroenterology Reports 2(1),* 55–60.

Sechser, A., Osorio, J., Freise, C., & Osorio, W. (2001). Artificial liver support devices for fulminant liver failure. *Clinics in Liver Disease, 5*(2), 415–430.

Starzl, T. E. (1990). The development of clinical renal transplantation. *American Journal of Kidney Diseases, 16*(6), 548–556.

United Network for Organ Sharing. *National organ transplant waiting list tops 75,000.* Retrieved October 15, 2001, from the UNOS Web Site: http://www.unos.org/Newsroom/archive_newsrelease_20010309_75000.htm.

United Network for Organ Sharing. *Number and type of organ transplant programs.* Retrieved October 15, 2001, from UNOS Web Site: http://www.unos.org/Newsroom/critdata_main.htm

United Network for Organ Sharing. *Number and type of UNOS members.* Retrieved October 15, 2001, from the UNOS Web Site: http://www.unos.org/Newsroom/critdata_main.htm

United Network for Organ Sharing. *Number of patients removed from the OPTN waiting list due to death: January 1, 1988–2000.* Retrieved October 15, 2001, from the UNOS Web Site: http://unos.org/Newsroom/critdata_wait.htm

United Network for Organ Sharing. *Online.* Retrieved April 8, 2001, from the UNOS Web Site: http://unos.org/Frame_Default.asp

United Network for Organ Sharing. *Patients on the UNOS national patient waiting list.* Retrieved April 8, 2001, from the UNOS Web Site: http://www.unos.org/Newsroom/critdata_main.htm

United Network for Organ Sharing. *Transplant patient survival in the U.S.: Longest living adult recipients.* Retrieved October 15, 2001, from the UNOS Web Site: http://www.unos.org/Newsroom/critdata_milestones.htm

United Network for Organ Sharing. *Transplant milestones.* Retrieved October 15, 2001, from the UNOS Web Site: http://www.unos.Newsroom/critdata_milestones.htm

United Network for Organ Sharing. *Transplant Milestones in the United States and Canada.* Retrieved October 15, 2001, from the UNOS Web Site: http://www.unos.org/Newsroom/critdata_milestones.htm.

United Network for Organ Sharing. *U.S. transplants by organ and donor type: 1988–December 2000*. Retrieved October 15, 2001, from the UNOS Web Site: http://www.unos.org/Newsroom/critdata_transplants_ustx.htm

U.S. Department of Health and Human Services. (1999). *Annual report of the U.S. Scientific Registry for Transplant Recipients and the Organ Procurement and Transplantation Network: Transplant data, 1989–1998*. Rockville, MD: Author.

U.S. Department of Health and Human Services. (2000). *Annual report of the U.S. Scientific Registry for Transplant Recipients and the Organ Procurement and Transplantation Network: Transplant data, 1990–1999*. Rockville, MD: Author.

Voronoy, U. (1937). Blocking the reticuloendothelial system in man in some forms of mercuric chloride intoxication and the transplantation of the cadaver kidney as a method of treatment for the anuria resulting from the intoxication. *Siglo Medico, 97*, 296–297.

2

Infectious Diseases in Transplant Recipients

Sandra A. Cupples and Daniel R. Lucey

Transplantation offers the best chance of survival and improved quality of life for many patients afflicted with end-stage organ disease. Despite the progress that has been made over the last 30 years, however, infection remains a significant cause of posttransplant morbidity and the leading cause of death in solid organ transplant recipients. Over two thirds of recipients will have at least one episode of infection during the first posttransplant year (Rubin, 1994). This chapter will discuss infection in terms of risk factors, etiology, occurrence, diagnosis, organ-specific considerations, prevention, and treatment, including drug interactions between immunosuppressive drugs and antimicrobial agents.

RISK FACTORS FOR INFECTION

Three factors determine the risk of infection in solid organ transplant recipients:

- Epidemiological exposure in the community or hospital environment
- Net state of immunosuppression
- Ongoing preventive antimicrobial therapy

The recipient's net state of immunosuppression is the combined effect of all of the factors that influence the patient's susceptibility to infection:

- The current immunosuppression regimen that depresses cell-mediated immunity, blunts antibody response, and induces leukopenia
- Any disruption of normal endothelial and epithelial barriers
- Any concurrent metabolic dysfunction (e.g., malnutrition, hyperglycemia, and uremia)
- Any concurrent immunomodulatory viruses (e.g., cytomegalovirus [CMV], Epstein-Barr virus [EBV]; hepatitis B and C, and human immunodeficiency virus [HIV])
- Defects in host defenses secondary to underlying disease (Fishman & Rubin, 1998; Patel & Paya, 1997; Tolkoff-Rubin & Rubin, 2000)

ETIOLOGY OF INFECTION

Transplant recipients can develop infections exogenously and endogenously. Exogenous sources of infection include the allograft, blood products, the community, and nosocomial transmission during episodes of increased antirejection therapy or immunomodulatory viremia. Endogenous infections are caused by reactivation of latent infection in the recipient (Love, 1996).

GENERAL PRINCIPLES

The diagnosis and management of infectious disease in transplant recipients can be guided by the following general principles:

1. Microorganisms that cause infection can be classified as
   - Pathogens that are associated with classic infections such as influenza, typhoid, and cholera
   - Pathogens that are typically benign (e.g., normal flora) but may cause lethal infections if the mucocutaneous barrier is breached
   - Pathogens that rarely cause infection in immunocompetent individuals but are associated with significant morbidity and mortality in transplant recipients
2. Immunosuppressive therapy alters the inflammatory response and mutes the clinical manifestations of invasive infection.
3. The most important determinants of survival are how quickly the diagnosis is made and how soon pathogen-specific therapy is begun.

4. It is better to prevent than treat infection; hence the rationale for prophylactic or preemptive therapy (Table 2.1).
5. Treatment of invasive infections is based on individual factors such as organism load, infection site(s), and net state of immunosuppression rather than standard courses of antimicrobial therapy.
6. The posttransplant infection timetable is useful to community health care providers in making a differential diagnosis and identifying and correcting sources of excessive environmental exposure (Tolkoff-Rubin & Rubin, 2000).

INFECTION TIMETABLE

As immunosuppression regimens have been standardized over the years, it has become evident that certain infections are more common at particular intervals posttransplant. Moreover, this pattern is typically the same for all types of solid organ transplantation procedures (see Table 2.2 and Figure 2.1).

DIAGNOSIS OF INFECTION

The two pillars of infection management are early diagnosis and prompt initiation of therapy. In transplant recipients, traditional diagnostic tests may lack sensitivity. Therefore, more sophisticated diagnostic tests must be used early on—even for seemingly benign and often vague symptoms. In addition, the typical inflammatory response to infection may be blunted due to immunosuppressive therapy (Patel & Paya, 1997).

The most important clinical presentations of infection in organ transplant recipients are

- Fever without any localizing findings
- Fever with headache, changes in state of consciousness, or other central nervous system (CNS) findings
- Unexplained skin lesions
- Febrile pneumonitis (Kontoyiannis & Rubin, 1995).

TABLE 2.1 Major Organisms Causing Posttransplant Infection: Clinical Manifestations, Prevention/Prophylaxis, Diagnostic Tests, and Treatment Options

Organism	May cause	Clinical manifestations	Prevention/ prophylaxis	Diagnostic tests	Treatment options
CMV	CMV syndrome Tissue invasive disease: Gastroenteritis Myocarditis Pneumonitis Hepatitis Retinitis (rare) Encephalitis (rare) Pancreatitis (rare)	CMV syndrome: Fever Fatigue Malaise Leukopenia Myalgias Thrombocytopenia Elevated LFTs Gastroenteritis: Anorexia, dysphagia Abdominal cramping Nausea, vomiting, diarrhea Ulceration, bleeding Pneumonitis: Fever Dyspnea (Avery, 1998a, 1998b; Dummer, 1995; Miller, 1991)	Use of CMV-negative, filtered, or leukocyte-poor blood products Ganciclovir Acyclovir Valacyclovir CMV hyperimmune globulin Unselected immunoglobulin Preemptive therapy for patients at high risk (e.g., IV ganciclovir during antilymphocyte antibody therapy) (Avery, 1998a, 1998b; Martin, 1995; Rubin 1994, 2000)	Serologic: Complement fixing assay Immunofluorescence ELISA Latex agglutination systems Virologic: Antigenemia assay Quantitative PCR Tissue culture Biopsy (Avery, 1998b; Rubin, 1994)	IV ganciclovir* followed by oral ganciclovir CMV hyperimmune globulin for tissue-invasive disease Immunoglobulin Foscarnet (for ganciclovir-resistant organisms or patients intolerant of ganciclovir) * Dose must be adjusted for renal dysfunction (Avery, 1998a, 1998b; Rubin 1994, 2000; Singh, 1997)

continued

TABLE 2.1 (continued)

Organism	May cause	Clinical manifestations	Prevention/prophylaxis	Diagnostic tests	Treatment options
Epstein-Barr virus	Mononucleosis PTLD: nodal or extranodal disease of the CNS, GI tract, lungs or bone marrow (Singh, 1997)	Mononucleosis: Lymph node hyperplasia Splenomegaly Atypical mononuclear leukocytes Abnormal LFTs Fever Pharyngitis PTLD: Mononucleosis-like syndrome Weight loss Fever of unknown origin Abdominal pain Anorexia Jaundice Bowel perforation GI bleeding Renal and hepatic dysfunction Pneumothorax Pulmonary infiltrates CNS findings (seizures, altered level of consciousness) Allograft involvement (Patel & Paya, 1997; Rubin, 1994)	Preemptive therapy for patients at high risk (e.g., IV ganciclovir during antilymphocyte antibody therapy) (Rubin, 1994)	Mononucleosis: CBC EBV antibody LFTs Heterophil agglutination antibody test PTLD: CT scan (Note: Absence of adenopathy does not rule out PTLD; disease can be entirely extranodal) (Rubin, 1994) Tissue biopsy	Mononucleosis: Acyclovir PTLD: Benign polyclonal polymorphic B-cell hyperplasia: Acyclovir Ganciclovir Decreased immunosuppression (possibly) Early malignant polyclonal polymorphic B-cell lymphoma: Acyclovir Ganciclovir Interferon-α Gamma globulin Anti-B-cell antibodies (anti-CD 20) Decreased immunosuppression (possibly)

TABLE 2.1 (continued)

Organism	May cause	Clinical manifestations	Prevention/ prophylaxis	Diagnostic tests	Treatment options
					Monoclonal polymorphic B-cell lymphoma: Chemotherapy Radiation Resection Decreased immunosuppression (Patel & Paya, 1997; Rubin, 1994)
Herpes simplex 1 Herpes simplex 2	Herpes labialis Herpetic esophagitis Anogenital lesions Visceral infection is rare (Singh, 1997)	HSV 1: Crusted ulcerations Verrucous lip lesions HSV-2: Coalescing ulcerations without clear-cut vesicles (Rubin, 1994)	Acyclovir Ganciclovir (Dummer, 1995; Rubin, 1994)	Viral culture Direct immunofluorescence studies Tzanck smear (Patel & Paya, 1997; Rubin, 1994)	Acyclovir Ganciclovir Famciclovir Valacyclovir (Sia & Paya, 1998) Foscarnet (Patel & Paya, 1997) (Rubin, 1994)

continued

TABLE 2.1 (*continued*)

Organism	May cause	Clinical manifestations	Prevention/ prophylaxis	Diagnostic tests	Treatment options
Varicella zoster	Localized dermatomal zoster	Localized dermatomal zoster that involves 2 or 3 adjoining dermatomes without visceral involvement (viral reactivation)	Seronegative recipients with significant exposure (same-room contact with diagnosed case of chicken pox or direct contact with skin lesions of shingles) (Love, 1996)	Characteristic unilateral vesicular lesions VZV antibody titer Tzanck smear Direct immunofluorescence studies	Localized infection: Acyclovir Famciclovir Valacyclovir (oral) (Sia & Paya, 1998)
	Disseminated infection	Primary, disseminated infection: associated with hemorrhagic pneumonia, skin lesions, encephalitis, pancreatitis, hepatitis, and disseminated intravascular coagulation (Rubin, 1994)	Varicella zoster hyperimmune globulin within 72 hours of significant exposure IV acyclovir within 24 hours of eruption of skin rash		Disseminated infection: Acyclovir (intravenous) VZV immune globulin (Patel & Paya, 1997; Rubin, 1994; Singh, 1997)
HHV-6	Bone marrow suppression Encephalitis Interstitial pneumonitis	Fever Malaise Rash Bone marrow dysfunction (Rubin, 1994)	None at present	Serologic testing PCR assay	Ganciclovir Foscarnet (Singh, 1997)

continued

TABLE 2.1 *(continued)*

Organism	May cause	Clinical manifestations	Prevention/prophylaxis	Diagnostic tests	Treatment options
Hepatitis viruses	Acute or chronic hepatitis Cirrhosis	Recurrent HBV infection: + HBsAg (typically 2–6 months posttransplant) Hepatocellular symptoms that can range from mild hepatitis to fulminant liver failure) HCV: Chronic hepatitis (Patel & Paya, 1997)	HBV vaccine for non-immune transplant candidates Perioperative anti-HBV immune globulin for liver transplant candidates with HBV infection	HBV: Serologic testing HCV: Detection of HCV-RNA by reverse transcriptase PCR Liver biopsy	HBV immune globulin HCV: Interferon + Ribavirin (Tolkoff-Rubin & Rubin, 2000)
Listeria monocytogenes	Bacteremia Meningitis Meningoencephalitis Myocarditis Cerebritis without meningitis Pneumonia (Love, 1996; Rubin, 1994)	Fever (1–5 days) Headache Decreased level of consciousness Focal neurological deficits Nuchal rigidity Spinal fluid: neutophils, lymphocytes; glucose may be normal Abdominal cramps, diarrhea (Dummer, 1995; Rubin, 1994)	TMP-SMZ Dietary precautions regarding milk, cheeses, under-cooked meats, and uncooked vegetables (Love, 1996; Rubin, 1994; Thaler & Rubin, 1996)	Blood, sputum cultures CT scan MRI CSF: cell count, Gram's stain, culture, and protein and sugar determination Note: Organism may be confused with diphtheroids in Gram's-stain smears of pus or sputum	Meningial doses of penicillin or ampicillin Gentamicin TMP-SMZ for penicillin-allergic patients (Dummer, 1995; Rubin, 1994)

continued

TABLE 2.1 *(continued)*

Organism	May cause	Clinical manifestations	Prevention/ prophylaxis	Diagnostic tests	Treatment options
Nocardia	Pulmonary and extrapulmonary infection (CNS, skin, and bone) (Dummer, 1995; Love, 1996)	Subacute symptoms: Fever Cough Chest pain Pulmonary nodules, abscesses, cavitating lesions, infiltrates, effusions (Dummer, 1995)	TMP-SMZ (Thaler & Rubin, 1996)	Cultures: sputum, BAL fluid Gram's stain Modified acid-fast stain (Dummer, 1995)	Sulfasoxazole TMP-SMZ Amikacin Imipenem Third-generation cephalosporins Minocycline Isolated pulmonary infection: 3–6 months therapy Disseminated disease: 12 months of therapy (Dummer, 1995)
Legionella	Pneumonia	Fever, chills Focal pulmonary infiltrate Headache Confusion Minimally productive cough Diarrhea Chest pain Malaise Dyspnea (Ampel & Wing, 1994)	Routine culture of hospital water supply Water treatment to control nosocomial infection	Cultures: sputum and BAL fluid Direct fluorescent antibody stain Urinary antigen detection (can only detect serogroup 1 of *Legionella pneumophila* species) Fine-needle aspiration of lung Open lung biopsy (Ampel & Wing, 1994; Dummer, 1995)	Quinolones (particularly levofloxacin or ciprofloxacin) Rifampin (may interact with other drugs via the hepatic cytochrome p450 system) Doxycycline

continued

TABLE 2.1 (continued)

Organism	May cause	Clinical manifestations	Prevention/ prophylaxis	Diagnostic tests	Treatment options
					Macrolides (azithromycin, erythromycin interact with immunosuppressive medications and should generally be avoided) TMP-SMZ (but side effects include bone marrow suppression, hepatitis, and rash)
Mycobacteria	Pulmonary and extrapulmonary infection (intestinal, skeletal, cutaneous, CNS) (Love, 1996)	Pulmonary: Nonproductive cough Mucopurulent secretions Hemoptysis Dyspnea Chest pain Fever Excessive sweating Weight loss Organ-specific manifestations	Test and treat before transplantation transplantation Isoniazid (controversial) (Dummer, 1995; Rubin, 1994)	Chest radiograph Bronchoscopy with BAL Transbronchial biopsy Pleural needle biopsy Tuberculin test: often negative Smears for acid-fast bacilli and mycobacterial culture	Isoniazid*† Rifampin*† Pyrazinamide Ethambutol *Increases catabolism of steroids and cyclosporine and tacrolimus; monitor levels of cyclosporine and tacrolimus

continued

TABLE 2.1 (continued)

Organism	May cause	Clinical manifestations	Prevention/ prophylaxis	Diagnostic tests	Treatment options
				Organ-specific histology	†Monitor renal and hepatic function (Rubin, 1994)
Aspergillus	Pulmonary and extrapulmonary infection	Pulmonary involvement: Nonproductive cough Pleuritic chest pain Pulmonary infiltrates or nodules Dyspnea Low-grade fever (Patel & Paya, 1997) Invasive/disseminated infection: Refractory fever Sinusitis Epistaxis; nasal pain Periorbital pain or swelling Cutaneous embolic lesions Progressive erythema or induration along tunneled venous catheter (Wheat, 1994)	Aerosolized Amphotericin B (Reichenspurner et al., 1997) Epidemiologic: Minimize contact with fungal spores; shield patient from nosocomial environmental hazards: high-efficiency particulate air filters; high-performance masks Preemptive: Amphotericin B if respiratory tract is colonized (Thaler & Rubin, 1996)	Chest radiography Note: May be normal BAL Transbronchial biopsy Open lung biopsy CT scan (e.g., lung, sinuses) Tissue biopsy Sputum cultures: Repeated positive sputum cultures suggest invasive disease Positive sputum cultures plus cavitary lung disease suggest invasive disease	Amphotericin B Itraconazole (Oral* or IV) *Absorption may be erratic, especially in patients with low gastric acidity; monitor plasma concentration of drug (Patel & Paya, 1997; Rubin, 1994; Wheat, 1994)

continued

TABLE 2.1 (continued)

Organism	May cause	Clinical manifestations	Prevention/ prophylaxis	Diagnostic tests	Treatment options
		CNS involvement: Headache Mental status changes Diffuse CNS depression Focal neurologic findings Seizures Evolving cerebral vascular accidents		Patients may have invasive disease with negative sputum culture (Patel & Paya, 1997; Wheat, 1994)	
Candida	Mucocutaneous candidiasis (oropharyngeal thrush, candidal esophagitis, vaginitis, intertrigo, paronychia, onychomycosis) Sternal wound infection Disseminated infection Intra-abdominal abscess	Thrush White patches or ulcers in mouth Vaginitis: White or yellow vaginal discharge Pruritus Intertrigo: Erythematous, papular skin rash Paronychia: Redness, swelling, suppuration around nail edge	Clotrimazole troches Mycostatin (Dummer, 1995; Love, 1996)	Localized infection: Cultures with Gram's stain Disseminated candidiasis: Blood cultures CT scan Biopsy of skin lesions Tissue biopsy (dePauw, 2000; Wheat, 1994)	Clotrimazole Mycostatin Fluconazole for esophagitis and refractory candidiasis*† *Monitor renal function and cyclosporine levels; adjust dose accordingly †Effective for most Candida species except Candida krusei and Candida glabrata

continued

TABLE 2.1 *(continued)*

Organism	May cause	Clinical manifestations	Prevention/ prophylaxis	Diagnostic tests	Treatment options
	UTI Endocarditis (Love, 1996; Rubin, 1994)	Onychomycosis: Thickened, discolored nails			Candidemia in unstable or critically ill patients: Amphotericin B followed by fluconazole if organism is sensitive to fluconazole Candidemia in stable patients: fluconazole if organism is sensitive to fluconazole (Avery, 1994; Love, 1996; Thaler & Rubin, 1996)
Cryptococcus neoformans	Primary pulmonary infection	Pulmonary infection: Cough Lung nodules CNS involvement: Progressive headache Memory or attention deficits		Lumbar puncture CT scan MRI Blood culture	Amphotericin B* Amphotericin B* with 5 Flucytosine† Fluconazole*

continued

TABLE 2.1 (continued)

Organism	May cause	Clinical manifestations	Prevention/ prophylaxis	Diagnostic tests	Treatment options
	Secondary seeding of skin, CNS, eye, urinary tract and skeletal system (Rubin, 1994)	Emotional disturbance Disorders of balance Cranial nerve dysfunction Fever Meningismus Confusion Dysphasia Muscle weakness, tremor Urinary incontinence Focal neurologic signs Seizures Cutaneous involvement: Ulcers Papules or pustules Subcutaneous swelling or tumors Ecchymoses Granulomata Abscesses Vesicles Palpable purpura or papules Necrotizing vasculitis Cellulitis (Dummer, 1995; Patel & Paya, 1997)		CSF analysis: cell count, protein and sugar; Gram's stain, acid-fast and fungal stains, and cultures (fungal, bacterial, and mycobacterial) Cryptococcal antigen test on blood, CSF, pleural fluid (Rubin, 1994; Wheat, 1994)	*Requires monitoring of renal function and cyclosporine levels †Requires monitoring of 5 Flucytosine levels to minimize hepatic and bone marrow toxicity (Dummer, 1995; Singh, 1997; Wheat, 1994)

continued

TABLE 2.1 (*continued*)

Organism	May cause	Clinical manifestations	Prevention/ prophylaxis	Diagnostic tests	Treatment options
Pneumocystis carinii	Pneumonitis (Love, 1996)	Fever Dry cough Dyspnea Hypoxemia Tachypnea Diffuse pulmonary infiltrates (Rickenbacher & Hunt, 1996; Thaler & Rubin, 1996)	TMP-SMZ Dapsone Aerosolized pentamidine Atovaquone (Dummer, 1995; Love, 1996; Thaler & Rubin, 1996)	Transbronchial lung biopsy Needle biopsy of lung BAL Chest radiograph (may be negative) (Fishman, 1994; Para-meshwar, 1996; Rickenbacher & Hunt, 1996; Tolkoff-Rubin & Rubin, 2000)	TMP-SMZ (high-dose)* Pentamidine Dapsone-trimethoprim Atovaquone (for mild PCP) Clindamycin-primaquine (if not G6PD-deficient) *Dose must be adjusted for renal dysfunction (Avery, 1994; Dummer, 1995; Fishman, 1994)
Coccidioides immitis	Disseminated infection Isolated pulmonary infection	Subacute respiratory illness with either focal or dis-seminated interstitial or miliary infiltrates Fever Nonproductive cough Arthritis Osteomyelitis		Tissue biopsy Culture: respiratory secretions, blood, urine, joint fluid Serologic tests (not always positive)	Amphotericin B* Fluconazole or itra-conazole† for main-tenance therapy *Requires monitoring of renal function and cyclosporine levels

continued

TABLE 2.1 *(continued)*

Organism	May cause	Clinical manifestations	Prevention/ prophylaxis	Diagnostic tests	Treatment options
	Extrapulmonary involvement: spleen, joints, liver, brain, thyroid, pancreas, peritoneum, muscle, myocardium, skin, CNS (Love, 1996; Patel & Paya, 1997)	Mucocutaneous or CNS manifestations (especially meningitis) (Rubin, 1994)		Complement fixation tests (Wheat, 1994)	†Absorption may be erratic, especially in patients with low gastric acidity; monitor plasma concentration of drug (Patel & Paya, 1997; Wheat, 1994)
Histoplasma capsulatum	Disseminated infection (Love, 1996)	Subacute respiratory illness with either focal or disseminated interstitial or miliary infiltrates Fever (+/-) Night sweats Chills Cough Headache Arthritis, myalgias CNS manifestations Hepatosplenomegaly Cutaneous, intestinal, oral mucosal lesions (Patel & Paya, 1997; Rubin, 1994)	Itraconazole for seropositive recipients (Patel & Paya, 1997)	Methenamine-silver stain Peripheral blood stains Cultures: blood, respiratory secretions, tissue Serology Antigen detection (urine, serum, CSF, BAL fluid) Chest radiography (may be normal) (Patel & Paya, 1997; Wheat, 1994)	Amphotericin B* Itraconazole for maintenance therapy *Requires monitoring of renal function and cyclosporine levels

continued

TABLE 2.1 (continued)

Organism	May cause	Clinical manifestations	Prevention/ prophylaxis	Diagnostic tests	Treatment options
Crypto-sporidium	Gastroenteritis Gallbladder infection (Fishman, 1994)	Profuse, watery diarrhea Abdominal pain Nausea and vomiting Fever Myalgias (Fishman, 1994)	Boil water for 5 minutes, or use distilled water Avoid ice cubes in restaurants Avoid soda fountain drinks	Stool testing Antibody detection assays Small or large bowel biopsy (Fishman, 1994)	Fluid and electrolytes Maintenance of nutritional status Spiramycin effective for some patients; adverse effects reported (increased stool output and volume loss) (Fishman, 1994)
Toxoplasma gondii	Myocarditis Pericarditis Pneumonitis Encephalitis Hepatitis Retinochoroiditis (Fishman, 1994; Love, 1996; Parameshwar, 1996)	Mononucleosis-like syndrome of fever and lymphadenopathy Myocardial dysfunction that mimics rejection Pulmonary: fever, dyspnea, cough, hemoptysis CNS involvement: multiple focal neurologic deficits; altered mental status; fever with headache (Fishman, 1994)	Particularly for serone-negative recipient/seropositive donor: Pyrimethamine Pyrimethamine + sulfonamide Pyrimethamine + folinic acid Co-trimoxazole Atovaquone TMP-SMZ Avoid changing cat litter boxes	Endomyocardial biopsy Antibody titers Lung lavage and/or biopsy CT scan of head Chest radiograph Tissue and/or blood culture Serologic assays (Fishman, 1994; Thaler & Rubin, 1996)	Pyrimethamine with folinic acid and sulfadiazine Clindamycin and pyrimethamine with folinic acid (Patel & Paya, 1997)

continued

TABLE 2.1 *(continued)*

Organism	May cause	Clinical manifestations	Prevention/ prophylaxis	Diagnostic tests	Treatment options
			Avoid raw or under-cooked meat (Dummer, 1995; Parameshwar, 1996; Singh, 1997; Thaler & Rubin, 1996)		
Strongyloides stercoralis	Ulcerating, hemorrhagic enterocolitis Hemorrhagic pneumonia Disseminated disease: Pulmonary CNS (Gram-negative meningitis) (Rubin, 1994)	GI: 　Abdominal pain and distention 　Diarrhea 　Nausea and vomiting 　Adynamic ileus 　Small bowel obstruction 　GI hemorrhage Pulmonary: 　Tachypnea 　Dyspnea 　Bronchospasm 　Cough 　Hemoptysis CNS: 　Headache 　Fever 　Eosinophilic meningitis 　Mental status changes 　Coma 　Focal neurologic deficits 　Gram-negative meningitis	Consider preemptive Ivermectin for transplant candidates who have traveled to or lived in endemic areas	Stool specimen for rhabditiform larvae (may be negative) Papanicolaou's stain of duodenal aspirates, urine, ascitic fluid, sputum, stool Jejunal biopsy Serologic testing Chest radiograph (frequently inconclusive)	Albendazole Ivermectin* Taper of immuno-suppressive agents Systemic antibacterial therapy for bacteremia or meningitis *Periodic retreatments may be necessary (Patel & Paya, 1997; Rubin, 1994)

continued

TABLE 2.1 *(continued)*

Organism	May cause	Clinical manifestations	Prevention/ prophylaxis	Diagnostic tests	Treatment options
		Skin manifestions: Migratory, puritic, raised, linear rash that may move at rate of 10 cm/hour Crops of urticarial eruptions: immediate hypersensitive reactions to migrating worms (especially on waist and buttocks) (Fishman, 1994; Patel & Paya, 1997)			

BAL = bronchoalveolar lavage; ELISA = enzyme-linked immunoabsorbent assay; CBC = complete blood count; CNS = central nervous system; EBV = Epstein-Barr virus; GI = gastrointestinal; LFT = liver function tests; PCR = polymerase chain reaction; PTLD = posttransplantation lymphoproliferative disease; TMP-SMZ = trimethoprim sulfamethoxazole; VZV = varicella zoster virus; UTI = urinary tract infection; MRI = magnetic resonance imaging; CMV = cytomegalovirus; CSF = cerebrospinal fluid; CT = computed tomography; HBV = hepatitis B virus; HBsAg = hepatitis B surface antigen; HCV = hepatitis C virus; HCV-RNA = hepatitis C virus-Ribonucleic acid; HHV-6 = human herpes virus-6; HSV = herpes simplex virus; IV = intravenous

TABLE 2.2 Infection Timetable

Time period	Major types of infection	Example
During first month • Bacterial and candidal infections account for > 90 percent of infections during this time period	Infection related to surgical incision, indwelling lines and catheters (incidence highest in liver and lung transplant recipients) Nosocomial infections Urinary tract infection Respiratory infection Infections present in recipient pretransplant (prime concern: pneumonia) Infections present in allograft (may lead to infection of vascular suture line, mycotic aneurysm, and rupture)	Infection caused by: Staphylococci Gram-negative bacilli Candida Rarely: *Aspergillus* species *Legionella* species *Nocardia asteroides*
Months 2–6 • Residual infection from the first time period may continue, especially in liver and lung transplant recipients	Opportunistic infections Immunomodulatory viral infections	Opportunistic: *Pneumocystis carinii* *Listeria monocytogenes* Fungal infections Immunomodulatory viruses: Cytomegalovirus Epstein-Barr virus Hepatitis viruses Human immunodeficiency virus
After 6 months Three categories of recipients: • 80% have satisfactory graft function and are on maintenance doses of immunosuppression: infections acquired are similar to those of general population	Community-acquired infection	Respiratory infections: Influenza Adenoviruses Parainfluenza Respiratory syncytial virus *Mycobacterium tuberculosis*

TABLE 2.2 *(continued)*

Time period	Major types of infection	Example
• 10% have chronic viral infections that can lead to graft failure, malignancy, or HIV infection		Infections caused by contaminated food/water: *Salmonella* species *Listeria monocytogenes*
• 10% fail to do well after transplant as a result of acute/chronic rejection and immunosuppression; they are at increased risk of developing opportunistic infections		Opportunistic infections: *Cryptococcus neoformans* *Aspergillus* species *Nocardia asteroides* *Pneumocystis carinii*
		Endemic mycotic infections: *Histoplasma capsulatum* *Coccidioides immitis* *Blastomyces dermatitidis*
		Strongyloides stercoralis

Source: Avery, 1998a; Dummer, 1995; Kontoyiannis & Rubin, 1995; Miller, 1991; Rubin, 1994.

HISTORY

In diagnosing infection, it is important to take the following into consideration:

- Time interval since transplantation: Certain infections are more common at particular intervals posttransplant.
- Rejection history (severity and treatment): Risk of infection is higher any time immunosuppressants are increased to treat rejection.

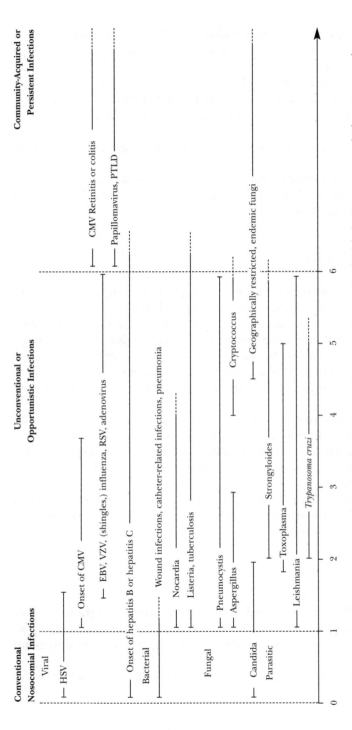

Exceptions to the usual sequence of infections after transplantation suggest the presence of unusual epidemiologic exposure or excessive immunosuppression.
HSV = herpes simplex virus   CMV = cytomegalovirus   EBV = Epstein-Barr virus   VZV = varicella-zoster virus
RSV = respiratory syncytial virus   PTLD = posttransplantation lymphoproliferative disease   Zero indicates the time of transplantation.
Solid lines indicate the most common period for the onset of infection; dotted lines and arrows indicate periods of continued risk at reduced levels. From Fishman, A.
Rubin, R. H., (1998). Medical progress: Infection in organ-transplant recipients. *New England Journal of Medicine*, 338(24), 1741–1751. Copyright © 1998, Massachusetts
Medical Society. All rights reserved. Used with permission.

Figure 2.1 Usual sequence of infections after organ transplantation.

- Current doses of immunosuppressants: Risk of infection is highest in the early postoperative period when immunosuppressive therapy is most intense.
- Current antimicrobial prophylaxis (if any)
- History of viremia: Certain viruses (e.g., CMV, EBV) are immunomodulatory viruses that can suppress the immune system.
- Pretransplant infection history
- Recent exposure to nosocomial, community, or geographic sources of infection
- Duration of symptoms: Bacterial infections usually manifest over a period of 24 to 48 hours, but can evolve over several (3–5) days (Avery, 1998a; Miller, 1991).

PHYSICAL EXAMINATION

- Pay particular attention to the sinuses, pharynx, lymph nodes, lungs, heart, abdomen, and skin (rashes and incisions).
- Although seemingly benign in appearance, metastatic skin lesions may be the first indication of a systemic infection due to opportunistic organisms such as *Cryptococcus neoformans, Candida,* and *Nocardia asteroides*; biopsies of unexplained skin lesions are essential.
- The most common type of tissue-invasive infection is pulmonary infection.
- Fever response may be blunted by high-dose corticosteroids or by severe end-organ dysfunction (e.g., uremia, advanced liver failure).
- Certain infections are not typically associated with fever (e.g., localized herpes simplex and herpes zoster infections, and mucosal candidal infections).
- Viral infections may have a subacute presentation (Avery, 1998a; Dummer, 1995; Fishman & Rubin, 1998; Kaye, Johnson, Wolfson, & Sober, 1994; Kontoyiannis & Rubin, 1995; Miller, 1991).

RADIOGRAPHY

- Radiography (conventional and/or computed tomography) is key to diagnosing infection of the chest and CNS—the two most important and common causes of life-threatening infection in transplant recipients.
- Chest films: Findings and onset (acute vs. subacute) may be useful (see Table 2.3).

- Single lung transplant recipients: Radiographic abnormalities in the native lung may make diagnosis of infection in the native lung difficult.
- Presence of new infiltrates necessitates an early, definitive diagnosis (Dummer, 1995; Rizk & Faul, 2000).

COMPUTED TOMOGRAPHY (CT)

- CT often provides more information than conventional radiography, especially in febrile patients with negative or subtle findings on chest radiography.
- CT is useful in determining which invasive diagnostic procedure would be indicated.
- Use of intravenous contrast material depends on patient's current renal function.
- In certain types of infection (e.g., pulmonary infections due to fungi or *Nocardia*), CT scans are more accurate than conventional radiography in determining the extent of infection and the patient's response to therapy.
- Fine-needle aspiration with CT guidance is indicated for focal, subsegmental, or nodular pulmonary disease.
- For patients with concurrent or sequential respiratory infections, CT is useful in identifying the second causative agent.
- CT scan of the sinuses: Patients taking cyclosporine may be predisposed to sinusitis; they may have acute sinusitis with minimal pain or tenderness.
- CT scan is better than magnetic resonance imaging (MRI) of the sinuses because only CT will show bony involvement (e.g., by invasion from the sinuses through the bone into the brain).
- Abdominal CT is useful for suspected abscesses or adenopathy. The majority of CNS infections in transplant recipients are caused by *Aspergillus* species, *C. neoformans,* and *Listeria monocytogenes*; therefore, patients with these infections require an MRI or CT scan of the brain.
- *Nocardial* infection of the lung always requires an MRI or CT scan of the head to rule out CNS nocardiosis. In general, MRI is more sensitive than head CT, even CT with contrast, in detecting brain and spinal cord lesions (Avery, 1998a; Dummer, 1995; Rizk & Faul, 2000; Tolkoff-Rubin & Rubin, 2000).

TABLE 2.3 Differential Diagnosis of Fever And Pulmonary Infiltrates in Organ Transplant Recipients According to the Abnormality on Chest Roentgenography and Rate of Progression of the Illness*

Radiographic Abnormality	*Cause*	
	Acute Illness†	*Subacute or Chronic Illness†*
Consolidation	Bacteria (including legionella) Thromboembolism Hemorrhage Pulmonary edema	Fungi *N. asteroides* Tumor Tuberculosis Viruses Drug reactions Radiation *P. carinii*
Peribronchovascular abnormality	Pulmonary edema Leukoagglutinin reaction Bacteria Viruses (influenza)	Viruses *P. carinii* Radiation Drug reactions (occasionally) *N. asteroides* Tumor Fungi Tuberculosis
Nodular infiltrate‡	Bacteria (including legionella) Pulmonary edema	Fungi *N. asteroides* Tuberculosis *P. carinii*

* From Fishman, A. Rubin, R. H. (1998). Medical progress: Infection in organ-transplant recipients. *New England Journal of Medicine,* 338(24), 1741–1751.Copyright © 1998, Massachusetts Medical Society. All rights reserved. Used with permission.

† An acute illness is defined as one that develops and requires medical attention in less than 24 hours. A subacute or chronic illness develops over a period of several days to weeks.

‡ A nodular infiltrate is defined as one or more focal defects more than 1 cm^2 in area on chest radiography with well-defined borders, surrounded by aerated lung. Multiple tiny nodules of smaller size are seen in a wide variety of disorders (e.g., cytomegalovirus and varicella zoster virus infections) and are not included here.

EARLY BRONCHOSCOPY

Early bronchoscopy is indicated for

- Unexplained dyspnea or hypoxemia, regardless of chest radiograph findings (pulmonary embolism should be considered if chest radiography is normal)
- Severe pulmonary illness
- Chest radiograph findings, particularly diffuse pulmonary infiltrates, that suggest opportunistic infection (Avery, 1998a; Dummer 1995)

ULTRASONOGRAPHY (US)

- Renal: useful for diagnosing obstructions or fluid collections (infected lymphoceles)
- Right upper quadrant US in liver transplant recipients: demonstrates patency of vessels (Avery, 1998a)

IMMUNOLOGICAL TECHNIQUES

- Skin tests or serological response tests may be of limited use for two reasons:
  - Immunosuppressive therapy may result in false-negative skin tests and serological response (circulating antibody).
  - Many pathogens such as *Candida* and *Aspergillus species* are so common in the environment that positive results may be obtained in the absence of the active disease.
- Antigen detection tests permit a quantitative assessment of microbial burden that can be used to guide therapy.
- Antigen tests (e.g., cryptococcus, histoplasma, legionella, and CMV antigen tests) signify active infection because they are based on the organism itself, and not the immune response to the organism (e.g., antibody-based tests).
- Polymerase chain reaction (PCR) assays can provide valuable information about some of the herpes family viruses (CMV, varicella zoster virus [VZV], EBV, herpes simplex virus [HSV]-1, HSV-2, and human herpesvirus [HHV]-6) with respect to diagnosis, viral load, prognosis, and therapeutic response (Tolkoff-Rubin & Rubin, 2000).

HISTOLOGICAL ASSESSMENT

Histological techniques are extremely important in the diagnosis of infection and should be used when possible because

- They facilitate rapid diagnosis and prompt initiation of therapy.
- They facilitate specific diagnosis, thereby decreasing the need for multidrug antimicrobial therapy—an important consideration given the number of interactions between antimicrobial agents and calcineurin inhibitors (cyclosporine and tacrolimus).
- Many opportunistic pathogens are difficult to grow in culture (Tolkoff-Rubin & Rubin, 2000).

INVASIVE GASTROINTESTINAL TESTS

Endoscopy, endoscopic retrograde cholangiopancreatography and colonoscopy are useful in diagnosing CMV infection, EBV-associated posttransplant lymphoproliferative disease (PTLD), *Clostridium difficile,* and *Helicobacter pylori* infections (Avery, 1998a).

BLOOD TESTS

- Serologic antibody tests (but not antigen tests) may be less sensitive because of the blunted inflammatory response to infection.
- Leukopenia may be caused by CMV infection or medications (e.g., ganciclovir, azathioprine, or mycophenolate mofetil).
- Liver enzyme levels may be elevated as a result of CMV infection, rejection, hepatitis A, B, or C infections, or medications (Avery, 1998a; Rubin, 1994).

URINALYSIS

Urinary tract infections in kidney transplant recipients may be asymptomatic. Therefore, urinalysis is an important diagnostic tool, particularly the more comprehensive urine cytodiagnostic tests (e.g., to demonstrate viral inclusions suggestive of BK virus or adenovirus).

CONSULTATIONS

Diagnosis and treatment of infection in transplant recipients is often challenging. Consultations with infectious disease physicians and/or pulmonologists are often required to identify causative organisms and to promptly initiate pathogen-specific therapy.

FEVER

The differential diagnosis of fever is complex. It is useful to consider the time period in which the fever occurs. The most common causes of fever for each time period are the following:

First Month after Transplantation
- Technical complications related to surgery, invasive lines, etc.
- Allograft rejection
- Antilymphocyte therapy, especially first few and last doses of a 10 to 14-day course
- (Note: Conventional drug fevers are uncommon.)

Months 2–6
- Viral infections (especially CMV)
- Antilymphocyte therapy

After 6 Months
- Occult opportunistic infections
- Antilymphocyte therapy (Kontoyiannis & Rubin, 1995)

FEVER OF UNKNOWN ORIGIN (FUO)

A challenging clinical situation is that of the transplant recipient who has had a fever of unknown origin for more than 7 days despite a comprehensive work-up and few other focal manifestations. Infections that may present in this fashion include

- Systemic viral syndromes due to CMV or EBV
- Disseminated tuberculosis
- Histoplasmosis
- Cryptococcosis
- Systemic toxoplasmosis

- Early *pneumocystis carinii* infection
- HIV infection (rarely) (Dummer, 1995)

Noninfectious causes of FUO include

- Rejection, especially in liver, kidney, and lung transplant recipients (Note: Allograft rejection is the most common cause of fever during the first posttransplant month.)
- Tissue ischemia
- Pulmonary emboli
- Drug reactions, particularly to antilymphocyte antibody therapy and antibiotics (Dummer, 1995; Rubin, 1994)

CNS INFECTIONS

The presentation of CNS infections in transplant recipients often differs from that in nonimmunosuppressed patients:

- Immunosuppressants may mask the signs of meningeal irritation
- The simultaneous presence of fever and headache is often the most reliable indication of the possibility of a CNS infection
- Transplant recipients who present with unexplained headache, with or without fever, should have a complete neurologic evaluation that includes
    - CT scan of the head to rule out a mass effect (e.g., cryptococcoma, tuberculoma, lymphoma, or brain abscess) or if there is papilledema, focal neurologic deficit, or altered state of consciousness
    - Lumbar puncture if there is no mass effect on head CT or MRI, papilledema, or focal neurologic deficit; cerebral spinal fluid (CSF) examination should include cell count, protein and sugar levels, Gram's stain, acid-fast and fungal stains, cultures (fungal, bacterial, and mycobacterial), and cryptococcal antigen testing
    - MRI for patients with spinal cord findings, focal neurologic findings, unexplained decrease in mental status, or unexplained CSF abnormalities (Rubin, 1994), even if a CT scan is normal

The four clinical syndromes that are typically observed in transplant recipients are

- Acute to subacute meningitis (common pathogen: *Listeria monocytogenes*)

- Subacute to chronic meningitis (common pathogens: *C. neoformans, Mycobacterium tuberculosis, Coccidioides immitis,* and *Histoplasma capsulatum*)
- Focal brain lesions (common pathogen: *Aspergillus* infection; occasionally: *Listeria, Toxoplasma, Nocardia,* or mucormycosis)
- Dementia due to progressive multifocal leukoencephalopathy caused by the polyomavirus JC) (Kontoyiannis & Rubin, 1995)

WHEN TO HOSPITALIZE

The diagnostic work-up of the solid organ transplant recipient can be challenging. Generally, it is recommended that the recipient be hospitalized for more aggressive testing if

- Chest infiltrates are present.
- Fevers above 38.5°C persist.
- The patient appears toxic.
- The patient cannot perform activities of daily living (Dummer, 1995).

INFECTIONS IN SPECIFIC ORGAN TRANSPLANT POPULATIONS

Although posttransplant infections typically occur at somewhat predictable time intervals, certain organ-specific differences do exist. Overall, infection morbidity and mortality are highest among liver and lung transplant recipients and lowest among kidney and heart transplant recipients (Dummer, 1995).

KIDNEY TRANSPLANT RECIPIENTS

- Urinary tract infection (UTI) is the most common bacterial infection. UTIs may be asymptomatic; patients with urosepsis typically do not have urgency, frequency, or dysuria. Asymptomatic candiduria can be serious because of the potential for development of obstructing candidal fungal balls, ascending candidal pyelonephritis, and sepsis, particularly in diabetic patients with bladder dysfunction.
- CMV infection is the most important pathogen among renal transplant recipients.
- Unilateral leg edema on the side of the kidney transplant may be a sign of a lymphocoele, either infected or not infected, near the kidney transplant.

- FUO may be associated with a deep wound infection; diagnosis requires needle aspiration of wound and US or CT scanning of both pelvic implantation and nephrectomy operative sites.
- Hepatitis infections are more common in renal transplant recipients than in any other types of solid organ recipients except liver transplant patients.
- Female recipients have an increased risk of intraepithelial and invasive squamous tumors of the cervix associated with human papillomavirus (Dummer, 1995; Grossman, 1998; Holochek, Agunod, Burrell-Diggs, & Darmody, 1995; Patel & Paya, 1997; Rubin, 1994; Sia & Paya, 1998).

HEART TRANSPLANT RECIPIENTS

The lung is the most common site of infection in heart transplant recipients (Patel & Paya, 1997).

Mediastinitis

Mediastinitis is most common during the first 2 to 4 weeks posttransplant. Initial symptoms of mediastinitis may be subtle (mild chest discomfort, slight edema, and/or erythema along the sternal incision). Some patients may present with fever and bacteremia (Dummer, 1995).

CMV

- CMV is the single most common and important pathogen that affects heart transplant recipients.
- The risk of CMV infection is 50% to 75% in seronegative patients who receive a seropositive allograft and in patients who require antilymphocyte antibody therapy to treat rejection.
- The risk of developing symptomatic CMV disease is significantly greater when the virus that is activated is of donor origin rather than recipient origin.
- The GI tract is the most common site of CMV infection.
- CMV pneumonitis has the highest morbidity and mortality of any CMV infection (Miller, 1991; Rubin, 2000; Thaler & Rubin, 1996).

Toxoplasmosis

- Toxoplasmosis is more common in heart and heart–lung transplant recipients than in any other transplant groups because these pathogens encyst in the heart muscle.

- The overall incidence of toxoplasmosis in heart transplant recipients ranges from 4% to 12%. However, the incidence increases to more than 50% for *toxoplasma*-seronegative recipients who receive allografts from seropositive donors.
- Symptoms of toxoplasmosis may appear from 3 weeks to 6 months posttransplant.
- Toxoplasmosis can mimic rejection; therefore, endomyocardial biopsy is required for a definitive diagnosis (Dummer, 1995; Singh, 1997; Thaler & Rubin, 1996).

HEART–LUNG AND LUNG TRANSPLANT RECIPIENTS

- Bacterial pathogens are the most common cause of pulmonary infections in lung transplant recipients; early pathogens include *Klebsiella pneumoniae, Pseudomonas aeruginosa, Escherichia coli, Staphylococcus aureus,* and *Enterobacter cloacae.*
- Fungal, viral, and pneumocystis infections occur more frequently in lung transplant recipients than in any other transplant group.
- CMV is the most lethal infection among lung transplant recipients.
- The donor lung is the only type of allograft that is frequently infected or colonized with bacterial pathogens.
- Infections involving bronchial or tracheal anastomoses may cause airway dehiscence. Nosocomial bacteria, *candida,* and *aspergillus* are commonly associated with anastomotic infections.
- The native lung of single lung transplant recipients is also susceptible to infection.
- Radiographic changes in the native lung (e.g., those caused by fibrosis) may make diagnosis difficult.
- Pseudomonas infections are particularly problematic among recipients who undergo lung transplantation for cystic fibrosis (Deusch et al., 1993; Dummer, 1995; Frost, 1999; Singh, 1997).

LIVER TRANSPLANT RECIPIENTS

- The abdomen is the most common site of bacterial infection.
- Of all solid organ transplant recipients, liver transplant recipients have the highest incidence of invasive fungal infections.
- Early after transplant, intra-abdominal and liver abscesses, peritonitis, wound infections, and cholangitis are common; therefore, abdominal scanning tests (CT scan or Doppler US), cholangiograms, and

hepatic angiography may be required for the febrile and/or bacteremic recipient.

- Infections often involve *Candida* and common microbial flora such as *E. coli, enterococcus,* and anaerobes. Other pathogens include coagulase positive and negative staphylococci and diphtheroids. Vancomycin-resistant enterococci (VRE) infections can also occur.
- Recipients with Roux-en-Y choledochojejunostomy anastomoses have a higher rate of abdominal infections than recipients with a choledochostomy (duct-to-duct) biliary anastamoses because the former technique is associated with the reflux of enteric organisms into the biliary system.
- Fever may not occur with some organisms (e.g., *Candida*). Elevated white count or lack of clinical improvement may be the only indication of infection.
- Almost all liver transplant recipients who had pretransplant hepatitis C virus (HCV) infections remain viremic after transplantation. Recurrent HCV occurs in 30% to 70% of these patients during the first posttransplant year.
- Without adequate immunoprophylaxis, hepatitis B virus (HBV) graft infection recurs in 80 to 100 percent of hepatitis B surface antigen-positive liver transplant recipients (Fontana et al., 2001). However, the recurrence rate is significantly reduced with the appropriate use of hepatitis B immune globulin and new antiviral agents such as lamivudine and adefovir (Bzowej & Wright, 1998; Keefe, 2000; Paya, 2001).

KIDNEY–PANCREAS TRANSPLANT RECIPIENTS

Wound infections and UTIs are more common in kidney–pancreas transplant recipients than in isolated kidney transplant recipients. Factors associated with an increased risk of UTI include

- Enzymatic digestion of the glycosaminoglycan layer that normally protects the urothelium
- Change in urinary pH secondary to pancreatic exocrine secretions
- Underlying glycosuria (Patel & Paya, 1997)

PANCREAS TRANSPLANT RECIPIENTS

Pancreas transplant recipients are particularly susceptible to candidiasis (due to underlying diabetes, indwelling bladder catheters, and drainage of exocrine secretions into the bladder). The most common bacterial infections are wound and intra-abdominal infections (Singh, 1997).

SMALL BOWEL TRANSPLANT RECIPIENTS

Recipients are at risk for intra-abdominal and wound infections. Bacterial translocation (from intestinal lumen to bloodstream) can occur as a result of either bacterial overgrowth or sloughing of the intestinal mucosa secondary to ischemic injury or rejection. Clinical manifestations of microbial migration include high fever, chills, and symptoms of septic shock (Abu-Elmagd et al., 1992; Funovits, Staschak-Chicko, Kovalak, & Altiere, 1995).

SPECIFIC TYPES OF INFECTIONS

HERPES VIRUS INFECTIONS

The major viral infections that affect transplant recipients are those caused by cytomegalovirus, Epstein-Barr virus, herpes simplex 1 and 2, varicella zoster virus, and human herpesvirus-6. Latency is a characteristic of all herpes viruses: Once the virus is present, the viral genome remains in infected host cells for life and immunosuppression can trigger replication of the latent virus. It is important to differentiate the terms *infection* and *disease.* *Infection* with herpes viruses indicates viral replication as evidenced by culture or serologic testing. The term *disease* indicates that the recipient has specific symptoms that can be attributed to herpes viruses (Singh, 1997).

Cytomegalovirus (CMV)

- Cytomegalovirus is the most important of the opportunistic pathogens because of its direct pathogenic effect, its role in allograft rejection, and its immunomodulatory ability to facilitate superinfection by other microbes.
- CMV occurs in 30% to 70% of all solid organ transplant recipients; approximately 50% of these recipients develop symptomatic disease.
- CMV infection and disease typically occur most frequently in heart–lung and lung transplant recipients, followed (in descending order) by small bowel, liver, heart, and kidney transplant recipients.
- The transplanted organ is more likely to be affected than a native organ; however, CMV pneumonitis can occur in all types of solid organ transplant recipients.
- Any factor that induces an inflammatory process or stress (e.g., sepsis, rejection, or augmented immunosuppressive therapy) is associated with the reactivation of latent CMV. Whether clinical disease develops depends on the relationship between viral load and host defenses.

- The relationship between CMV and rejection is bidirectional: CMV can cause rejection, and the rejection-mediated inflammatory response can increase CMV viral replication.
- Recipients who present with lower GI bleeding within 4 months of transplantation should be worked up for CMV colitis (Fishman & Rubin, 1998; Patel & Paya, 1997; Singh, 1997; Tolkoff-Rubin & Rubin, 2000).

Epstein-Barr Virus (EBV)

- Approximately 90% of adults are seropositive for Epstein-Barr virus. Therefore, most EBV infections in transplant recipients are reactivation infections. Reactivation infections occur in approximately 30% to 40% of EBV seropositive recipients.
- EBV seronegative recipients can acquire primary EBV infection from the community or from the allograft or blood products. Primary EBV infections occur in approximately 70% to 80% of EBV seronegative transplant recipients.
- Although EBV infection may be asymptomatic, its consequences range from mononucleosis to posttransplant lymphoproliferative disease (PTLD). Risk factors for PTLD include
  - High EBV viral load
  - Primary EBV infection
  - CMV infection
  - High-dose antilymphocyte antibody therapy, high-doses of cyclosporine or tacrolimus, or pulse corticosteroid therapy, particularly if used in combination.
  - Type of organ transplanted (Fishman & Rubin, 1998; Tolkoff-Rubin & Rubin, 2000).
- The incidence of EBV is highest in small bowel transplant recipients, followed, in decreasing order, by heart-lung, lung, heart, liver, and renal transplant recipients (Fishman & Rubin, 1998; Rubin, 1994; Singh, 1997; Tolkoff-Rubin & Rubin, 2000).

Herpes Simplex Virus (HSV)

- Virtually all HSV infections in transplant recipients result from reactivation of a latent virus.
- HSV infections occur in 25% to 40% of transplant recipients.
- Herpes labialis is the most common clinical manifestation of HSV-1. These lesions may bleed, interfere with nutritional intake, and require local analgesia to control pain.

- Squamous cell carcinoma must be ruled out in verrucous lip lesions that do not respond to acyclovir therapy.
- HSV may cause hepatitis, especially in liver transplant recipients (Patel & Paya, 1997, Rubin, 1994; Singh, 1997).

Varicella Zoster Virus (VZV)

- Approximately 10% of all solid organ transplant recipients will develop clinical zoster as a result of reactivation of dormant VZV in the dorsal root ganglia.
- Although VZV infection may occur at any time, it typically occurs between 3 months and 3 years posttransplant.
- VZV seronegative recipients are advised to report any exposure to VZV so that zoster immune globulin may be promptly administered; Patients should be observed closely so that clinical manifestations can be promptly treated (Avery, 1994).
- Cutaneous manifestations may be muted, especially if immune globulin is given; therefore, watch for primarily visceral manifestations.
- Chickenpox in a transplant recipient constitutes a medical emergency and requires hospitalization for intravenous antiviral therapy (Avery, 1994; Dummer, 1995; Rubin, 1994).

Human Herpesvirus-6 (HHV-6)

- Most posttransplant HHV-6 infections result from endogenous reactivation of latent virus in the recipient.
- Onset is typically between 2 and 4 weeks posttransplant.
- Coinfection with CMV is common (Rubin, 1994; Singh, 1997).
- HHV-6 can cause meningoencephalitis, pneumonitis, and bone marrow suppression.

HEPATITIS INFECTIONS

Approximately 10% to 15% of transplant recipients are subject to the morbidity and mortality associated with chronic liver disease. Liver disease may be the result of drug-induced hepatotoxicity or virus-induced disease. Hepatotoxic drugs include

- Certain immunosuppressive agents, particularly azathioprine and cyclosporine

- Antimicrobial agents, particularly antituberculous medications such as isoniazid (INH), pyrazinamide, rifampin, trimethoprim-sulfamethoxazole, alpha-methyl-dopa, and azole antifungal agents
- Antihypertensive agents
- Diuretics (Rubin, 1994).

Hepatitis C Virus (HCV)

- HCV is a leading cause of posttransplant hepatitis.
- At 10 years posttransplant, 10% to 20% of recipients with HCV infection will have end-stage liver disease and/or hepatocellular carcinoma.
- The combination of interferon and ribavirin is the most effective therapy, but often patients cannot tolerate this regimen. This combination is effective in less than half of patients with HCV infection who have the most common genotype found in the United States (genotype 1) (Singh, 1997; Tolkoff-Rubin & Rubin, 2000).

Hepatitis B Virus (HBV)

- HBV is associated with the development of hepatitis, cirrhosis, and hepatocellular carcinoma in transplant recipients.
- Immunosuppressive therapy may blunt liver function abnormalities and histologic evidence of HBV activity.
- At 10 years posttransplant, approximately 50% of recipients with HBV infection will have end-stage liver disease and/or hepatocellular carcinoma (Rubin, 1994; Tolkoff-Rubin & Rubin, 2000).

HUMAN IMMUNODEFICIENCY VIRUS (HIV)

- Most transplant-related HIV infections were acquired before 1985, when HIV screening became routine.
- Among recipients with primary transplant-related HIV infections, the mean time to the development of acquired immune deficiency syndrome is approximately 3 years (Rubin, 1994; Singh, 1997).

BACTERIAL INFECTIONS

Unusual bacterial pathogens of major concern include *Listeria monocytogenes, Nocardia asteroides, Legionella pneumophila,* and typical and atypical mycobacteria. Bacteria are responsible for 40 to 80 percent of posttransplant pneumonias. Significant nosocomial pathogens associated with early posttransplant pneumonia include *Pseudomonas aeruginosa,* Enterobacteriaceae, and *Staphylococcus aureus* (Singh, 1997). Staphylococci are a significant cause of nosocomial bacteremia (Singh, 1997).

Listeriosis

- *Listeria monocytogenes* is one of the most frequent causes of CNS infection in transplant recipients.
- Listeriosis that causes meningitis can have a 25% mortality rate (Dummer, 1995; Rubin, 1994).

Nocardiosis

- Infection is acquired through inhalation into the lungs or inoculation into the skin.
- Patients typically have subacute onset of symptoms; however, some may present with disseminated infection. Common sites of dissemination include the CNS, skin, and bone (Dummer, 1995).

Legionellosis

- A contaminated hospital water supply is the most commonly implicated source of legionellosis. Transmission has also been linked to drinking water, contaminated ventilators, nebulizers, water heaters, room humidifiers, and water aerosolization sources.
- The possibility of legionella infection should be considered whenever a transplant recipient presents with pneumonia-like symptoms. Simultaneous infection by other pulmonary pathogens may occur. The mortality rate of legionella pneumonia in transplant recipients often exceeds 50% (Ample & Wing, 1994; Dummer, 1995).
- The urine antigen test for legionella only detects *Legionella pneumophilia* serotype 1.

Tuberculosis

- The forms of tuberculosis that have been seen in transplant recipients include cavitary disease of the lung as well as miliary, bowel, skeletal, renal, bone marrow, liver, skin, and CNS disease.
- Tuberculin tests are positive in approximately one fourth to one third of recipients with tuberculosis.

- Isoniazid prophylaxis in transplant candidates and recipients is controversial and should be discussed with the transplant center (Patel & Paya, 1997; Rubin, 1994). Active tuberculosis must be ruled out before giving prophylaxis with either isoniazid alone or the combination of rifampin plus pyrazinamide, so as to prevent the development of resistance to these drugs.

FUNGAL INFECTIONS

Fungal infections may be categorized as opportunistic infections (e.g., aspergillosis, candidiasis, cryptococcosis, and pneumocystis) and infection with geographically restricted mycoses (histoplasmosis, coccidioidomycosis, and blastomycosis) (Rubin, 1994).

General Considerations

- Risk factors for fungal infections include older age, poor allograft function, leukopenia, hyperglycemia, high doses of corticosteroids, and multiple or recent episodes of rejection.
- Although the incidence of fungal infection among transplant recipients is lower than that of bacterial or viral infections, mortality associated with fungal infections ranges between 27% and 77%.
- The clinical manifestations of fungal infections are often nonspecific and frequently overlap with other processes (infectious and noninfectious).
- Once a fungal infection is diagnosed, the clinician should look for metastatic infection, particularly to the skin, skeleton, and CNS (Patel & Paya, 1997).
- It is important to determine if the fungal infection represents a therapeutic emergency or a subacute process:
  - In the case of a therapeutic emergency, amphotericin B is the treatment of choice until the process is under control; follow-up therapy with a less toxic agent is then indicated. Either traditional amphotericin B deoxycholate or the newer lipid-containing formulations of amphotericin B, which are less nephrotoxic, can be used.
  - If a subacute process is involved, less toxic therapy (e.g., with fluconazole) is indicated until microbiological control is achieved (Tolkoff-Rubin & Rubin, 2000).

Aspergillosis

- From 15% to 20% of all fungal infections are due to aspergillosis.
- Aspergillosis is associated with extremely high morbidity and mortality. Infections with CNS involvement or disseminated disease are almost always fatal.
- Risk factors for invasive disease include prolonged surgical time, laparotomy, neutropenia, elevated serum creatinine level, CMV infection, and augmented immunosuppressive therapy.
- The lung is the most common site of primary infection. Clinical manifestations of invasive pulmonary disease are nonspecific.
- Tissue infection is followed by invasion of blood vessels, which in turn leads to tissue infarction, hemorrhage, and metastatic seeding (Dummer, 1995; Patel & Paya, 1997; Rickenbacher & Hunt, 1996; Singh, 1997).

Candidiasis

- Mucocutaneous infections and candiduria (urinary tract infection) are the most common manifestations of candidiasis and do not necessarily indicate systemic disease. However, deep skin lesions and/or candidemia are usually indicative of systemic disease.
- Candidemia is associated with more than a 50% incidence of visceral seeding. Therefore, these patients require systemic chemotherapy.
- Recipients with even a single blood culture positive for *Candida* species must have systemic therapy for 10 to 14 days or longer and be evaluated for line-related infection (Patel & Paya, 1997; Rubin, 1994; Tolkoff-Rubin & Rubin, 2000).

Cryptococcosis

Cryptococcoccis typically occurs more than 6 months after transplantation. Among transplant recipients, *Cryptococcus neoformans* is the most common cause of fungal CNS infection (Rubin, 1994).

Pneumocystis pneumonia

Pneumocystis infection typically occurs between 2 and 6 months posttransplant. A number of diseases may mimic pneumocystis, including CMV and adenovirus infection, influenza, respiratory syncytial virus, adult respiratory distress syndrome, miliary tuberculosis, and disseminated fungal infections (Dummer, 1995).

Endemic Disease

- Endemic mycoses should be considered in symptomatic patients who have traveled to or lived in Central or South America, Southeast Asia, or the Midwest or southwestern U.S.
- The pathogenesis of histoplasmosis, coccidioidomycosis and blastomycosis is similar to that of tuberculosis. The following clinical presentations should prompt consideration of endemic disease in the differential diagnosis:
  - Subacute respiratory illness with focal or disseminated infiltrates on chest radiograph (interstitial or miliary)
  - Non-specific febrile illness
  - Illness in which metastatic aspects predominate (e.g., mucocutanous manifestations in histoplasmosis or blastomycosis; CNS manifestations in coccidioidomycosis) (dePauw, 2000; Rubin, 1994).

PROTOZOAL INFECTIONS

Protozoal infections common among transplant recipients are those caused by *Toxoplasma gondii* and *Cryptosporidium parvum*.

Toxoplasmosis

The incidence of toxoplasmosis is highest in *Toxoplasma* seronegative recipients who receive allografts from seropositive donors. (See Section on Heart Transplantation).

Cryptosporidiosis

- Diarrhea caused by *cryptosporidium* is frequently fatal in immunocompromised patients. Hospitalization may be required to reverse dehydration and wasting.
- Infection of the proximal small bowel is common; however, organisms can also be harbored in the hepatobiliary tree.
- Organisms shed by patients are infectious; therefore universal precautions are mandatory.
- This disease is transmitted by fecal-oral contamination or water transmission. Transplant recipients whose water supplies may be contaminated with *cryptosporidium* are instructed to take special precautions (Table 2.2) (Fishman, 1994).

HELMINTHIC (WORM) PARASITES

Strongyloidiasis

- *Strongyloides stercoralis,* an intestinal nematode, is endemic in many areas and has been found in 36 states.
- This organism can live in the GI tract for decades.
- Transplant candidates who have lived in endemic areas should have Papanicolaou's smears of sputum, duodenal aspirates, and purged stool specimens to look for larvae.
- Eosinophilia, a typical marker for parasitic infection, may be absent due to immunosuppressive therapy and concurrent systemic bacterial infection (Rubin, 1994).

PREVENTION OF INFECTION

Nonpharmacological measures to prevent infection are listed in Table 2.4. Pharmacological measures to prevent infection include prophylactic and preemptive antimicrobial therapy when immunosuppression therapy is most intense (Table 2.2), routine American Heart Association prophylaxis against infective endocarditis, and vaccinations.

- Prophylactic therapy is the administration of antimicrobial agents to an entire population in order to prevent the occurrence of a given infection (e.g., low-dose trimethoprim-sulfamethoxazole (TMP-SMZ) administered for 6 months to heart transplant recipients).
- Preemptive therapy is the administration of antimicrobial agents to a particular subset of patients at highest risk for infection (e.g., intravenous ganciclovir administered concurrently with a 10 to 14-day course of antilymphocyte therapy) (Kontoyiannis & Rubin, 1995).

VACCINES

Standard vaccine protocols for solid organ transplant recipients have not been determined. There is some concern that vaccine-induced stimulation of the immune system may trigger rejection. The transplant recipient's immune response to vaccines may be variable. Several of the Centers for Disease Control and Prevention guidelines for preventing infection among hematopoietic stem cell transplant recipients *may* be considered for solid organ transplant recipients. These include the pneumococcal

TABLE 2.4   Nonpharmacological Measures to Prevent Infection

- Frequent and thorough hand washing by patient and family members
- Avoidance of people with obvious signs of illness
- Use of leukocyte-depleted or cytomegalovirus-negative blood products; use of high-efficiency leukocyte filters
- Periodic infection surveillance: serologic titers for cytomegalovirus, Epstein-Barr virus, herpes simplex, hepatitis, human immunodeficiency virus, and other viruses; annual chest radiography
- Avoidance of close contact with infants and others who have recently received live virus vaccines such as the oral polio, varicella, or measles-mumps-rubella vaccines
- Avoidance of potential animal sources of infection (e.g., cat litter boxes, bird cages, and aquariums)
- Avoidance of raw or partially cooked foods of animal origin
- Avoidance of cross-contamination between raw and cooked foods
- Washing raw fruits and vegetables thoroughly before eating (Love, 1996)

vaccine and the *Haemophilus influenzae* type B vaccine ("Guidelines," 2000). Some transplant centers prefer to treat tetanus-related wounds with tetanus immune globulin alone (Avery, 1994).

Influenza Vaccine

Administration of an annual influenza vaccination remains controversial. According to the Centers for Disease Control and Prevention (1993, p. 7), "Because influenza may result in serious illness and complications for immunocompromised persons, vaccination is recommended and may result in protective antibody levels in many immunocompromised recipients." Some transplant centers prefer to make patient-specific decisions regarding the influenza vaccine based on the interval since transplant and the recipient's rejection history and current level of immunosuppression. However, all household contacts of the transplant recipient should obtain an annual influenza vaccine unless otherwise contraindicated (Patel & Paya, 1997).

Hepatitis B Vaccine

This vaccine is generally recommended for HBV seronegative recipients; however, serologic response (hepatitis B surface antibody) may be variable (Avery, 1994).

Live Attenuated Vaccines

Transplant recipients should not receive live attenuated viruses because viral replication may be facilitated in immunocompromised individuals. Specific live viruses to avoid include

- Oral polio vaccine (OPV)
- Measles-mumps-rubella vaccine
- Bacillus Calmette-Guerin
- Smallpox vaccine
- TY21a typhoid vaccine
- Yellow fever vaccine, if severely immunosuppressed (Centers for Disease Control and Prevention, 1993)

In addition, the OPV should not be administered to household contacts of transplant recipients. The Centers for Disease Control and Prevention (1993, p. 5) recommend that "[i]f OPV is inadvertently administered to a household or intimate contact (regardless of prior immunization status) of an immunocompromised patient, close contact between the patient and the recipient of the OPV should be avoided for approximately one month after vaccination, the period of maximum excretion of the virus." Poliovirus can be shed in the stool of individuals who receive the live OPV. If a household contact must receive a polio vaccine, the enhanced inactivated polio vaccine is recommended.

TREATMENT OF INFECTION

GENERAL PRINCIPLES

There are several general principles that guide the management of infection in transplant recipients:

1. Antimicrobial agents can be prescribed in a therapeutic, prophylactic, or preemptive mode (Table 2.2).
2. Regardless of specific mode, antimicrobial therapy is linked to the type and dose of immunosuppression agents the recipient is currently taking.
3. Antimicrobial therapy is not prescribed for "fixed" courses, but rather is based on "microbial burden." The greater the burden, the longer and more intense the therapy. Therapy is continued until clinical and laboratory evidence demonstrates that active infection has been eradicated.

4. For patients whose source of infection is linked to an anatomical or technical abnormality, surgical correction of the abnormality is mandatory; otherwise, antimicrobial therapy will fail.
5. In general, pathogen-specific antimicrobial therapy is preferred over broad-spectrum, empiric antibiotics (Table 2.2).
6. Antimicrobial therapy is based on the history and physical examination and guided by the results of Gram's stains and other diagnostic tests (Table 2.2).
7. The goals of antimicrobial therapy are
   • Eradication of active infection
   • Limitation of any pathologic effect
   • Prevention of recurrence
8. Certain antimicrobial agents can significantly interact with cyclosporine and tacrolimus. Macrolide antibiotics, in particular, should be avoided whenever possible because they elevate levels of calcineurin inhibitors (Miller, 1991; Rubin, 2000; Tolkoff-Rubin, 2000).

DRUG INTERACTIONS

Antimicrobial agents can cause both pharmacokinetic and idiosyncratic drug interactions (Table 2.5). Pharmacokinetic interactions occur because cyclosporine and tacrolimus are metabolized via the cytochrome p450 hepatic enzyme system. Antimicrobial agents that down-regulate this system increase cyclosporine or tacrolimus levels. Down-regulation can result in nephrotoxicity, overimmunosuppression, and infection. Other antimicrobials upregulate the cytochrome p450 system and can cause inadequate immunosuppression and graft rejection (Dummer, 1995; Rubin, 1994). Idiosyncratic nephrotoxicity can occur in patients with normal renal function. Because of the potential for drug interactions and nephrotoxicity, the patient's transplant center should be contacted for specific recommendations regarding antimicrobial therapy.

REFERENCES

Abu-Elmagd, K., Fung, J. J., Reyes, J., Casavilla A., Van Thiel, D. H., Iwaki, Y., Warty, V., Nikolaidis, N., Block J., & Nakamura, K. (1992). Management of intestinal transplantation in humans. *Transplantation Proceedings, 24*(3), 1243–1244.

Ampel, N. M., & Wing, E. J. (1994). Legionellosis in the compromised host. In R. H. Rubin & L. S. Young (Eds.), *Clinical approach to infection in the compromised host* (3rd ed., pp. 335–353). New York: Plenum.

TABLE 2.5 Antimicrobial Agents: Pharmacokinetic and Idiosyncratic Drug Interactions

Increase cyclosporine or tacrolimus levels	Decrease cyclosporine or tacrolimus levels	Potential to cause additive nephrotoxicity
Azithromycin	Imipenem	Acyclovir
Clarithromycin	Isoniazid	Aminoglycosides
Erythromycin	Nafcillin	Amphotericin B
Fluconazole	Rifampin	Ciprofloxacin (high dose)
Itraconazole	Sulfamethoxazole	Erythromycin
Josamycin		Foscarnet
Ketoconazole		Ketoconazole
		Pentamidine
		Trimethoprim-sulfamethoxazole (IV and high doses)
		Quinolones (high doses)
		Vancomycin

Source: Avery 1998a; Sollinger & Pirsch, 1996; Tolkoff-Rubin & Rubin, 2000; Wagoner, 1997.

Avery, R. K. (1994). Infections and immunizations in organ transplant recipients: A preventive approach. *Cleveland Clinic Journal of Medicine, 61*(5), 386–392.

Avery, R. K. (1998a). Infectious disease and transplantation: Messages for the generalist. *Cleveland Clinic Journal of Medicine, 65*(6), 305–314.

Avery, R. K. (1998b). Prevention and treatment of cytomegalovirus infection and disease in heart transplant recipients. *Current Opinion in Cardiology, 13,* 122–129.

Bzowej, N. H., & Wright, T. L. (1998). Viral hepatitis in the transplant patient. In R. A. Bowden, P. Ljungman, & C. V. Paya (Eds.), *Transplant infections* (pp. 309–324). Philadelphia: Lippincott-Raven.

Centers for Disease Control and Prevention. (1993). Recommendations of the Advisory Committee on Immunization Practices (ACIP): Use of vaccines and immune globulins in persons with altered immunocompetence. *Morbidity and Mortality Weekly Report, 43*(No. RR-4), 1–18.

dePauw, B. E. (2000). Advances in the management of invasive fungal infections in organ transplant recipients: Step by step. *Transplant Infectious Disease, 2,* 48–50.

Deusch, E., End, A., Grimm, M., Graninger, W., Klepetko, W., & Wolner, E. (1993). Early bacterial infections in lung transplant recipients. *Chest, 104*(5), 1412–1416.

Dummer, S. (1995). Infections in transplantation. In L. Makowa & L. Sher (Eds.), *Handbook of organ transplantation* (pp. 305–335). Austin, TX: Landes Bioscience.

Fishman, J. A. (1994). *Pneumocystis carinii* and parasitic infections in the immuno-compromised host. In R. H. Rubin & L. S. Young (Eds.), *Clinical approach to infection in the compromised host* (3rd ed., pp. 275–334). New York: Plenum.

Fishman, J. A., & Rubin, R. H. (1998). Medical progress: Infection in organ transplant recipients. *New England Journal of Medicine, 338*(24), 1741–1751.

Fontana, R. J., Hann, H. L., Wright, T., Everson, G., Baker, A., Schiff, E. R., Riely, C., Anscheutz, G., Riker-Hopkins, M., & Brown, N. (2001). A multicenter study of lamivudine treatment in 33 patients with hepatitis B after liver transplantation. *Liver Transplantation, 7*(6), 504–510.

Frost, A. E. (1999). Role of infections, pathogenesis, and management in lung transplantation. *Transplantation Proceedings, 31,* 175–177.

Funovits, M., Staschak-Chicko, S. M., Kovalak, J. A., & Altieri, K. A. (1995). Transplantation of the small intestine. In M. T. Nolan & S. M. Augustine (Eds.), *Transplantation nursing: Acute and long-term management* (pp. 319–345). Norwalk, CT: Appleton & Lange.

Grossman, R. A. (1998). Care of the renal transplant recipient: A field guide for the generalist. *Disease-A-Month, 44*(6), 269–282.

Guidelines for preventing opportunistic infections among hematopoietic stem cell transplant recipients. *Morbidity and Mortality Weekly Report,* (2000, October 20). pp. 97–125.

Holechek, M. J., Agunod, M. O., Burrell-Diggs, D., & Darmody, J. K. (1995). Renal transplantation. In M. T. Nolan & S. M. Augustine (Eds.), *Transplantation nursing: Acute and long-term management* (pp. 210–237). Norwalk, CT: Appleton & Lange.

Kaye, E. T., Johnson, R. A., Wolfson, J. S., & Sober, A. J. (1994). Dermatologic manifestations of infection in the compromised host. In R. H. Rubin & L. S. Young (Eds.), *Clinical approach to infection in the compromised host* (3rd ed., pp. 105–119). New York: Plenum.

Keefe, E. B. (2000). End-stage liver disease and liver transplantation: Role of lamivudine therapy in patients with chronic hepatitis B. *Journal of Medical Virology, 61,* 403–408.

Kontoyiannis, D. P., & Rubin, R. H. (1995). Infection in the organ transplant recipient. *Infectious Disease Clinics of North America, 9*(4), 811–822.

Love, K. (1996). Prevention and prophylaxis of infection in thoracic transplantation. In R. W. Emery & L. W. Miller (Eds.), *Handbook of cardiac transplantation* (pp. 17–30). Philadelphia: Hanley & Belfus.

Martin, M. (1995). Prophylactic cytomegalovirus management strategies. *Transplantation Proceedings, 27*(5, Suppl. 1), 23–27.

Miller, L. W. (1991). Long-term complications of cardiac transplantation. *Progress in Cardiovascular Diseases, 33*(4), 229–282.

Parameshwar, J. (1996). Follow-up after cardiac transplantation. *British Journal of Hospital Medicine, 56*(7), 350–354.

Patel, R., & Paya, C. V. (1997). Infections in solid organ transplant recipients. *Clinical Microbiology Reviews, 10,* 86–124.

Paya, C. V. (2001). Prevention of fungal and hepatitis virus infections in liver transplantation. *Clinical Infectious Diseases, 33,* (Suppl. 1), S47–S52.

Reichenspurner, H., Gamberg, M., Nitschke, H., Valantine, H., Hunt, S., Oyer, P. E., & Reitz, B. A. (1997). Significant reduction in the number of fungal infections after lung, heart–lung, and heart transplantation using aerosolized Amphotericin B prophylaxis. *Transplantation Proceedings, 29,* 627–628.

Rickenbacher, P. R., & Hunt, S. A. (1996). Long-term complications of transplantation. In R. W. Emery & L. W. Miller (Eds.), *Handbook of cardiac transplantation* (pp. 201–216). Philadelphia: Hanley & Belfus.

Rizk N. W., & Faul, J. L. (2000). Diagnosis and natural history of pulmonary infections in transplant recipients. *Chest, 117*(2), 303–305.

Rubin, R. H. (1994). Infection in the organ transplant recipient. In R. H. Rubin & L. S. Young (Eds.), *Clinical approach to infection in the compromised host* (3rd ed., pp. 629–705). New York: Plenum.

Rubin, R. H. (2000). Prevention and treatment of cytomegalovirus disease in heart transplant patients. *Journal of Heart and Lung Transplantation, 19*(8), 731–735.

Sia, I. G., & Paya, C. V. (1998). Infectious complications following renal transplantation. *Surgical Clinics of North America, 78*(1), 95–112.

Singh, N. (1997). Infections in solid-organ transplant recipients. *American Journal of Infection Control, 25,* 409–417.

Sollinger, H., & Pirsch, J. (1996). *Transplantation drug pocket reference guide* (2nd ed.). Austin, TX: Landes Bioscience.

Thaler, S. J., & Rubin, R. H. (1996). Opportunistic infections in the cardiac transplant patient. *Current Opinion in Cardiology, 11,* 191–203.

Tolkoff-Rubin, N. E., & Rubin, R. H. (2000). Recent advances in the diagnosis and management of infection in the organ transplant recipient. *Seminars in Nephrology, 20*(2), 148–163.

Wagoner, L. E. (1997). Management of the cardiac transplant recipient: Roles of the transplant cardiologist and primary care physician. *American Journal of the Medical Sciences, 314*(3), 173–184.

Wheat, J. (1994). Fungal infections in the immunocompromised host. In R. H. Rubin & L. S. Young (Eds.), *Clinical approach to infection in the compromised host.* (3rd ed., pp. 211–237). New York: Plenum.

3

Nutritional Issues in Adult Organ Transplantation

Jeanette Hasse

Nutrition therapy is vital in the care of organ transplant recipients. Appropriate pretransplant nutritional interventions treat symptoms of end-stage organ failure and help patients maintain adequate nutritional status. Acute posttransplant nutrition treatments focus on preventing infection, promoting wound healing, supporting metabolic demands, replenishing depleted nutrient stores, and mediating the immune response (Hasse, 2001). Nutrition goals in the chronic posttransplant phase are aimed at preventing or treating nutrition-related comorbid conditions such as obesity, hyperlipidemia, diabetes mellitus, hypertension, and osteoporosis.

The acute posttransplant phase is transient and nutrition interventions during this phase are managed by the transplant team at a transplant center. However, nutrition therapy during the pretransplant and chronic posttransplant phases must often be provided by the transplant patient's community health care providers. This chapter will focus on the nutrition therapy that should be provided to organ transplant patients while they are awaiting a transplant and during the chronic posttransplant time period.

ASSESSMENT

NUTRITION SCREENING AND ASSESSMENT

Organ transplant candidates and recipients are at high risk for nutritional deficiencies. A screening program should be implemented by health care providers to identify patients at risk of nutritional depletion. Screening tools such as those developed by the Nutrition Screening Initiative (http://www.aafp.org/nsi) are useful in identifying patients at risk who would benefit from a full nutritional assessment. Table 3.1 reviews components of a comprehensive nutritional assessment for an adult organ transplant candidate/recipient. There are two categories of patients at highest risk of perioperative complications—the severely malnourished and the severely or morbidly obese.

PRETRANSPLANT

MALNUTRITION

Malnourished patients tend to have more perioperative complications than well-nourished recipients. Hypoalbuminemia (< 3.5 mg/dL) increases risk of cytomegalovirus infection, renal graft failure, and pancreas graft failure in kidney–pancreas transplant recipients (Becker et al., 1999). Malnutrition in liver transplant patients has been related to increased rates of bacterial infections (Harrison, McKiernan, & Neuberger, 1997) and mortality (Harrison et al., 1997; Hasse et al., 1998; Lautz, Selberg, Körber, Bürger, & Müller, 1992; Pikul, Sharpe, Lowndes, & Chent, 1994; Selberg et al., 1997; Stephenson, Moretti, El-Maolem, Clavien, & Tuttle-Newhall, 2000).

The cause of pretransplant malnutrition is multifactorial and may include any of the following (Hasse & Roberts, 2000):

- Anorexia
- Gastrointestinal symptoms (nausea, vomiting, diarrhea, constipation)
- Dysgeusia
- Dysphagia
- Hypermetabolism
- Drug-nutrient interactions
- Poor nutrient delivery to tissues
- Psychosocial factors (limited access to food, inability to prepare food)
- Restricted diets

TABLE 3.1 Components of a Comprehensive Nutritional Assessment for an Adult Organ Transplant Recipient

Component	Purpose	Specific elements
Physical assessment	Determine general nutrition condition including fat and muscle stores and fluid retention.	Initial overview: • Is the patient of appropriate weight for stature? • Does patient have noticeable ascites or fluid retention? • Is muscle wasting apparent? • Does the patient require oxygen, wheelchair, or other assistive device? • Is the patient jaundiced? • Is the patient alert?
	Assess the degree and distribution of deficiencies.	Detailed physical examination: • Evaluate degree and distribution of fat and/or muscle loss and fluid retention. • Examine skin for color, texture, ecchymoses, telangectasias, etc. • Examine nail beds and hair for symptoms of nutrient deficiencies. • Assess the oral cavity for dental problems or signs of vitamin deficiencies.
History	Determine cause, degree, and duration of nutrient deficiencies.	• Obtain medical history of the type, degree, duration, and treatment of organ failure and associated complications. • Evaluate the patient's physical function. • Obtain accurate dietary history to determine adequacy of current dietary intake.

continued

TABLE 3.1 *(continued)*

Component	Purpose	Specific elements
		• Note gastrointestinal symptoms (e.g., nausea, vomiting, diarrhea, and early satiety) and other factors affecting appetite or intake. • Evaluate medications for drug-nutrient interactions. • Question patient thoroughly about use of nutrition supplements, vitamin or mineral supplements, and herbal preparations. • Assess psychosocial and economic conditions to determine patient's ability to comply with prescribed dietary regimen.
Anthropometric measurements	Provide objective measurements to evaluate and monitor progress.	• Fluid retention may have least effect on upper arm measurements. • Anthropometric measurements have limitations in sensitivity and reliability but may be useful if monitored serially over time. • Reliability is improved if all serial measurements are made by a single observer. • Other functional measurements such as hand grip strength may be helpful as indirect measures of protein stores.

continued

TABLE 3.1 *(continued)*

Component	Purpose	Specific elements
Laboratory tests	Provide detailed information; must be used selectively to avoid tests confounded by nonnutritional factors.	• Serum protein concentrations are affected by many nonnutritional factors (e.g., fluid status, liver and kidney function, and vitamin status). • Urinary tests (e.g., nitrogen balance and creatinine-height index) are also influenced by many nonnutritional factors (e.g., fluid status and liver and kidney function). • Immunocompetence tests (e.g., skin test antigens and total lymphocyte count) are influenced by immunosuppressive drugs.

Sources: Reprinted with permission from Hasse, J. M. (2001). Nutrition assessment and support of organ transplant recipients. *Journal of Parenteral and Enteral Nutrition, 25*(3), 120–131.

- Altered mental status
- Malabsorption
- Early satiety

Of these factors, unnecessarily restricting patients' diets is an iatrogenic cause of malnutrition. For example, restricting dietary protein in diets of patients with cirrhosis is generally discouraged. Protein restriction does little to improve a patient's condition and often results in further muscle and weight loss.

Likewise, there are many guidelines to help patients attain optimal dietary intake:

- Oral diets are preferred if possible.
- Patients should be encouraged to eat small, frequent meals containing high-calorie, high-protein foods.

- Dietary restrictions should be limited or avoided if at all possible.
- Drinking oral liquid nutritional supplements may help patients meet nutrient goals.
- Vitamin and mineral supplementation may be necessary to provide adequate micronutrient intake.
- If a medication interferes with food intake or absorption, consider altering medication type, dose, or administration times.
- If nausea, diarrhea, or constipation prevail, treat with medications to relieve symptoms or cause.
- Help patient obtain assistance with food procurement and preparation when necessary.

If oral intake is not adequate, nutrition support should be initiated. Tube feeding is the preferred route unless the gut is not functioning (such as severe ileus or pancreatitis). Tube feeding can be provided at home while a patient is awaiting transplantation and can be administered continuously or cyclically depending on how much oral intake the patient can consistently sustain. Specific nutrient recommendations are summarized in Table 3.2.

OBESITY

Obesity has been identified as a risk factor associated with delayed kidney graft function (Drafts et al., 1997; Holley et al., 1990; Meier-Kriesche et al., 1999; Moreso et al., 1998; Pirsch et al., 1995) and reduced kidney graft survival (Gill, Hodge, Novick, Steinmuller, & Garred, 1993; Halme, Eklund, Kyllonen, & Salmela, 1997; Holley et al., 1990; Meier-Kriesche et al., 1999; Pirsch et al., 1995; Wilson et al., 1995). Severe obesity is associated with increased rates of wound infection in liver transplant patients (Braunfeld et al., 1996; Keeffe, Gettys, & Esquivel, 1994; Sawyer, Pelletier, & Pruett, 1999; Testa et al., 1998). For these reasons, safe weight loss should be attempted prior to transplantation, and even sometimes prior to acceptance for transplantation.

Success with weight loss is usually enhanced when therapy and follow-up is provided by qualified professionals. Initially, it must be determined if a patient is motivated and willing to make changes to result in weight loss. If the patient is willing to make changes, a coordinated team approach addressing dietary requirements, exercise regimen, and psychosocial/behavioral factors should be implemented to assist a patient in obtaining a healthy weight loss. Follow-up is essential (as it is in dealing with substance abuse) to achieve long-term success and compliance.

TABLE 3.2 Pretransplant Nutrient Recommendations

Nutrient		Considerations and Recommendations
Calories	*Weight Maintenance*	• 1.2–1.3 × BEE (basal energy expenditure by Harris Benedict equation) depending on activity level or 30 calories/kg
	Weight gain	• 1.5 × BEE or 35–40 calories/kg
	Weight loss	• Deficit of 500 to 1,000 calories/day depending on current intake, anticipated time until transplant, and ability to exercise
Protein	*Maintenance*	• 0.8–1.2 g/kg/day
	Repletion	• 1.3–2.0 g/kg/day
	Dialysis	• Hemodialysis: 1.2–1.5 g/kg/day
		• Peritoneal: 1.5 g/kg/day
	Hepatic encephalopathy	• True protein-induced hepatic encephalopathy is rare. See above guidelines for protein recommendations.
		• Consider use of branched-chain amino acid–enriched supplements.
Vitamins	*A*	• Deficiency can be caused by steatorrhea, neomycin, cholestyramine, alcoholism, and inadequate retinol-binding protein production by the liver.
		• Levels are often increased with renal failure.
	B_6	• Deficiency can be caused by alcoholism.
	B_{12}	• Deficiency can be caused by alcoholism, cholestyramine.
	Niacin	• Deficiency can be caused by alcoholism.
	Thiamine	• Deficiency can be caused by alcoholism, high-carbohydrate diet.
	C	• Low plasma and leukocyte levels may be a result of dietary restrictions of fruits and vegetables and losses during dialysis in renal transplant patients.

continued

TABLE 3.2 *(continued)*

Nutrient		Considerations and Recommendations
	D	• Deficiency can be caused by poor diet, steatorrhea, glucocorticoids, cholestyramine, and inadequate 25-hydroxylation of cholecalciferol and ergocalciferol in the cirrhotic liver. • Renal transplant patients may lack the active form of vitamin D.
	E	• Deficiency can be caused by steatorrhea, antibiotics, cholestyramine.
	K	• Deficiency can be caused by steatorrhea, antibiotics, cholestyramine.
	Folate	• Deficiency can be caused by alcoholism, antibiotics. • Level may be depressed in dialysis patients.
Minerals/ electrolytes	*Calcium*	• Urinary excretion increased by glucocorticoids. • Gastrointestinal loss with steatorrhea. • In renal transplant patients, low serum levels result from abnormal vitamin D, calcium, and phosphorus metabolism.
	Copper	• In liver transplant patients, decreased excretion occurs with biliary obstruction or Wilson's disease.
	Iron	• Deficiency can be caused by chronic bleeding. • In renal transplant patients, deficiency may be due to decreased erythropoietin, decreased red blood cell production, and dialysis losses. • In liver transplant patients, excess iron stores occur in hemochromatosis.
	Magnesium	• Deficiency can be caused by diuretics, alcoholism, immunosuppressants. • Decreased excretion can be caused by renal failure.

continued

TABLE 3.2 *(continued)*

Nutrient		Considerations and Recommendations
	Phosphorus	• Deficiency can be caused by anabolism, alcoholism, glucocorticoids. • Increased levels are seen with renal failure.
	Potassium	• Hypokalemia can be caused by potassium-wasting diuretics, anabolism, insulin use. • Hyperkalemia can be caused by decreased renal function, potassium-sparing diuretics.
	Sodium	• Sodium may need to be restricted depending on fluid status and blood pressure.
	Zinc	• Deficiency can be caused by diarrhea, diuretics, alcoholism. • Decreased excretion can be caused by renal failure. • Low levels may be seen in dialysis patients.

Source: Adapted with permission from Hasse, J. M. (1998). Solid organ transplantation. In L. E. Matarese & M. M. Gottschlich (Eds.), *Contemporary nutrition support practice: A clinical guide* (pp. 547–560). Philadelphia: W. B. Saunders.

POSTTRANSPLANT

ACUTE POSTTRANSPLANT—HOSPITALIZATION

During the acute posttransplant phase, when a patient cannot eat adequate amounts to support requirements of metabolic demands, activity, and replenishment, nutrition support is indicated. Enteral feeding is preferred over parenteral feeding whenever the gut is functional. Immediate postoperative tube feeding may be beneficial for some organ recipients such as liver transplant patients. Oral diets are usually implemented 1 to 3 days after most transplants, with the exception of intestinal, pancreas, and kidney–pancreas transplant recipients, who may need additional time for gut rest. Nutrition support is weaned based on adequacy of oral intake. It is during this phase that nutrition-related side effects of immunosuppressive medications first manifest themselves (see Table 3.3).

CHRONIC POSTTRANSPLANT

The community health care provider is more likely to deal with chronic posttransplant problems of overnutrition rather than the acute posttransplant problems of undernutrition and repletion. Chronic posttransplant complications linked to nutrition include

- Obesity
- Hyperlipidemia
- Diabetes mellitus
- Hypertension

These chronic posttransplant complications contribute to cardiovascular disease and other conditions that affect long-term survival (Aker, Iven, Grabensee, & Heering, 1998; Brann, Bennett, Keck, & Hosenpud,1998; Canzanello et al., 1997; Löcsey, Asztalos, Kincses, Berczi, & Paragh, 1998). Together with osteoporosis, these complications have the potential to adversely affect quality of life. Attention to appropriate therapies to reduce these complications is therefore vital. The causes of these comorbid conditions are multifactorial, with nutrition being a common link. The suggested treatments for these conditions also overlap.

Obesity

Obesity, whether preexisting or developed after transplantation, adversely affects other posttransplant comorbid complications. Therefore, achievement or maintenance of a healthy weight is paramount posttransplant. There are many factors that contribute to obesity (Everhart et al., 1998; Hasse, 1997; Johnson et al., 1993; Mathe et al., 1992; Merion et al., 1991; Palmer, Schaffner, & Thung, 1991):

- Excess calorie intake due to hyperphagia, unhealthy eating behaviors, and resolution of malabsorption
- Inadequate calorie expenditure due to a sedentary lifestyle and lack of exercise
- Genetic predisposition to weight gain
- Age, gender, and race also influence body weight

Weight loss is possible posttransplant (Lopes, Martin, Errasti, & Martinez, 1999; Patel, 1998). There are multiple components to a healthy weight loss program. These include

TABLE 3.3 Immunosuppressive Medications, Nutritional Side Effects, and Interventions

Drug	Nutritional side effect	Suggested nutrition therapy
Anti-lymphocyte globulin (ATGAM, thymoglobulin)	• fever and chills • increased risk of infection, profound leukopenia, thrombocytopenia	• Provide nutrient-dense foods patient will eat. • Ensure patient is receiving adequate protein.
Azathioprine (Imuran)	• nausea, vomiting • diarrhea • mucositis • macrocytic anemia • pancreatitis	• Try antiemetic medications; if vomiting does not subside, consider tube feeding or TPN. • Review drugs and substitute for those that may be causing diarrhea; make sure that patient is receiving adequate fluid to replace losses. • Provide foods that won't irritate throat. • Make sure folate intake is adequate. • Initiate parenteral nutrition if pancreatitis is severe.
Basiliximab (Simulect)	• none reported	
Corticosteroids (Prednisone, prednisolone, solu-cortef, solu-medrol, methylpre-dnisolone)	• hyperglycemia • sodium retention • ulcers • osteoporosis • hyperphagia	• Monitor blood sugar and need for long-term diabetic diet and hypoglycemic agents. • Avoid high-sodium foods. • Ensure adequate calcium and vitamin D intake; consider need for calcitriol, fluoride, or estrogen. • Behavior modification to to prevent overeating

continued

TABLE 3.3 *(continued)*

Drug	Nutritional side effect	Suggested nutrition therapy
	• impaired wound healing and increased infection risk	• Ensure adequate protein intake; consider need for vitamin A or C or zinc.
	• hypertension	• Avoid high-sodium foods; maintain a healthy weight.
	• pancreatitis (rare)	• Initiate parenteral nutrition if pancreatitis is severe.
Cyclosporine (Neoral, Gengraf, Sandimmune)	• hyperkalemia	• Restrict high-potassium foods.
	• hypomagnesemia	• Supplement with high-magnesium foods or supplements.
	• hypertension	• Avoid high-sodium foods; maintain a healthy weight.
	• hyperglycemia	• Monitor blood sugar and need for long-term diabetic diet and hypoglycemic agents.
	• hyperlipidemia	• Limit fat intake to < 30% calories as fat during long-term phase; maintain a healthy weight.
Daclizumab (Zenapax)	• none reported	
Muromonab-CD3 (OKT3)	• nausea, vomiting	• Try antiemetic medications; if vomiting does not subside, consider tube feeding or TPN.
	• diarrhea	• Review drugs and substitute for those that may be causing diarrhea; make sure that patient is receiving adequate fluid to replace losses.

continued

TABLE 3.3 *(continued)*

Drug	Nutritional side effect	Suggested nutrition therapy
	• anorexia	• Offer frequent meals of nutrient-dense foods.
	• fever, chills, myalgias	
Mycophenolate mofetil (CellCept)	• diarrhea	• Review drugs and substitute for those that may be causing diarrhea; make sure that patient is receiving adequate fluid to replace losses.
Sirolimus (Rapamycin, Rapamune)	• hyperlipidemia • GI disorders (constipation, diarrhea, nausea/ vomiting, dyspepsia)	• Limit fat intake to < 30% calories as fat during long-term phase; maintain a healthy weight. • Monitor oral intake; consider alternate methods of nutrition support if intake is suboptimal.
Tacrolimus (Prograf, FK506)	• nausea, vomiting • hyperkalemia • hyperglycemia • abdominal distress	• Try antiemetic medications; if vomiting does not subside, consider tube feeding or TPN. • Avoid high-potassium foods. • Monitor blood sugar and need for long-term diabetic diet and hypoglycemic agents. • Monitor oral intake; consider alternate methods of nutrition support if intake is suboptimal.

GI = gastrointestinal
TPN = total parenteral nutrition
Source: Adapted with permission from Hasse, J. (1991). Role of the dietitian in the nutrition management of adults after liver transplantation. *Journal of the American Dietetic Association, 91*(4), 473–476.

- Calorie reduction
- Behavior modification
- Exercise
- Reduction of corticosteroid dose when possible and/or switching to a tacrolimus- versus cyclosporine-based immunosuppression regimen (Canzanello et al., 1997)

Just as in the pretransplant phase, patients will be successful with weight loss if they are psychologically ready and motivated to make changes and participate in long-term weight management interventions. Psychological aspects of weight loss include

- Screening patients for readiness and motivation before attempting treatment
- Counseling patients who are not willing to make changes; counseling should focus on identifying and removing barriers and motivating the patient to change
- Establishing realistic goals (a sustained weight loss of 10% to 15% is more desirable than a 25% weight loss that is not maintained)

Goals should focus on better health:

- Decreased cholesterol
- Decreased glucose levels
- Improved blood pressure

Patients should be referred to a weight loss program so that the complexities of weight management may be addressed.

The use of weight loss medications has not been tested for safety or efficacy in this population. Sibutramine (Meridia) is contraindicated in conditions that may occur in transplant recipients, such as congestive heart failure, coronary artery disease, severe liver impairment, severe renal impairment, and uncontrolled or poorly controlled hypertension (*Drug Facts and Comparisons,* 2000). Orlistat (Xenical) can alter cyclosporine levels (*Drug Facts and Comparisons, 2000*).

Hyperlipidemia

Posttransplant hyperlipidemia is a risk factor for coronary artery disease as well as posttransplant vasculopathy. Vasculopathy may lead to coronary artery disease in heart transplant recipients, chronic rejection in kidney transplant recipients, and vanishing bile duct syndrome in liver transplant recipients (Kobashigawa & Kasiske, 1997). There are many potential factors contributing to hyperlipidemia (Brown et al., 1997; Donahoo, Kosmiski, & Eckel, 1998; Kobashigawa & Kasiske, 1997; Lye, Hughes, Leong, Tan, & Lee, 1995; Mathe et al., 1992; McCune et al., 1998; Moore et al., 1993; Palmer et al., 1991; Perez, 1993). These include

- Obesity
- Genetic predisposition
- Diabetes mellitus
- High-fat, high-saturated fat diet
- Sedentary lifestyle
- Renal dysfunction
- Antihypertensive drugs
- Proteinuria
- Cyclosporine: binds to low-density lipoprotein (LDL)–cholesterol receptor; decreases bile acid synthesis from cholesterol and transport of cholesterol to intestines; increases hepatic lipase activity; decreases lipoprotein lipase activity
- Corticosteroids: inhibit lipoprotein lipase; increase hepatic synthesis of very low-density lipoprotein (VLDL)–cholesterol; enhance activity of acetyl-coenzyme A carboxylase and free fatty synthetase; decrease LDL-receptor activity; increase 3-hydroxy-3-methylglutaryl coenzyme A [HMG-CoA] reductase activity
- Sirolimus (Rapamune)

Treatment of hyperlipidemia includes appropriate diet, exercise, alteration in immunosuppressive drug regimen, and, potentially, lipid-lowering medication (Arnadottir & Berg, 1997; Arnadottir, Eriksson, Germershausen, & Thysell, 1994; Kobashigawa & Kasiske, 1997; Lopes et al., 1999; Lye et al., 1995; Martinez-Castelao et al., 1999; Palmer et al., 1991; Salen et al., 1994). Specific recommendations may include

- Calorie-appropriate diet to achieve healthy weight
- < 300 mg cholesterol, < 30% of calories from fat, 7%–10% of calories from saturated fat (American Heart Association Step 1 Diet)
- Aerobic exercise
- Reduction of corticosteroid dose
- Change from cyclosporine-based immunosuppression to tacrolimus-based immunosuppression
- A lipid-lowering medication (the HMG-CoA reductase inhibitors are preferred)

- Omega-3 fatty acids (fish oil) may decrease triglyceride concentrations and reduce platelet aggregation and blood pressure, but more trials are necessary before they can be recommended

Finally, hyperhomocysteinemia is another risk factor for the development of atherosclerosis. Hyperhomocysteinemia has been documented in cyclosporine-treated kidney transplant recipients (Arnadottir, Hultberg, Vladov, Nilsson-Ehle & Thysell, 1996; Arnadottir, Hultberg, Wahlberg, Fellström, & Dimény, 1998; Bostom et al., 1997a, 1997b). Supplementation with folate and vitamins B_6 and B_{12} may be helpful in treating hyperhomocysteinemia (Bostom et al., 1997a, 1997b).

Diabetes Mellitus

The prevalence of posttransplant diabetes mellitus is variable depending on the type of organ transplant, the type and dose of immunosuppression, and the criteria used to diagnose diabetes. Immunosuppressive drugs are a major cause of posttransplant diabetes; therefore, when the immunosuppressive drugs are reduced, hyperglycemia often improves. Potential risk factors for posttransplant diabetes mellitus include (Ekstrand, Eriksson, Gronhagen-Riska, Ahonen, & Groop, 1992; Jindal, 1994; Jindal et al., 1996; Jindal, Sidner, & Milgrom, 1997; Mor et al., 1995; Pirsch, Miller, Deierhoi, Vincenti, & Filo, 1997):

- Corticosteroids (reduces number of insulin receptors, decreases insulin receptor affinity, impairs uptake of peripheral glucose and ability of insulin to suppress hepatic glucose production)
- Cyclosporine (inhibits insulin secretion)
- Tacrolimus (may be more diabetogenic than cyclosporine because posttransplant diabetes occurs at the same or higher rate with tacrolimus than cyclosporine despite a lower dose of corticosteroids)
- Positive family history of diabetes mellitus
- Obesity
- Increased age
- Ethnicity (highest rates of diabetes are found in African-American, Native American, and Hispanic people)

Management of diabetes typically includes

- Carbohydrate-controlled diet
- Self-blood glucose monitoring
- Exercise

- Insulin or oral hypoglycemic agent
- Reduction in corticosteroid dose (if possible)

Hypertension

Aside from genetic factors and increased body weight, the most common cause of posttransplant hypertension is immunosuppressive medications (Moreso et al., 1998). Cyclosporine- or tacrolimus-induced vasoconstriction causes systemic hypertension and decreased renal blood flow (Luke, 1991; Miller, 1991; Monsour et al., 1995; Textor, Canzenello, Taler, Schwartz, & Augustine, 1995). However, patients maintained on cyclosporine have a significantly higher rate of posttransplant hypertension compared with patients maintained on tacrolimus (Canzanello et al., 1997). Therapy for posttransplant hypertension includes

- 2 to 4 g daily dietary sodium restriction
- Maintenance or achievement of healthy body weight
- Regular aerobic exercise
- Antihypertensive medications

Osteoporosis

Increased bone turnover, decreased bone mass, microarchitectural deterioration of bone tissue, and increased bone fragility characterize posttransplant osteopenic bone disease (Neuhaus et al., 1995). As with the other posttransplant comorbid conditions, there are multiple risk factors for posttransplant osteoporosis (Katz and Epstein, 1992; Nisbeth, Lindh, Ljunghall, Backman, & Fellström, 1999; Porayko et al., 1991; Trautwein, et al., 2000; Vedi et al., 1999; Westeel et al., 2000). These include

- Certain disease states: Patients with primary biliary cirrhosis, sclerosing cholangitis, hemochromatosis, chronic renal failure, or intestinal failure requiring long-term parenteral nutrition have increased rates of posttransplant osteoporosis.
- Corticosteroids: Increase bone resorption and suppress osteoblastic function; affect sex hormone secretion, intestinal calcium absorption, renal excretion of calcium and phosphate, and the vitamin D system
- Cyclosporine: May cause bone resorption to exceed bone formation.
- Decreased activity
- Alcohol abuse
- Diuretic use

- Decreased estrogen levels
- Gender (female > male)
- Type 1 diabetes mellitus
- Hyperparathyroidism
- Cigarette smoking

Therapy to prevent or treat osteoporosis should include

- Calcium (1,000–1,500 mg daily) and vitamin D supplementation
- Estrogen replacement in estrogen-deficient women (unless otherwise contraindicated)
- Weight-bearing exercise
- Cessation of smoking
- Minimization of corticosteroids
- Moderate sodium intake
- Possibly fluoride supplement or bone-modulating medications

DIETARY SUPPLEMENTS

There is very little scientific research about positive or negative effects of transplant recipients taking nutritional supplements. Vitamin supplementation is probably appropriate for transplant recipients, especially when pretransplant malnutrition existed. A general multivitamin and mineral preparation meeting 100% of the recommended dietary allowance is usually a safe recommendation. Of course, supplementation prescriptions must be individualized (see Table 2).

Ingestion of dietary supplements including herbal products has gained popularity. In the United States, standardization and quality control standards in the production of these supplements is not included in the Dietary Supplement Health and Education Act of 1994 (Chang, 1998).

- Because of the lack of regulation, one cannot be certain of the content or form of the supplement claimed to be in the package.
- Many herbal preparations and other supplements have not been tested in transplant recipients; patients are taking a risk by consuming these products.
- Herbal medications (such as Saint John's wort) may interact with immunuosuppressants and increase the need for high doses to maintain therapeutic drug levels.
- Some herbal medications are designed to boost the immune system; this may increase the risk of rejection.

FOOD SAFETY

Immunosuppressed individuals are at increased risk of complications from foodborne infections. Therefore, food handling, preparation, and storage methods should follow these food safety guidelines (Partnership for Food Safety Education 2000):

- Wash hands with warm soapy water before preparing or eating food and after touching raw meat, poultry, fish, and eggs.
- Use all meat, fish, and poultry within 1 to 2 days of purchase, or freeze for later use.
- Always use pasteurized milk, cheese, and other dairy products.
- Never buy dented cans of food.
- Wash all fruits and vegetables before eating, slicing, or cooking.
- Keep cooked meats and other foods away from surfaces that have touched raw meat or eggs.
- After use, sanitize preparation area, appliances, cutting boards, counters, sponges, and dish towels.
- Do not eat raw or undercooked meats, eggs, poultry, and fish or shellfish. Appropriate temperatures:
  - Red meats—160°F
  - Poultry pieces—170°F
  - Whole poultry—180°F (or until the juices run clear and there is no pink)
  - Fish and seafood—140°F (or white and flaky throughout)
- Freeze or refrigerate foods promptly after meals.
- When eating out, choose fruits with removable skins, such as bananas and oranges.
- Be wary of buffets because foods are often held too long at inappropriate temperatures.
- Drinking water should be from a safe, treated source (well water can be safe if treated).
- If water source is not reliably safe, boil drinking water for 3 minutes and store in a clean, covered container.

RESOURCES

Nutrition counseling will enhance a patient's ability to follow nutrition guidelines and prevent nutrition-related complications (Patel, 1998). The transplant team and dietitian can be a resource, but if the patient cannot easily visit the center for a nutrition consult, a local registered dietitian should be consulted. Names of registered dietitians listed by geographic area are available on the American Dietetic Association Web site (www. eatright.org/find.html).

CONCLUSION

Providing appropriate nutrition therapy to transplant candidates and recipients improves transplant outcomes and patients' quality of life. Timely intervention can also prevent costlier medical treatments for complications associated with malnutrition, obesity, diabetes mellitus, hyperlipidemia, hypertension, and osteoporosis. A transplant candidate's/recipient's primary health care provider must be the gatekeeper for identifying needs and referring patients to the transplant team or qualified nutrition professionals for treatment.

REFERENCES

Aker, S., Ivens, K., Grabensee, B., & Heering, P. (1998). Cardiovascular risk factors and diseases after renal transplantation. *International Urology and Nephrology, 30*(6), 777–788.

Arnadottir, M., & Berg, A. L. (1997). Treatment of hyperlipidemia in renal transplant recipients. *Transplantation, 63*(3), 330–345.

Arnadottir, M., Eriksson, L. O., Germershausen, J. I., & Thysell, H. (1994). Low-dose simvistatin is a well-tolerated and efficacious cholesterol-lowering agent in ciclosporin-treated kidney transplant recipients: Double-blind, randomized, placebo-controlled study in 40 patients. *Nephron, 68*(1), 57–62.

Arnadottir, M., Hultberg, B., Vladov, V., Nilsson-Ehle, P., & Thysell, H. (1996). Hyperhomocysteinemia in cyclosporine-treated renal transplant recipients. *Transplantation, 61*(3), 509–512.

Arnadottir, M., Hultberg, B., Wahlberg, J., Fellström, B., & Dimény, E. (1998). Serum total homocysteine concentration before and after renal transplantation. *Kidney International, 54*(4), 1380–1384.

Becker, B. N., Becker, Y. T., Heisey, D. M., Leverson, G. E., Collins, B. H., Odorico, J. S., D'Alessandro, A. M., Knechtle, S. J., Pirsch, J. D., & Sollinger, H. W. (1999). The impact of hypoalbuminemia in kidney–pancreas transplant recipients. *Transplantation, 68*(1), 72–75.

Bostom, A. G., Gohh, R. Y., Beaulieu, A. J., Nadeau, M. R., Hume, A. L., Jacques, P. F., Selhub, J., & Rosenberg, I. H. (1997a). Treatment of hyperhomocysteinemia in renal transplant recipients: A randomized, placebo-controlled trial. *Annals of Internal Medicine, 127*(12), 1089–1092.

Bostom, A. G., Gohh, R. Y., Tsai, M. Y., Hopkins-Garcia, B. J., Nadeau, M. R., Bianchi, L. A., Jacques, P. F., Rosenberg, I. H., & Selhub, J. (1997b). Excess prevalence of fasting and postmethionine-loading hyperhomocysteinemia in stable renal transplant recipients. *Arteriosclerosis, Thrombosis and Vascular Biology, 17*(10), 1894–1900.

Brann, W. M., Bennett, L. E., Keck, B. M., & Hosenpud, J. D. (1998). Morbidity, functional status, and immunosuppressive therapy after heart transplantation: An analysis of the Joint International Society for Heart and Lung Transplantation/United Network for Organ Sharing Thoracic Registry. *Journal of Heart and Lung Transplantation, 17*(4), 374–382.

Braunfeld, M. Y., Chan, S., Pregler, J., Neelakanta, G., Sopher, M. J., Busuttil, R. W., & Scete, M. (1996). Liver transplantation in the morbidly obese. *Journal of Clinical Anesthesia, 8,* 585–590.

Brown, J. H., Murphy, B. G., Douglas, A. F., Short, C. D., Bhatnagar, D., Mackness, M. I., Hunt, L. P., Doherty, C. C., & Durrington, P. N. (1997). Influence of immunosuppressive therapy on lipoprotein(a) and other lipoproteins following renal transplantation. *Nephron, 75*(3), 277–282.

Canzanello, V. J., Schwartz, L., Taler, S. J., Textor, S. C., Wiesner, R. H., Porayko, M. K., & Krom, R. A. F. (1997). Evolution of cardiovascular risk after liver transplantation: A comparison of cyclosporine A and tacrolimus (FK506). *Liver Transplantation and Surgery, 3*(1), 1–9.

Chang, R. (1998). Quality and standards in dietary supplements. *Support Line, 20*(4), 3–4.

Donahoo, W. T., Kosmiski, L. A., & Eckel, R. H. (1998). Drugs causing dyslipoproteinemia. *Endocrinology and Metabolism Clinics of North America, 27*(3), 677–697.

Drafts, H. H., Anjum, M. R., Wynn, J. J., Mulloy, L. L., Bowley, J. N., & Humphries, A. L. (1997). The impact of pretransplant obesity on renal transplant outcomes. *Clinical Transplantation, 11,* 493–496.

Drug facts and comparisons. (2000). St. Louis: Wolters Kluwer.

Ekstrand, A. V., Eriksson, J. G., Gronhagen-Riska, C., Ahonen, P. J., & Groop, L. C. (1992). Insulin resistance and insulin deficiency in the pathogenesis of posttransplantation diabetes in man. *Transplantation, 53,* 563–569.

Everhart, J. E., Lombardero, M., Lake, J. R., Wiesner, R. H., Zetterman, R. K., & Hoofnagle, J. H. (1998). Weight change and obesity after liver transplantation: Incidence and risk factors. *Liver Transplantation and Surgery, 4*(4), 285–296.

Gill, I. S., Hodge, E. E., Novick, A. C., Steinmuller, D. R., & Garred, D. (1993). Impact of obesity on renal transplantation. *Transplantation Proceedings, 25,* 1047–1048.

Halme, L., Eklund, B., Kyllonen, L., & Salmela, K. (1997). Is obesity still a risk factor in renal transplantation? *Transplant International, 10,* 284–288.

Harrison, J., McKiernan, J., & Neuberger, J. M. (1997). A prospective study on the effect of recipient nutritional status on outcome in liver transplantation. *Transplant International, 10,* 369–374.

Hasse, J. (1991). Role of the dietitian in the nutrition management of adults after liver transplantation. *Journal of the American Dietetic Association, 91*(4), 473–476.

Hasse, J. M. (1997). Diet therapy for organ transplantation: A problem-based approach. *Nursing Clinics of North America, 32*(4), 863–880.

Hasse, J. M. (1998). Solid organ transplantation. In L. E. Matarese & M. M. Gottschlich (Eds.), *Contemporary nutrition support practice: A clinical guide* (pp. 547–560). Philadelphia: W. B. Saunders.

Hasse J. M. (2001). Nutrition assessment and support of organ transplant recipients. *Journal of Parenteral and Enteral Nutrition, 25*(3), 120–131.

Hasse, J. M., Gonwa, T. A., Jennings, L. W., Goldstein, R. M., Levy, M. F., Husberg, B. S., & Klintmalm, G. B. (1998). Malnutrition affects liver transplant outcomes [Abstract]. *Transplantation, 66*(8), S53.

Hasse, J. M. & Roberts, S. (2000). Transplantation. In J. L. Rombeau & R. H.

Rolandelli (Eds.), *Parenteral nutrition.* (3rd ed., pp. 529–561). Philadelphia: W. B. Saunders.

Holley, J. L., Shapiro, R., Lopatin, W. B., Tzakis, A. G., Hakala, T. R., & Starzl, T. E. (1990). Obesity as a risk factor following cadaveric renal transplantation. *Transplantation, 49,* 387–389.

Jindal, R. M. (1994). Posttransplant diabetes mellitus—a review. *Transplantation, 58*(12), 1289–1298.

Jindal, R. M., Sidner, R. A., Hughes, D., Pescovitz, M. D., Leapman, S. B., Milgrom, M. L., Lumeng, L., & Filo, R. S. (1996). Metabolic problems in recipients of liver transplants. *Clinical Transplantation, 10,* 213–217.

Jindal, R. M., Sidner, R. A., & Milgrom, M. L. (1997). Post-transplant diabetes mellitus: The role of immunosuppression. *Drug Safety, 16*(4), 242–257.

Johnson, C. P., Gallagher-Lepak, S., Zhu, Y. R., Hartz, A. J., Roza, A. M., & Adams, M. B. (1993). Factors influencing weight gain after renal transplantation. *Transplantation, 56,* 822–827.

Katz, I. A., & Epstein, S. (1992). Posttransplant bone disease. *Journal of Bone and Mineral Research, 7,* 123–126.

Keeffe, E. B., Gettys, C., & Esquivel, C. O. (1994). Liver transplantation in patients with severe obesity. *Transplantation, 57,* 309–311.

Kobashigawa, J. A., & Kasiske, B. L. (1997). Hyperlipidemia in solid organ transplantation. *Transplantation, 63,* 331–338.

Lautz, H. U., Selberg, O., Körber, J., Bürger, M., & Müller, M. J. (1992). Protein-calorie malnutrition in liver cirrhosis. *The Clinical Investigator, 70,* 478–486.

Löcsey, L., Asztalos, L., Kincses, Z., Berczi, C. S., & Paragh, G. Y. (1998). The importance of obesity and hyperlipidaemia in patients with renal transplants. *International Urology and Nephrology, 30*(6), 767–775.

Lopes, I. M., Martin, M., Errasti, P., & Martínez, J. A. (1999). Benefits of a dietary intervention on weight loss, body composition, and lipid profile after renal transplantation. *Nutrition, 15*(1), 7–10.

Luke, R. G. (1991). Pathophysiology and treatment of posttransplant hypertension. *Journal of American Society of Nephrology, 2*(Suppl. 1), S37–S34.

Lye, W. G., Hughes, K., Leong, S. O., Tan, C. C., & Lee, E. J. C. (1995). Abnormal lipoprotein(a) and lipid profiles in renal allograft recipients: Effects of treatment with pravastatin. *Transplantation Proceedings, 27*(1), 977–978.

Martinez-Castelao, A. Grinyó, J. M., Fiol, C., Castiñeiras, M. J., Hurtado, I., Gil-Vernet, S., Serón, D., Porta, I., Miñarro, A., Villarroya, A., & Alsina, J. (1999). Fluvastatin and low-density lipoprotein oxidation in hypercholesterolemic renal transplant patients. *Kidney International, 56*(Suppl. 71), S231–234.

Mathe, D., Adam, R., Malmendier, C., Gigou, M., Lontie, J. F., Dubois, D., Martin, C., Bismuth, H., & Jacotot, B. (1992). Prevalence of dyslipidemia in liver transplant recipients. *Transplantation, 54,* 167–170.

McCune, T. R., Thacker, L. R. II, Peters, T. G., Mulloy, L, Rohr, M. S., Adams, P. A., Yium, J., Light, J. A., Pruett, T., Gaber, A. O., Selman, S. H., Jonsson, J., Hayes, J. M., Wright, F. H., Armata, T., Blanton, J., & Burdick, J. F. (1998). Effects of tacrolimus on hyperlipidemia after successful renal transplantation: A Southeastern Organ Procurement Foundation multicenter clinical study. *Transplantation, 65*(1), 87–92.

Meier-Kriesche, H. U., Vaghalea, M., Thambuganipalle, R., Friedman, G., Jacobs, M., & Kaplan, B. (1999). The effect of body mass index on long-term renal allograft survival. *Transplantation, 68*(9), 1294–1297.

Merion, R. M., Twork, A. M., Rosenberg, L., Ham, J. M., Burtch, G. D., Turcotte, J. G., Rocher, L. L., & Campbell, D. A. (1991). Obesity and renal transplantation. *Surgery Gynecology & Obstetrics, 172,* 367–376.

Miller, L. W. (1991). Long-term complications of cardiac transplantation. *Progress in Cardiovascular Diseases, 33,* 229–282.

Monsour, H. P., Wood, R. P., Dyer, C. H., Galati, J. S., Ozaki, C. F., & Clark, J. H. (1995). Renal insufficiency and hypertension as long-term complications in liver transplantation. *Seminars in Liver Disease, 15,* 123–132.

Moore, R., Thomas, D., Morgan, E., Wheeler, D., Griffin, P., Salaman, J., & Rees, A. (1993). Abnormal lipid and lipoprotein profiles following renal transplantation. *Transplantation Proceedings, 25,* 1060–1061.

Mor, E., Facklam, D., Hasse, J., Sheiner, P., Emre, S., Schwartz, M., & Miller, C., for the U.S. Multicenter FK506 Study Group. (1995). Weight gain and lipid profile changes in liver transplant recipients: Long-term results of the American FK506 multicenter study. *Transplantation Proceedings, 27*(1), 1126.

Moreso, R., Serón, D., Anunciada, A. I., Hueso, M., Ramón, J. M., Fulladosa, X., Gil-Vernet, S., Alsina, J., & Grinyó, J. M. (1998). Recipient body surface area as a predictor of posttransplant renal allograft evolution. *Transplantation, 65*(5), 671–676.

Neuhaus, R., Lohmann, R., Platz, K. P., Guckelberger, O., Schon, M., Lang, M., Hierholzer, J., & Neuhaus, P. (1995). Treatment of osteoporosis after liver transplantation. *Transplantation Proceedings, 27*(1), 1226–1227.

Nisbeth, U., Lindh, E., Ljunghall, S., Backman, U., & Fellström B. (1999). Increased fracture rate in diabetes mellitus and females after renal transplantation. *Transplantation, 67*(9), 1218–1222.

Palmer, M., Schaffner, F., & Thung, S. N. (1991). Excessive weight gain after liver transplantation. *Transplantation, 51,* 797–800.

Partnership for Food Safety Education. (2001). Foodborne illness. Retrieved January 19, 2002 from the Partnership for Food Safety Education Web site: www.fightbac.org

Patel, M. G. (1998). The effect of dietary intervention on weight gains after renal transplantation. *Journal of Renal Nutrition, 8*(3), 137–141.

Perez, R. (1993). Managing nutrition problems in transplant patients. *Nutrition in Clinical Practice, 8*(1), 28–32.

Pikul, J., Sharpe, M. D., Lowndes, R., & Chent, C. N. (1994). Degree of preoperative malnutrition is predictive of postoperative morbidity and mortality in liver transplant recipients. *Transplantation, 57,* 469–472.

Pirsch, J. D., Armbrust, M. J., Knechtle, S. J., D'Alessandro, A. M., Sollinger, H. W., Heisey, D. M., & Belzer, F. O. (1995). Obesity as a risk factor following renal transplantation. *Transplantation, 59,* 631–633.

Pirsch, J. D., Miller, J., Deierhoi, M. H., Vincenti, F., & Filo, R. S. for the FK506 Kidney Study Group. (1997). A comparison of tacrolimus (FK506) and cyclosporine for immunosuppression after cadaveric renal transplantation. FK506 Kidney Transplant Study Group. *Transplantation, 63*(7), 977–983.

Porayko, M. K., Wiesner, R. H., Hay, J. E., Krom, R. A. F., Dickson, E. R., Beaver, S., & Schwerman, L. (1991). Bone disease in liver transplant recipients: Incidence, timing, and risk factors. *Transplantation Proceedings, 23,* 1462–1465.

Salen, P., de Lorgenril, M., Boissonnat, P., Monjaud, I., Guidollet, P., Dureau, G., & Renaud, S. (1994). Effects of a French Mediterranean diet on heart transplant recipients with hypercholesterolemia. *American Journal of Cardiology, 73,* 825–827.

Sawyer, R. G., Pelletier, S. J., & Pruett, T. L. (1999). Increased early morbidity and mortality with acceptable long-term function in severely obese patients undergoing liver transplantation. *Clinical Transplantation, 13,* 126–130.

Selberg, O., Böttcher, J., Tusch, G., Pichlmayr, R., Henkel, E., & Müller, M-J. (1997). Identification of high- and low-risk patients before liver transplantation: A prospective cohort study of nutritional and metabolic parameters in 150 patients. *Hepatology, 25,* 652–657.

Stephenson, Jr., G. R., Moretti, E. W., El-Moalem, H., Clavien, P. A., & Tuttle-Newhall, J. E.. (2000). Malnutrition in liver transplant patients: Pre-operative subjective global assessment (SGA) is predictive of outcome following liver transplantation. [Abstract]. *Journal of Parenteral and Enteral Nutrition, 24,* S10.

Testa, G., Hasse, J. M., Jennings, L. W., Levy, M. F., Brkic, B., Cook, B., Obiekwe, S., Husberg, B., Goldstein, R. M., Gonwa, T. A., & Klintmalm, G. B. (1998). Morbid obesity is not an independent risk factor for liver transplantation. [Abstract] *Transplantation, 66,* S53.

Textor, S. C., Canzenello, V. J., Taler, S. J., Schwartz, L., & Augustine, J. (1995). Hypertension after liver transplantation. *Liver Transplantation and Surgery, 1*(5, Suppl. 1), 20.

Trautwein, C., Possienke, M., Schlitt, H-J., Böker, K. H. W., Horn, R., Raab, R., Manns, M. P., & Brabant, G. (2000). Bone density and metabolism in patients with viral hepatitis and cholestatic liver diseases before and after liver transplantation. *American Journal of Gastroenterology, 95,* 2343–2351.

Vedi, S., Greer, S., Skingle, S. J., Garrahan, N. J., Ninkovic, M., Alexander, G. A., & Compston, J. E. (1999). Mechanism of bone loss after liver transplantation: A histomorphometric analysis. *Journal of Bone and Mineral Research, 14*(2), 281–287.

Westeel, F. P., Mazouz, K., Ezaitouni, F., Hottelart, C., Ivan, C., Fardellone, P., Brazier, M., El Esper, I., Petit, J., Achard, J. M., Pruna, A., & Fournier, A. (2000). Cyclosporine bone remodeling effect prevents steroid osteopenia after kidney transplantation. *Kidney International, 58,* 1788–1796.

Wilson, G. A., Bumgardner, G. L., Henry, M. L., Elhammas, E. A., Qiu, W., Davies, E. A., & Ferguson, R. M. (1995). Decreased graft survival rate in obese pancreas/kidney recipients. *Transplantation Proceedings, 27,* 3106–3107.

4

Transplantation Pharmacotherapy

Daniele K. Gelone and
Kathleen D. Lake

Today's immunosuppressive strategies are focused on achieving a delicate balance among the primary transplant goals of preventing acute rejection, maintaining long-term graft function and survival, and minimizing drug-induced side effects. Despite the complexities of these goals, advances in the understanding of the mechanisms responsible for rejection continue and have been paralleled by the development of novel, more effective immunotherapies.

Current maintenance immunosuppressive regimens consist of combinations of immunosuppressive agents that are utilized for the lifetime of the graft, such as

- Cyclosporine, USP (Sandimmune)
- Cyclosporine, USP [modified] (Neoral, generic formulations)
- Tacrolimus (Prograf)
- Mycophenolate mofetil (Cellcept)
- Azathioprine (Imuran, USP generic)
- Corticosteroids
- Sirolimus (Rapamune).

In addition to maintenance therapy, a number of centers use either monoclonal or polyclonal induction agents, including

- IL-2 receptor blockers (e.g., Basiliximab [Simulect] or Daclizumab [Zenapax])
- Antithymocyte globulins (e.g., Thymoglobulin and Atgam)
- Muromonab-CD3 (OKT3)

These monoclonal and polyclonal agents typically are used for short periods of time immediately posttransplant (e.g., induction therapy) in high-risk patients (e.g., African American patients, patients with high panel reactive antibody [PRA] levels, or patients undergoing retransplantation) or to spare the kidney from early exposure to nephrotoxic agents.

High-dose pulse corticosteroids remain the primary treatment for acute rejection; however, tacrolimus and mycophenolate mofetil have also been used for this purpose (Kelly, Burckart, & Venkataramanan, 1995; Klein, 1999; Mele & Halloran, 2000). Thymoglobulin, Atgam or OKT3 are used for the treatment of delayed graft function and steroid-resistant rejection episodes (Burk & Matuszewski, 1997; Hong & Kahan, 2000).

The newer immunotherapy regimens are quite effective at reducing the incidence of acute rejection in renal transplantation. The recent phase III multicenter kidney trials have reported incidences well under 30% (Brennan et al., 1999; European Mycophenolate Mofetil Cooperative Study Group, 1995; Johnson et al., 2000; Kahan, 2000; Miller, Mendez, Pirsch, & Jensik, 2000; Sollinger, 1995; Tricontinental Mycophenolate Mofetil Renal Transplantation Study Group, 1996; Vincenti et al., 1998). It is important to recognize that these trials have been designed to evaluate safety and efficacy of the new agents, but in some studies, the new agents have been compared to control therapy (e.g., cyclosporine and prednisone alone) that is not considered the standard of care at most U.S. transplant centers. Nor do the trials adequately assess the utility of these agents in high-risk populations.

MAINTENANCE IMMUNOSUPPRESSIVE MEDICATIONS

CALCINEURIN INHIBITORS (CYCLOSPORINE, TACROLIMUS)

The addition of cyclosporine (CSA) to the armamentarium of immuno-suppressive agents significantly changed the face of transplantation. Cyclosporine-based regimens markedly improved 1-year graft survival and rejection rates in kidney transplant recipients, which resulted in general-ized acceptance among other organ transplants shortly thereafter (Kahan, 1989). Compared to regimens including polyclonal antilymphocyte agents, azathioprine, and high-dose corticosteroids, the availability of CSA in the early 1980s and tacrolimus in the early 1990's provided more selective immunosuppression while preserving host defenses. Although structurally dissimilar, cyclosporine and tacrolimus exhibit many analogous properties, including mechanism of action, efficacy, side effects and drug interactions. Tacrolimus has long been considered the drug of choice for liver and kidney-pancreas transplantation, while tacrolimus and cyclosporine share the market for kidney, heart, and lung transplantation (Shapiro, 1999, 2000; Taylor et al., 1999, Taylor et al., 2000).

Cyclosporine (Sandimmune, Neoral, USP generics)

CSA, a fat soluble cyclic polypeptide of fungal origin, actively inhibits production of interleukin-2 (IL-2) from CD4+ cells while sparing CD8+ cells, B cells, macrophages, and granulocytes. CSA binds to cyclophilin, an immunophilin, forming the cyclosporine–cyclophilin complex; this complex subsequently binds calcineurin, resulting in impaired cytokine gene transcription responsible for promotion of T-cell activation (Matsuda & Koyasu, 2000). Cytokines impaired by this process include IL-2, interleukin-4 (IL-4), and tumor necrosis factor-alpha (TNF-alpha).

Several oral formulations of CSA are commercially available. The first formulation of CSA introduced on the market was Sandimmune, which was followed by Neoral modified solution. Because of unique differences between the Sandimmune and Neoral formulations, these agents exhibit distinct pharmacokinetic profiles. Therefore, Sandimmune is not bioequivalent to Neoral or its AB-rated generic equivalents. (Christians, First, & Benet, 2000). Generic formulations of Neoral have been available since 1999, and there are currently three AB-rated CSA modified solutions. Available generic preparations include Gengraf Cyclosporine Capsules, USP [Modified] (Abbott Laboratories), Cyclosporine capsules USP [Modified] (Eon Laboratories), and Cyclosporine Soft Gelatin Capsules [Modified] (Sidmak Laboratories). The SangCya liquid modified solution was withdrawn from the market in July 2000 when it was found to be non-bioequivalent to Neoral when diluted in apple juice (Food and Drug Administration, 2000).

CSA is distributed extensively in the blood, approximately 58% bound to red blood cells (RBCs) and 33% in plasma bound primarily to lipoproteins (90%). The oral bioavailability of Sandimmune cyclosporine is highly variable, ranging from 10% to 90%, with an overall absorption of approximately 30% (Kahan, 1989). Additionally, oral absorption of Sandimmune is highly bile dependent, resulting in greater variability among patients with diarrhea, biliary diversion, diabetic gastroparesis, or malabsorption

(Kahan, 1989). Consequently, Neoral has now largely replaced Sandimmune, based on Neoral's improved bioavailability (30%–45%), more consistent oral absorption, less variability in CSA pharmacokinetics, and less dependence on bile for absorption (Kahan et al., 1995). However, a number of long-term patients are still maintained on the Sandimmune formulation.

The pharmacokinetic inter/intrapatient variabilities exhibited by these products may be explained by inherent polymorphisms expressed by metabolic enzymes (CYP3A4) and countertransport proteins (p-glycoprotein) located in the gut. Both formulations are available as an oral solution (100 mg/ml) and as 25 mg and 100 mg gelatin capsules. The Sandimmune solution may be administered in milk, chocolate milk, or orange juice. The Neoral solution should be administered in apple or orange juice, as it results in an unpalatable mixture when mixed with milk. Gengraf modified solution has been reported to have improved palatability.

Tacrolimus (Prograf)

Tacrolimus, a macrolide antibiotic compound derived from *Streptomyces tsukabaensis,* shares a similar mechanism of action to that of CSA; however, tacrolimus is 10 to 100 times more potent (Plosker & Foster, 2000). Tacrolimus binds specifically to tacrolimus binding protein (FKBP), a cytoplasmic immunophilin, resulting in calcineurin inhibition, and ultimately inhibition of IL-2. Like CSA, it also induces transforming growth factor (TGF-beta 1). TGF-beta 1 possesses potent immunosuppressive activity and fibrogenic potential that are thought to contribute to the immunosuppressive and nephrotoxic properties of these agents.

Tacrolimus is available in an intravenous (IV) formulation as well as 0.5 mg, 1 mg, and 5 mg capsules. Oral tacrolimus is also erratically and incompletely absorbed but its absorption is independent of bile. Oral bioavailability of tacrolimus is approximately 20% to 25%; food may reduce the rate and extent of absorption. Because of this food effect, it is recommended that patients be consistent with respect to how they take tacrolimus. Like CSA, tacrolimus is also subject to inter/intrapatient bioavailability alterations mediated by p-glycoprotein and metabolic enzymes (CYP3A4) in the gut. Tacrolimus is also widely distributed in the blood; approximately 75% to 80% is bound to erythrocytes. Thus, whole blood concentrations can be expected to be 15 to 30 times greater than plasma concentrations. One difference from CSA is that it does not bind to lipoproteins and this may contribute to its lower incidence of hyperlipidemia. The half-life of tacrolimus is approximately 12 hours in liver transplant recipients and approximately 19 hours in kidney transplant recipients (Plosker & Foster, 2000).

Both tacrolimus and CSA are metabolized to multiple metabolites by the cytochrome p450 3A isoenzyme system in the liver and gut (Christians & Sewing, 1993; Plosker & Foster, 2000). Both agents are primarily excreted in the bile and have minimal renal elimination (Hong & Kahan, 2000). Consequently, drug dosage modifications are unnecessary with hemodialysis or renal dysfunction. Both tacrolimus and CSA are subject to pharmacokinetic variability; thus, pediatric and African American patients may require increased dosages. Elderly patients or those with liver dysfunction may require longer intervals of administration (Canafax, 1995; Kahan, 1989). Like CSA, tacrolimus is also susceptible to many clinically significant pharmacokinetic or pharmacodynamic drug interactions associated with its metabolism through the cytochrome p450 3A4 isoenzyme system (Lake & Canafax, 1995). Therefore, as additional drugs are added or discontinued from the patient's drug regimen, drug concentrations should be monitored if the agents have the potential to interact. Inhibitors and inducers are listed in Table 4.1. It is important to note that over-the-counter herbal preparations, such as Saint John's Wort, can interfere with the metabolism of calcineurin inhibitors (Barone, Gurley, Ketel, Lightfoot, & Abul-Ezz, 2000; Fugh-Burman, 2000). New agents should also be evaluated for their potential additive side effects, such as nephrotoxicity, neurotoxicity, hepatoxicity, hyperlipidemia, and hyperglycemia, as well as their effects on the metabolism of CSA, tacrolimus, and sirolimus.

CSA and tacrolimus exhibit similar side effects; however, the incidence varies between the two agents. Nephrotoxicity, neurotoxicity, electrolyte imbalances, headaches, bruising, hepatotoxicity, infection, nausea, vomiting, and diarrhea seem to occur to a similar degree among patients treated with tacrolimus or CSA. Hyperlipidemia, hypertension, and increased uric acid or gout occur more frequently with CSA. Alopecia, hyperglycemia, and mental status changes have been reported more frequently with tacrolimus as compared to CSA. However, CSA is associated with several unique side effects including acne, hirsutism, gingival hyperplasia, increased appetite, and pancreatitis. Many of these side effects are dose and serum concentration dependent and are also affected by other immunosuppressive agents (e.g., prednisone) the patient is receiving.

The calcineurin inhibitors, CSA and tacrolimus, have served as the cornerstone of solid organ transplant immunosuppressive therapy for the past decade. However, with the introduction of newer, more potent immunosuppressive agents, the concept of calcineurin-sparing or calcineurin-free regimens is gaining in popularity, and studies are under way to evaluate their potential utility and place in transplantation.

TABLE 4.1 Major Transplant Immunosuppressive Agents: Indications, Dosage, Administration, Pharmacokinetics, Interactions, Side Effects, and Therapeutic Drug Monitoring (TDM)

Azathioprine	Indications and Mechanism of Action	Dosage	Administration	Pharmacokinetics	Interactions	Side effects	TDM/miscellaneous
Available preparations Imuran Glaxo Wellcome Roxane Laboratories **Tablets:** 50 mg scored Parenteral: 100 mg as azathioprine, 20mL vial **Class** Antimetabolite Immunosuppressive agent	**Indication** Adjunctive therapy for prevention of rejection in solid organ transplants **Mechanism of action** Azathioprine, a prodrug that is converted into 6-mercaptopurine in the body, is thought to competitively antagonize, via the de novo and salvage pathways, nucleotide synthesis through alteration of DNA/RNA synthesis and function, thereby inhibiting T-cell activation.	**IV** Initially 3–5 mg/kg/day beginning at the time of transplant Given as a single daily dose on the day of transplant or in some cases 1–3 days prior to transplant **Oral** Initially 3–5 mg/kg/day Maintenance: 1–3 mg/kg/day **Renal failure** Dosage adjustments may be necessary in patients experiencing oliguria or tubular necrosis immediately status post-cadaveric renal transplant secondary to delayed elimination.	Administration rate is dependent on final volume of product. Average IV infusion time ~ 30–60 minutes.	**Absorption** F_{oral} = 41–47% **Protein binding** ~ 30% **Metabolism** Liver Undergoes derivative oxidation and methylation **Half-life** $t_{1/2}$ = ~ 3 hours (end-stage renal disease: expect prolonged $t_{1/2}$) **Excretion** Minor amounts excreted through kidney	**Increased toxicity** **Allopurinol** Requires AZA dose reduction to 25–35% previous dose **ACE Inhibitors** ↑ risk of leukopenia Agents causing myelosuppression, including sulfonamides, ganciclovir, cyclophosphamide, methotrexate, and mycophenolate mofetil Decreased efficacy of warfarin	Dose reduction or withdrawal for reversal **Most common side effects** Leukopenia Chills Thrombocytopenia Anemia Nausea Vomiting Diarrhea Anorexia Fever **Other side effects** Hypotension Arthralgias Macular papular rash Dyspnea Retinopathy Alopecia Immunosuppressive agents ↑ the risk of infection as well as certain types of cancer, including PTLD	Dose adjustments may be necessary based on patient renal function and WBC Discontinue in the presence of severe hematologic toxicity

continued

TABLE 4.1 (*continued*)

Azathioprine	Indications and Mechanism of Action	Dosage	Administration	Pharmacokinetics	Interactions	Side effects	TDM/ miscellaneous
		GFR > 50 mL/min: no adjustment necessary					
		GFR 10–50mL/min: 75% of the normal dose					
		GFR <10mL/min: 50% of the normal dose					

continued

TABLE 4.1 *(continued)*

Cyclophosphamide	Indications and Mechanism of Action	Dosage	Administration	Pharmacokinetics	Interactions	Side effects	TDM/ miscellaneous
Available preparations Cytoxan Bristol Meyers Squibb Neosar Pharmacia Upjohn **Tablets:** 25 mg, 50 mg **Parenteral:** injectable lyophilized cake 100 mg, 200 mg, 500 mg, 1 g, 2 g Class Antineoplastic alkylating agent Immunosuppressant	**Indication:** Prophylaxis of rejection in solid organ transplantation **Mechanism of action** Possesses alkylating properties that disrupt DNA replication, RNA transcription, and nucleic acid function; also exerts very significant immunosuppressive activity	1.5 mg–2 mg/kg/day **Renal failure** GFR > 50 mL/min: no adjustment necessary GFR 10–50 mL/min: 75% of the normal dose GFR < 10mL/min: 50% of the normal dose	**IV** Follow institution guidelines for administration of antineoplastic agents	**Absorption:** F$_{(oral)}$ ~ 75% **Protein binding:** 24% **Metabolism** Liver Prodrug converted to active metabolite through cytochrome p450 mixed function oxidase hepatic enzyme system. **Excretion** Renal: 5–25% unchanged drug **Half Life** Oral: 1.3–6.7 hours IV: 4.1–16 hours	**Increased toxicity** Allopurinol Hydrochlorothiazide: Enhanced myelosuppression **Decreased efficacy** Chloramphenicol Phenobarbital ↓ efficacy cyclophosphamide Ciprofloxacin Possible ↓ efficacy quinolone antibiotics	**Most common side effects** Alopecia Possible sterility Nausea Vomiting Anorexia Stomatitis Hemorrhagic cystitis **Other side effects** Headache Skin rash Facial flushing Myelosuppression Thrombocytopenia **Side effects that occur most commonly with high doses** Cardiotoxicity Dizziness Darkening skin/fingernails	

continued

TABLE 4.1 (continued)

Cyclophosphamide	Indications and Mechanism of Action	Dosage	Administration	Pharmacokinetics	Interactions	Side effects	TDM/ miscellaneous
					Digoxin ↓ efficacy digoxin secondary to ↓ absorption	Syndrome of inappropriate antidiuretic hormone secretion Hyperkalemia Renal tubular necrosis Hepatic toxicity Pulmonary fibrosis Immunosuppressive agents ↑ the risk of infection as well as certain types of cancer, including PTLD	

continued

TABLE 4.1 (continued)

Daclizumab	Indications and Mechanism of Action	Dosage	Administration	Pharmacokinetics	Interactions	Side effects	TDM/ miscellaneous
Available preparations Zenapax Hoffman LaRoche Parenteral: 5 mg/mL solution for injection (5 mL–25 mg single-use vial) **Class** IL-2 receptor antagonist Immunosuppressant Humanized monoclonal antibody	**Indication** Prophylaxis of rejection in solid organ transplantation **Mechanism of action** Specifically binds the alpha subunit of the IL-2 receptor, effectively inhibiting IL-2 mediated T-lymphocyte activation	**IV** 1 mg/kg diluted with 0.9% normal saline solution administered every 14 days for a total of 5 doses **1st dose:** Should be administered no more than 24 hours posttransplant	Infuse dose over 15–30 minutes Administer in facilities with appropriately equipped medical support Potential for anaphylactic reactions exists, although none have been reported.	Limited data exist **Half-life** $t_{1/2}$ = 44–360 hours Average $t_{1/2}$ = 90–100 hours	There have been no documented drug interactions	**Most common side effects** Gastrointestinal disturbance Nausea Vomiting Diarrhea Abdominal pain/distention Dyspepsia Epigastric pain Side effects were similar to those experienced by patients receiving placebo Immunosuppressive agents ↑ the risk of infection as well as certain types of cancer, including PTLD	

continued

TABLE 4.1 (*continued*)

Antithymocyte globulin	Indications and Mechanism of Action	Dosage	Administration	Pharmacokinetics	Interactions	Side effects	TDM/ miscellaneous
Available preparations Thymoglobulin Sangstat Medical Corporation **Parenteral:** intravenous lyophilized powder 25 mg/vial **Class** Immunosuppressant Polyclonal immunoglobulin derived from rabbits (IgG/IgM)	**Indication** Treatment of allograft rejection; used in conjunction with other immunosuppressant therapies **Mechanism of action** The manner by which Thymoglobulin produces its immunosuppressive action has yet to be fully elucidated. It is theorized that the antibody binds to cell receptors reducing the number of circulating T lymphocytes	**IV** 1.5 mg/kg/day for 5–14 days using high-flow vein, central venous catheter/brachial arteriovenous fistula or peripherally	**Rate of administration** Administer 1st infusion over a minimum of 6 hours Administer the remaining doses over a minimum of 4 hours subsequently Administer the medication through an in-line 0.22 micron filter Ensure that appropriate medical staff monitor patient for signs and symptoms of adverse reactions during and after the infusion	**Limited data exist** **Half-life** $t_{1/2} = \sim 30$ days Range 14–45 days	Has been used in conjunction with other immunosuppressive therapies. Potential for overimmunosuppression exists Some patients may produce antibody to this agent, causing a cross-reaction with the immune globulins	**Most common side effects** Fever/chills Thrombocytopenia Leukopenia Myalgia Hypertension Tachycardia Peripheral edema Bronchospasm/dypsnea Headache Dizziness Weakness Nausea Vomiting Diarrhea Abdominal pain Skin rash ↑ risk malignancy ↑ risk of infection **Other side effects** Nephrotoxicity in presence of serum sickness Transient ↑ in liver function tests Gastritis Immunosuppressive agents ↑ the risk of infection as well as certain types of cancer, including PTLD	

continued

TABLE 4.1 (*continued*)

Lymphocyte immune globulin	Indications and Mechanism of Action	Dosage	Administration	Pharmacokinetics	Interactions	Side effects
Available preparations Atgam Pharmacia Upjohn 50 mg/mL sterile solution horse gamma globulin (5 mL ampules) **Class** Immunosuppressant Polyclonal anti-lymphocyte globulin derived from horses	**Indication** Prevention/treatment of solid organ rejection **Mechanism of action** Lymphocyte selective immunosuppressant Exerts immunosuppressive action by depleting circulating T lymphocytes through alterations in cell-mediated immunity and humoral immune response	**IV** 10–15 mg/kg IV infusion (in normal saline solution) for 14 days with optional additional 7 doses on an every other day schedule if needed	**Route of administration** Administer via IV infusion over 4–6 hours via central vein or other large vein because risk of phlebitis Incompatability with dextrose and acidic solutions Extravasation should be avoided as patients will experience severe local reactions: severe pain, tissue necrosis, nerve damage	**Limited data exist** **Half-life** $t_{1/2} = \sim 5.7$ days **Excretion** Renal 1%	Has been used in conjunction with other immunosuppressive therapies. Potential for overimmunosuppression exists	**Most common side effects** Thrombocytopenia Leukopenia Chills Fever Pruritis Urticaria Nephrotoxicity Rash Apnea Dyspnea Back pain Chest pain **Other side effects** Anaphylaxis Viral hepatitis Hypotension Hypertension Tachycardia Congestive heart failure Thrombophlebitis Vasculitis Confusion Dizziness

continued

TABLE 4.1 (continued)

Lymphocyte immune globulin	Indications and Mechanism of Action	Dosage	Administration	Pharmacokinetics	Interactions	Side effects	
						Syncope Paresthesia Seizures Hyperglycemia Diaphoresis Diarrhea Nausea Vomiting Acute renal failure	
						Immunosuppressive agents ↑ the risk of infection as well as certain types of cancer, including PTLD	

continued

TABLE 4.1 (continued)

Basiliximab	Indications and Mechanism of Action	Dosage	Administration	Pharmacokinetics	Interactions	Side effects	TDM/ miscellaneous
Available preparations Simulect Norvartis Pharmaceuticals **Parenteral:** injectable lyophilized powder 20 mg/vial **Class** Immunosuppressant IL-2 receptor antagonist Murine–human chimeric monoclonal antibody	**Indication** Prevention of rejection in solid organ transplantation **Mechanism of action** Specifically binds the alpha subunit of IL-2 receptor complex, competitively inhibiting interleukin-2 mediated T-lymphocyte activation	**IV** **Day 0** 20 mg (IV) 2 hours prior to transplant **Day 4** 20 mg (IV) on posttransplant day 4	**Rate of administration** Administer IV infusion over 20–30 minutes once it has been reconstituted with 50 mL diluent (0.9% normal saline solution or D5W)	Limited data exist **Half-life** $t_{1/2} = \sim 5\text{–}10$ days	There have been no reported drug interactions	Side effects were similar to those with placebo Immunosuppressive agents ↑ the risk of infection as well as certain types of cancer, including PTLD	

continued

TABLE 4.1 (continued)

Muromonab-CD3	Indications and Mechanism of Action	Dosage	Administration	Pharmacokinetics	Interactions	Side effects
Available preparations Orthoclone OKT3 Ortho-Biotech Inc. McNeil Pharmaceuticals **Parenteral:** 5 mL-ampule Muromonab-CD-3 1 mg/mL **Class** Immunosuppressant agent Murine monoclonal antibody	**Indication** Treatment of acute allograft rejection unresponsive to standard protocols **Mechanism of action** Murine monoclonal antibody targeted to alter the function of T cells by binding to CD3 T-cell glycoprotein	**IV** 5 mg/day for 10–14 days (variable regimens used)	**Premedications** Many centers administer steroids, antihistamines, and acetaminophen to diminish early reactions Following the initial administration of the medication, patients should be closely monitored in an area appropriately equipped and staffed to handle emergency care Administer through IV bolus Do not administer through IV infusion Do not administer in conjunction with other drug solutions	Limited data exist **Half-life** $t_{1/2} = \sim 18$ hours	There have been no reported drug interactions	**Most common side effects reported after initial infusion** Fever Wheezing Chest pain Nausea Vomiting Diarrhea Nephrotoxicity Pulmonary edema Chills Pediatric patients: cerebral edema has also been reported. **Other side effects** Tremors Tachycardia Dizziness Nausea Vomiting Dyspnea Itching Headache Chest tightness

continued

TABLE 4.1 (continued)

Muromonab-CD3	Indications and Mechanism of Action	Dosage	Administration	Pharmacokinetics	Interactions	Side effects
						Chest pain Seizures Arthralgias Pancytopenia Hypotension Hypertension Anaphylactic reactions Immunosuppressive agents ↑ the risk of infection as well as certain types of cancer, including PTLD

continued

TABLE 4.1 (continued)

Cyclosporine	Indications and Mechanism of Action	Dosage	Administration	Pharmacokinetics	Interactions	Side effects	TDM/ miscellaneous
Available preparations *Neoral *Sandimmune †Gengraf ⊗ Cyclosporine, Modified USP *Novartis Pharmaceuticals †Abbott Laboratories ⊗ Eon Labs ⊗ Sidmak Labs **Parenteral:** 50 mg/mL (50 mL) **Capsule:** 25 and 100 mg **Oral solution:** 100 mg/mL **Class** Immunosuppressant Calcineurin inhibitor Cyclic polypeptide Neoral and Gengraf preparations are not bioequivalent to Sandimmune	**Indication** Prevention of acute rejection **Mechanism of action** Inhibits T-lymphocyte response by binding cyclophilin. It also inhibits IL-2 production, T-cell activation, and proliferation.	**Initial** **IV:** 2–4 mg/kg/day as continuous infusion (or lower) **Maintenance** **PO:** 5–15 mg/kg/day given as a divided dose every 12 hours Available blood assays include: high-performance liquid chromatography, monoclonal antibody RIAs, monoclonal antibody fluorescence polarimetry immunoassay, and microparticulate enzyme immunoassay Dose to maintain blood concentrations within therapeutic range	IV dose should be administered over 2 to 6 hours or as continuous infusion Pediatric recipients: require a significantly higher dosage than adults to achieve similar blood levels (~ 2–4 times higher) Administer oral preparation at 12-hour intervals Draw trough level within 1 hour prior to dose Avoid drawing trough level from the same line used for cyclosporine administration	**Absorption** F$_{oral}$; 30% (range variable: 10–89%) Bioavailability is highly dependent on bile. The oral modified solutions (e.g., Neoral) contain surfactant to improve absorption **Protein binding** ~ 90% lipoproteins Blood: plasma ratio = 2:1 (lower) **Half-life** t$_{1/2}$ = ~ 8 hrs (range: 5–18 hours) **Metabolism** Liver: largely undergoes metabolism via cytochrome p450 3A4 system	**Decreased cyclosporine level** (increase cyclosporine metabolism and decrease cyclosporine efficacy) Phenobarbital Phenytoin Carbamazepine Rifampin Nafcillin Saint John's Wort Rifabutin **Increased cyclosporine level** The following agents inhibit metabolism of cyclosporine and increase the risk of cyclosporine toxicity (not a complete list): Amiodarone Fluconazole Itraconazole Ketoconazole Diltiazem Nicardipine Verapamil	**Most common side effects** Nephrotoxicity Gingival hyperplasia Hirsutism Hypertension Hypercholesterolemia Hypomagnesemia Tremor Hypokalemia Hyperuricemia Other side effects Nausea Vomiting Diarrhea Abdominal pain Hyperkalemia Acne Seizure Headache Immunosuppressive agents ↑ the risk of infection as well as certain types of cancer, including PTLD	**Trough level** Whole blood assay therapeutic range: 100–400 mcg/L Plasma assay therapeutic range: 50–200 mcg/L Target goal trough level may vary according to organ type, transplant center, concomitant immunosuppression, and patient status **Monitoring** Blood pressure Serum creatinine Liver function tests Potassium Magnesium Fasting blood glucose

continued

TABLE 4.1 (continued)

Cyclosporine	Indications and Mechanism of Action	Dosage	Administration	Pharmacokinetics	Interactions	Side effects	TDM/ miscellaneous
			Clamping the T tube may increase absorption Cyclosporine is not removed by hemodialysis	Intestine and kidney: small extent **Excretion** Biliary, primarily 6% of dose (parent drug and metabolites) excreted in urine	Erythromycin Clarithromycin Cimetadine Cisapride Metoclopramide Danazol Bromocriptine Ciprofloxacin Grapefruit juice **Increased risk of nephrotoxicity** Aminoglycosides Amphotercin B Vancomycin Acyclovir Ganciclovir Nonsteroidal anti-inflammatory drugs **Increased risk of rhabdomyolysis** HMG-Co A inhibitors Gemfibrozil		

continued

TABLE 4.1 (continued)

Tacrolimus	Indications and Mechanism of Action	Dosage	Administration	Pharmacokinetics	Interactions	Side effects	TDM/ miscellaneous
Available preparations **Prograf** Fujisawa **Parenteral:** 5 mg/mL (1 mL) **Capsules:** 0.5, 1, and 5 mg Exptemp. Oral suspension: 0.5 mg/mL **Class** Immunosuppressant Calcineurin inhibitor Macrolide	**Indication** Prevention and treatment of acute rejection **Mechanism of action** Inhibits T-lymphocyte response by binding cyclophilin. It also inhibits IL-2 production, T-cell activation, and proliferation	**Initial** **IV:** 0.05–0.10 mg/kg/day continuous infusion (or lower) **Maintenance** **PO:** 0.1–0.3 mg/kg/day given as a divided dose every 12 hours Available blood assays include: microparticulate enzyme immunoassay, enzyme-linked immunoabsorbent assay Dose to maintain blood concentrations within therapeutic range	Observe patient for at least 30 minutes after initiation of IV infusion Administer oral preparation at 12-hour intervals Maintain consistency with respect to administration of tacrolimus and meals. Pediatric patients require a significantly higher dosage than adults to achieve similar blood levels (~ 2–4 times higher) Do not administer oral preparation with antacids or magnesium or calcium supplements	**Absorption** $F_{oral} = 14–32\%$ Oral absorption highly variable. Food may reduce absorption. Bioavailablity is not influenced by bile **Protein binding** ~ 99% bound to plasma proteins (albumin and alpha 1-acid glycoprotein) **Half-life** $t_{1/2} = $ ~ 12 hours **Metabolism** Liver: largely but also small intestine Undergoes metabolism via the cytochrome p450 3A4 enzyme system.	**Decreased tacrolimus level** (increase tacrolimus metabolism and decrease tacrolimus efficacy) Phenobarbital Antacids Phenytoin Carbamazepine Saint John's Wort Rifampin Rifabutin **Increased tacrolimus level** The following agents inhibit metabolism of tacrolimus and increase the risk of tacrolimus toxicity (not a complete list): Amiodarone Fluconazole Itraconazole Ketoconazole Diltiazem Nicardipine Verapamil	**Most common side effects** Nephrotoxicity Tremor Headache Diarrhea Nausea Peripheral edema Hypertension **Other side effects** Pleural effusion Hyperkalemia Pruritis Hypomagnesemia Vomiting Abdominal pain Paresthesia Insomnia Hyperglycemia Anemia Leukocytosis Abnormal liver function tests Atelectasis Ascites Weakness Seizures Rash Urinary tract infection Arthralgia	**Trough level** Whole blood assay therapeutic range: 5–20 mcg/L Plasma assay therapeutic range: 0.1–0.5 mcg/L Target goal trough level may vary according to organ type, transplant center, concomitant immunosuppression, and patient status **Kidney** Range: 5–20 ng/mL Months 1 to 3: 7–20 ng/mL Months 4 to 12: 5–15 ng/mL **Liver** Range: 5–20 ng/mL Months 1 to 12: 5–20 ng/mL

continued

TABLE 4.1 (continued)

Tacrolimus	Indications and Mechanism of Action	Dosage	Administration	Pharmacokinetics	Interactions	Side effects	TDM/ miscellaneous
			Draw trough level within 1 hour prior to dose Avoid drawing blood for trough level from the same line used for tacrolimus administration Tacrolimus is not removed by hemodialysis	**Excretion** Bile: extensive Kidney: minimal Less than 1% of dose excreted unchanged in urine	Erythromycin Cisapride Danazol Clarithromycin Cimetadine Metoclopramide Bromocriptine Ciprofloxacin Grapefruit juice **Increase risk of nephrotoxicity** Aminoglycosides Amphotercin B Cyclosporine Vancomycin Nonsteroidal anti-inflammatory drugs **Increase risk of rhabdomyolysis** HMG-Co A inhibitors Gemfibrozil	Myalgia Expressive aphasia Constipation Headache Immunosuppressive agents ↑ the risk of infection as well as certain types of cancer including PTLD	**Monitor** Blood pressure Serum creatinine Potassium Magnesium Fasting blood glucose Liver function tests

continued

TABLE 4.1 (continued)

Steroids	Indications and Mechanism of Action	Dosage	Administration	Pharmacokinetics	Interactions	Side effects	TDM/miscellaneous
Available Preparations Methylprednisolone Solu-Medrol Pharmacia & Upjohn	**Indication** Prevention and treatment of acute rejection	**Treatment of acute rejection** Adults: Administer 250 mg–1000 mg methylprednisolone IV daily for up to 3 days. May be followed by standard taper or taper per institution protocol	Methylprednisolone (1 g) may be administered via IV push over several minutes Alternatively, may also administer methylprednisolone via IV infusion over 10 to 20 minutes once reconstituted with 50 mL normal saline	**Absorption** F_{oral} = 74–99% **Protein binding** ~ 80% concentration dependent	Steroids undergo metabolism through the cytochrome p450 (3A4) enzyme system	**Most common side effects** Insomnia Nervousness Mood swings ↑ appetite Gastrointestinal upset	**Monitor** Blood pressure Potassium Fasting blood glucose Liver function tests
A-methapred Abbott Labs	**Mechanism of action** Nonspecific potent anti-inflammatory agents that exert activity through several mechanisms:			**Metabolism** Liver (extensive) **Half-life** $t_{1/2}$ = 2–3 hours	**Increased level of steroids** (increased toxicity) Ketoconazole	Peptic ulcer Glucose intolerance Hyperglycemia	**Approximate steroid conversion equivalents**
Various generic manufacturers				**Excretion** Renal (largely)	Itraconazole Clarithromycin	Hypertension Edema	Cortisone 25 mg
						Acne	Hydrocortisone 20 mg
Parenteral Methylprednisolone sodium succinate powder for injection: 40 mg; 125 mg; 500 mg; 1 g and 2 g	Decrease cytokines, including IL-1, IL-2, and IL-6	**Prevention of rejection** Per institution protocol	Closely monitor fasting blood sugar and blood pressure		**Decreased efficacy of steroids** (increase the metabolism of steroids)	Hirsutism Myopathy Arthralgia Osteoporosis Leukocytosis	Methylprednisolone 4 mg Prednisolone 5 mg
Depo-Medrol Pharmacia & Upjohn	Decrease monocyte cell surface molecule gene transcription	Taper per institution protocol			Phenytoin Phenobarbital Rifampin	Delayed wound healing Infections	Prednisone 5 mg
DepMedalone Forest Pharmaceuticals Aslone UAD	Down-regulation of endothelial cell adhesion molecule expression				Steroids reduce the response to skin test antigens	Cataracts Glaucoma Growth impairment	Triamcinolone 4mg
Methylprednisolone acetate injection: 20 mg/mL,						Cushingoid syndrome Sodium and water retention	Betamethasone 0.6–0.75 mg Dexamethasone 0.75 mg

continued

TABLE 4.1 *(continued)*

Steroids	Indications and Mechanism of Action	Dosage	Administration	Pharmacokinetics	Interactions	Side effects	TDM/ miscellaneous
40 mg/mL, and 80 mg/mL Medrol Pharmacia & Upjohn Various generic manufacturers' tablets: 2 mg, 4 mg, 8 mg, 16 mg, 24 mg, and 32 mg **Class** Immunosuppressant Corticosteroid	Inhibit phospholipase A2 enzyme activity Inhibit lymphocyte proliferation					Immunosuppressive agents ↑ the risk of infection as well as certain types of cancer, including PTLD	

continued

TABLE 4.1 (continued)

Mycophenolate mofetil (MMF)	Indications and Mechanism of Action	Dosage	Administration	Pharmacokinetics	Interactions	Side effects	TDM/ miscellaneous
Available preparations **CellCept** Roche Laboratories **Parenteral:** 25 mg/mL (20 mL) **Capsule:** 250 mg **Tablets:** 500 mg **Oral suspension:** 200 mg/mL (100 mL) **Class** Immunosuppressant Antimetabolite	**Indication** Prevention of acute rejection. **Mechanism of action** Mycophenolate mofetil is metabolized in the body to its active metabolite MPA. It blocks de novo synthesis of purine guanosine required for DNA synthesis. It also selectively and reversibly inhibits inosine monophosphate dehydrogenase, blocking T-and B-cell proliferation.	**Adult:** 2–3 g daily divided every 12 hours or every 8 hours **Pediatric:** 15 mg/kg twice daily or 1,200 mg/m² body surface area/day divided every 12 hours or every 8 hours Use lower dosage in patients with end-stage renal disease	Avoid administration of antacids or calcium or magnesium supplements in combination with the oral preparation. Separate administration of oral preparation by at least 2 hours from administration of ferrous sulfate or products containing calcium, magnesium, or antacids (e.g., calcium carbonate, Amphogel, Carafate) Available blood assays include high-performance liquid chromatography and ultrafiltration assays that measure MPA in plasma	**Absorption** F_{oral} = ~ 94% **Protein binding** ~ 97% **Half-life** $t_{1/2}$ = 16 to 18 hours **Metabolism** Liver: extensive **Excretion** Renal ~ 93% Feces ~ 6% Enterohepatic recirculation of active metabolite may occur	**Decreased level of MMF** (decreased efficacy) Antacids and oral magnesium reduce MMF absorption Metronidazole and cholestramine reduce bioavailability of MMF Acyclovir and ganciclovir levels may increase in the presence of MMF Probenecid may increase MPA or MPAG level Cyclosporine decreases MPA level	**Most common side effects** Abdominal pain Diarrhea Nausea Drug-induced fever Vomiting Peripheral edema Leukocytosis Leukopenia Thrombocytopenia **Other side effects** Hematuria Dyspnea Cough Infections Acne Pneumonia Back pain Headache Chest pain Constipation Insomnia Dizziness Tremor	**TDM** Monitor: CBC with differential Renal function Hepatic function Consider dose reductions in patients who exhibit severe hematologic toxicity.

continued

TABLE 4.1 (continued)

Mycophenolate mofetil (MMF)	Indications and Mechanism of Action	Dosage	Administration	Pharmacokinetics	Interactions	Side effects	TDM/ miscellaneous
					Uremic patients may exhibit signs and symptoms of MMF toxicity at normal doses. If applicable, consider dose reduction at that time.	Anemia Renal tubular necrosis Urinary tract infection Immunosuppressive agents ↑ the risk of infection as well as certain types of cancer, including PTLD	For gastrointestinal toxicities: Consider increasing frequency of administration (e.g., from every 12 hours to every 6 hours) or reducing dose

continued

TABLE 4.1 (continued)

Sirolimus	Indications and Mechanism of Action	Dosage	Administration	Pharmacokinetics	Interactions	Side effects	TDM/miscellaneous
Available preparation Rapamune Wyeth-Ayerst Laboratories **Oral Solution:** 1 mg/ml Tablets: 1 mg Rapamune (povidone) **Tablets:** 1 mg Rapamune (povidone) **Class** Immunosuppressant agent Macrolide antibiotic	**Indication** Prevention of solid organ transplant rejection **Mechanism of action** Blocks response to T-and B-cell cytokines resulting in antiproliferative effect Inhibits B-cell proliferation and differentiation to immunoglobulin secreting cells Promotes apoptosis Inhibits smooth muscle cell proliferation and arterial intimal thickening	**Load dose** 6 mg (or 3 times the maintenance dose) **Maintenance dose** 2 mg–5 mg/day African American patients may require higher dosages (5 mg/day)	**Oral solution** Dilute solution with 2 fluid ounces water or orange juice in glass or plastic container Do not mix with grapefruit juice or any other liquid Mix solution thoroughly and take immediately Then fill container with 4 ounces of fluid. Stir vigorously and take remainder immediately Administer consistently with or without food Administer sirolimus 4 hours after cyclosporine oral solution or capsule	**Absorption** $F_{oral} = 15\%$ Rate and extent of absorption is reduced in African American patients **Lipoprotein binding** ~ 40% lipoprotein ~ 60% non-lipoprotein Plasma: 3% RBCs: 95% **Metabolism** Liver: extensively Some extent small intestine Metabolized via the cytochrome p450 3A4 isoenzyme **Half-life** $t_{1/2}$ = 57–63 hours **Excretion** Bile extent unknown	**Increased sirolimus level** (Increased toxicity) Bromocriptine Cimetidine Clarithromycin Clotrimazole Danazol Diltiazem Erythromycin Erythromycin/sulfisoxazole Fluconazole Ketoconazole Itraconazole Nicardipine Metoclopramide Grapefruit juice **Ketoconazole** Inhibitor p450 3A4; should not be used in combination **Increased absorption of sirolimus** Cyclosporine **Increased risk of hyperlipidemia** Cyclosporine Prednisone Beta blockers	**Most common side effects** Anemia Thrombocytopenia Leukopenia Hypertension Hypertriglyceridemia Hypercholesterolemia Hypophosphatemia Hypokalemia Constipation Diarrhea Dyspepsia Nausea Vomiting Urinary tract infection Dyspnea **Other side effects** Nephrotoxicity Arthralgia Immunosuppressive agents ↑ the risk of infection as well as certain types of cancer, including PTLD	**TDM** **Trough:** Draw level 1 hour prior to next dose **Trough level:** whole blood assay therapeutic range: 3–36ng/mL (12 hour) **Steady state concentration:** achieved in 5–7 days post initiation or dosage adjustment Target goal trough level may vary according to organ type, transplant center, concomitant immunosuppression, and patient status **Monitor** Whole blood trough level CBC with differential

continued

TABLE 4.1 *(continued)*

Sirolimus	Indications and Mechanism of Action	Dosage	Administration	Pharmacokinetics	Interactions	Side effects	TDM/ miscellaneous
			Available blood assays include high-performance liquid chromatography: electro-spray tandem mass spectroscopy		**Increased risk of nephrotoxicity** Cyclosporine Aminoglycosides Amphotericin B **Decreased sirolimus level** (decreased efficacy*) Carbamazepine Fosphenytoin Rifapentine Phenobarbital Phenytoin Rifabutin Rifampin *Monitor sirolimus level and symptoms of rejection		Lipid/lipoprotein panels Liver function tests Blood glucose Routine blood work (electrolytes, renal function tests, etc.)

AZA = azathioprine
GFR = glomerular filtration rate
MPA = mycophenolic acid
MPAG = mycophenolic acid glucoronide
PTLD = posttransplant lymphoproliferative disease
RIA = radioimmune assay
WBC = white blood cell

INHIBITOR OF LATE T-CELL INHIBITION (TOR INHIBITORS)

SIROLIMUS (RAPAMUNE)

Approved in 1999, sirolimus is the most recent addition to the arsenal of immunosuppressive therapies. Although it is structurally related to tacrolimus, sirolimus exhibits a novel mechanism of action and distinct side effect profile. Sirolimus, a macrolide antibiotic isolated from *Streptomyces hygroscopius,* was originally studied for potential antifungal properties; its immunosuppressive activities were discovered later. Like CSA and tacrolimus, sirolimus binds to immunophilin, forming the sirolimus-FK binding protein (FKBP) complex. In contrast to CSA and tacrolimus, sirolimus does not inhibit calcineurin. Rather, sirolimus inhibits the activity of mammalian target of rapamycin (mTOR), a kinase enzyme. mTOR inhibition blocks cytokine mediated cell proliferation between phase G1 and S, and ultimately inhibits T- and B-cell proliferation (Ingle, Sievers, & Holt, 2000). It appears that FKBP, the binding protein for both sirolimus and tacrolimus, is ubiquitously available in vivo; thus, competition for the receptor is unlikely, and the two agents can be used together.

Following oral administration, sirolimus is poorly but rapidly absorbed with a bioavailability of approximately 15%. It exhibits a long half-life of approximately 57 to 62 hours; however, the half-life is shorter in some patients, including pediatric patients (Yatscoff, 1996). Sirolimus also exhibits highly variable pharmacokinetics, as do CSA and tacrolimus (Zimmerman & Kahan, 1997). Sirolimus is highly lipophilic and is approximately 95% bound to RBCs. It undergoes metabolism into multiple metabolites in the small intestine and liver mediated by the cytochrome p4503A enzyme system. Like calcineurin inhibitors, sirolimus is also substrate for p-glycoprotein, a countertransport efflux pump that is found in the gut. Approximately 2% of sirolimus is eliminated in the urine; the remaining 91% is eliminated in feces. Dosage adjustments are unnecessary in renal dysfunction. It is unlikely that hemodialysis will remove sirolimus given its high lipophilicity and large volume of distribution. Dosage adjustments are required when hepatic dysfunction is present. Patients with mild to moderate hepatic dysfunction should be administered one third the recommended dose.

Considering their shared metabolic pathway, drug interactions that may occur with CSA and tacrolimus should also be expected with sirolimus until proven otherwise. Clinically significant drug interactions may be expected of agents metabolized through the cytochrome p450 (3A4) isoenzyme system (Mignat, 1997). Inhibitors or inducers of the CYP450 (3A4) isoenzyme system should be added cautiously to the patient's regimen (see Table 4.1). The potential magnitude of these interactions is clearly demonstrated by sirolimus's interaction with rifampin and ketoconazole. Rifampin reduced sirolimus concentrations by 92%; after multiple doses of ketoconazole and sirolimus, a 990% increase in sirolimus level was observed (Ingle, Sievers, and Holt, 2000).

Compared to other agents, side effects associated with sirolimus are commonly dose dependent as well as unique. Sirolimus rarely causes nephrotoxicity, neurotoxicity, or hyperglycemia. Hyperlipidemia, including hypertriglyceridemia and hypercholesterolemia, is the most notable side effect of sirolimus and is magnified when used in combination with cyclosporine and prednisone. The hyperlipidemia should be managed appropriately utilizing exercise, diet modifications, and/or drug treatment with 3-hydroxy-3-methylglutaryl coenzyme A (HMG-CoA) reductase inhibitors. Clinicians should monitor patients closely when using HMG-CoA reductase inhibitors with sirolimus, as they are metabolized through the same pathway in the liver (CYP450 3A4) and the possibility for competitive metabolism exists. These patients may be at an increased risk for myopathy or rhabdomyolysis especially if prescribed other agents sharing the same metabolic pathway (e.g., gemfibrozil, niacin, or Ca^{++} channel blockers.) Other side effects include bone marrow suppression and liver dysfunction. Side effects may be ameliorated with dosage alterations (Ingle et al., 2000). Sirolimus does not cause nephrotoxicity by itself, but it appears to potentiate cyclosporine's nephrotoxicity when the two agents are administered concomitantly. Current recommendations are to use lower doses and levels of CSA when the two agents are used simultaneously. The area under the curve (AUC) of sirolimus increases by 230% when both agents are given concomitantly, whereas only an 80% increase was measured when CSA and sirolimus administration was separated by 4 hours (Kaplan, Meier-Kriesche, Napoli, & Kahan, 1998). Consequently, the manufacturer package information recommends that sirolimus should be taken 4 hours after CSA. The investigational agent RAD (40-O-[2-hydroxeythyl]-rapamycin) is administered concomitantly with CSA and is dosed twice a day. It is important to note that tacrolimus and sirolimus do not appear to have a significant interaction. In fact, a slight decrease in tacrolimus concentrations has been reported at the 2 mg as compared to the 1 mg sirolimus dose (Hariharan et al., 2001).

DRUG CONCENTRATION MONITORING

Therapeutic drug monitoring is used routinely for cyclosporine, tacrolimus, and sirolimus because of the high inter- and intra-patient pharmacokinetic variability for these agents and potential for serious consequences if levels occur outside the therapeutic range. Drug concentrations can be measured in different media (e.g., whole blood vs. plasma) and by various techniques (HPLC (high-performance liquid chromatography), enzyme immunoassays such as FPIA (fluorescence polarization immunoassay), RIA (radioimmunoassay), etc.). Practitioners cannot make an interpretation of the drug concentration without knowing the method or the media due to the different therapeutic ranges. In addition, therapeutic ranges typically differ depending on the type of organ transplant, the rejection history of the patient, time interval following transplantation, and the immunosuppressive regimen (e.g., lower cyclosporine concentrations are recommended for regimens including sirolimus or the investigational rapamycin derivative, RAD).

Trough concentration monitoring is routinely used for cyclosporine, tacrolimus and sirolimus. This technique appears to be a reasonably good approximation for drug exposure with tacrolimus, however it is less reliable for cyclosporine. Over the past decade, other strategies for cyclosporine abbreviated Area Under the Curves (AUCs) with two to four levels at one to four hours following the dose, single drug concentrations at two or three hours after the dose to approximate peak levels (e.g., C_2 or C_3, etc.) have been evaluated to identify a method that produces a better relationship between drug concentration and patient outcome (Dumont & Ensom, 2000) These techniques have not achieved widespread implementation due to the cost, inconvenience, and lack of clear cut data supporting their use. Peak concentrations must be drawn exactly on schedule whereas trough concentrations can be drawn up to 30 minutes before the dose and still provide reliable and reproducible results. A number of centers are currently studying the use of drug concentrations at two hours post dose in kidney transplant patients whereas it has recently been reported that levels drawn at one and/or three hours after the dose are more reliable for lung transplant recipients (Dumont, Partovi, Levy, Fradet, & Ensom, 2001). These methods have not been validated in populations known to have absorption problems (e.g., African American, diabetic, pediatric, or elderly recipients).

INHIBITORS OF T-CELL PROLIFERATION

Inhibitors of T-cell proliferation include mycophenolate mofetil (CellCept), azathioprine (Imuran), and cyclophosphamide (Cytoxan).

MYCOPHENOLATE MOFETIL (MMF) (CELLCEPT)

Mycophenolic acid (MPA), the active metabolite of mycophenolate mofetil, also inhibits T-cell proliferation. MPA competitively and reversibly inhibits inosine monophosphate dehydrogenase (IMPDH), resulting in blockade of de novo synthesis of guanosine nucleotides, which are necessary substrates of DNA (deoxyribonucleic acid) and RNA (ribonucleic acid) synthesis (Fulton & Markham, 1996). Consequently, both T- and B-lymphocyte proliferation are selectively inhibited because they are reliant upon de novo pathway for synthesis of guanosine (Sievers et al., 1997).

Three pivotal multicenter clinical trials in kidney transplant recipients demonstrated improved efficacy with MMF as compared to azathioprine-based regimens. Acute rejection rates were reduced significantly from over 40% with azathioprine-based regimens to 20% to 25% with MMF-based therapy (European Mycophenolate Mofetil Cooperative Study Group, 1995; Mathew, 1998; Sollinger, 1995; Tricontinental Mycophenolate Mofetil Renal Transplantation Study Group, 1996). Based on these studies, MMF has largely replaced azathioprine at most transplant centers because of its improved efficacy and minimal effects on other organ systems.

Following oral administration, MMF is rapidly absorbed and hydrolyzed to its active form, MPA, in the liver, then glucuronidated to its inactive metabolite, mycophenolic acid glucuronide (MPAG). Compared to patients immediately posttransplant, MPA peak plasma concentrations are approximately 50% higher in stable renal transplant recipients who are more than 3 months posttransplant (Fulton & Markham, 1996). MPA is eliminated primarily in the urine as MPAG; however, enterohepatic recirculation of the inactive metabolite MPAG may occur. Additionally, MPAG accumulation and reconversion via beta-glucuronidation to MPA may occur in patients with renal dysfunction. These mechanisms could possibly contribute to overimmunosuppression or toxicity (Fulton & Markham,1996). Although there are no current dosing guidelines, it is generally recommended that patients with renal dysfunction receive a total daily dose of 2 grams or less.

Both MPA and MPAG are highly protein bound to albumin—approximately 99% and 82%, respectively. Therefore, clinicians should cautiously use other highly protein-bound pharmacotherapeutic agents such as phenytoin, as these may result in increased free fraction of MPA or phenytoin. Concomitant disease states such as uremia, hyperbilirubinemia, and hypoalbuminemia may also alter protein binding and result in increased free fraction MPA (Kaplan et al., 1999). MMF should not be administered with antacids, magnesium, or iron-containing products, as they may decrease its absorption (Bullingham, Shah, Goldblum, & Schiff, 1996; Morii et al.,

2000). MPA enterohepatic recirculation and reabsorption may also be affected by bile acid sequestrants or antibiotics. Cyclosporine also interferes with this process, resulting in lower MPA concentrations as compared to those achieved with tacrolimus (Glaneman et al., 2000; Smak Gregoor et al., 1999; Van Gelder, Klupp, Barten, Christians, & Morris, 1999). MPAG elimination may be competitively inhibited by agents that undergo renal tubular secretion, including probenecid, acyclovir, and ganciclovir (Bullingham, Nicholls, & Kamm, 1998). MMF and azathioprine should not be used in combination because of the potential for additive bone marrow suppression.

MMF generally is a well-tolerated agent; however, side effects are more frequent with increased dosages ($\geq$ 3g/day) (Sollinger, 1995) (see Table 4.1). Side effects associated with MMF include gastrointestinal disturbances, hematologic abnormalities, infection, and malignancy. Diarrhea is one of the most frequently occurring adverse events (31%) experienced by patients. Other gastrointestinal side effects that occur slightly less frequently (< 25%) include constipation, nausea, dyspepsia, and vomiting. Strategies often employed by clinicians to help combat these side effects may include a change in the frequency of MMF administration (e.g., 1g PO BID to 500mg PO QID) or a decrease in the total daily MMF dosage. The most common hematologic side effects include leukopenia, anemia, thrombocytopenia, and leukocytosis. Dose adjustments may be warranted in patients experiencing these side effects as well. Immunosuppressive agents, including MMF, are associated with an increased risk of opportunistic infections and malignancy (lymphoproliferative disorders).

AZATHIOPRINE (IMURAN)

Although it was introduced nearly 30 years ago, azathioprine (AZA), an imidazole derivative of the antimetabolite 6-mercaptopurine, has played an important role in triple-drug therapy regimens throughout the years. AZA has been largely replaced by newer immunosuppressive therapies, initially by CSA and more recently by MMF or sirolimus. AZA is a prodrug that is rapidly converted in the liver and RBCs into 6-mercaptopurine (6-MP), which is then incorporated into cellular DNA, whereby it inhibits purine nucleotide synthesis (Chan, Canafax, & Johnson, 1987). It interferes with metabolism of RNA, thereby effectively inhibiting gene replication and consequent T-cell activation. Because AZA does not affect gene activation, it is not effective for treating rejection.

AZA exhibits rapid and incomplete oral absorption with a bioavailability of approximately 40%. Although both AZA and 6-MP have relatively short half-lives, the affect on purine inhibition is significant and may last for several days. Given its bioavailability, some recommend reducing the intravenous dose to one half of the oral dose (Chan et al., 1987). Others have suggested that it is not relevant to use the bioavailability of azathioprine, given that it is the prodrug, and have administered the full dose intravenously. The latter may be appropriate as long as the patient's complete blood count is normal.

AZA is also a broad-acting myelosuppressive agent. The primary toxicity of this agent is dose-related bone marrow suppression manifested as leukopenia, thrombocytopenia or macrocytic anemia. This usually appears 7 to 14 days after initiation of the agent (Lennard, Murphy, & Maddocks, 1984). Dosage adjustments or discontinuation of the agent should be based on CBC and platelet counts. AZA may cause gastrointestinal side effects, including diarrhea, hepatitis, or cholestasis, that would be reflected in abnormal liver function tests, including elevated bilirubin or transaminases. Alopecia is also more common with azathioprine and is partially responsible for the alopecia reported in the initial tacrolimus, azathioprine, and prednisone regimens (Shapiro et al., 1998; Ushigome et al., 1999).

Among transplant recipients, gout is a common posttransplant complication that may be treated with xanthine-oxidase inhibitors such as allopurinol. AZA is metabolized to 6-xanthine oxidase thiouric acid. The metabolism of AZA is blocked by xanthine-oxidase inhibitors, resulting in decreased metabolism of 6-MP and increased 6-MP blood levels. This may result in a life-threatening and costly drug interaction manifested by pancytopenia if not appropriately recognized and managed (Brooks, Dorr, & Durie, 1982; Kennedy, Hayney, & Lake, 1996). The addition of allopurinol to a regimen containing AZA requires an initial AZA dose reduction of 50% to 80%, followed by frequent monitoring of complete blood counts with platelets for approximately 4 weeks (Coffey, White, Lesk, Rogers, & Serpeck, 1972). In patients with gout, MMF is the preferred agent, as it does not interact with allopurinol.

CYCLOPHOSPHAMIDE (CYTOXAN)

Cyclophosphamide, an alkylating agent, is one of the most potent immunosuppressive agents ever derived. It inhibits both cell-mediated and humoral immune response. Cyclophosphamide has been infrequently used as an alternative agent in transplant recipients experiencing hepatotoxicity or leukopenia associated with AZA (Starzl, Halgrimson, & Penn, 1971). Generally, cyclophosphamide utilization is limited to rare instances in solid organ transplantation including severe, refractory, and extended rejection episodes resistant to standard therapies (Evrard, Miller, Schwartz, Thung, & Mayer, 1990).

Following oral administration, cyclophosphamide is well absorbed, as reflected by a bioavailability of approximately 75%. Approximately 25% is protein-bound with a volume of distribution of 0.34 to 1.2 L/kg. Cyclophosphamide is extensively metabolized by the liver with approximately 5% to 25% of drug excreted unchanged in the urine. Following oral or intravenous administration, the half-life of cyclophosphamide ranges from 1.3 to 6.8 hours and 4.1 to 16 hours, respectively. Dosage adjustments are not necessary with renal or hepatic dysfunction. Hemodialysis removes approximately 72% of cyclophosphamide from the bloodstream following a 6-hour dialysis treatment; thus, dosage adjustments may be necessary (Cunningham et al., 1988).

Cyclophosphamide is metabolized by cytochrome p450 mixed function oxidase enzymes into its active metabolite aldophosphamide and 4-hydroxycyclophosphamide. The active metabolites are cleaved at the tissue level into phosphoramide mustard and acrolein. The primary active metabolite of cyclophosphamide, phosphoramide mustard, exhibits cytotoxic effects through inhibition of DNA cross-linkage. At lower dosages, cyclophosphamide exhibits toxic effects on natural killer cells, macrophage activation, and precursors to suppressor T cells.

Adverse effects include bone marrow suppression manifested most frequently as leukopenia but thrombocytopenia or anemia may also occur. Clinicians should monitor white blood cell (WBC) counts with expectant nadir occurring within 1 to 2 weeks after initiation of therapy. Dosages should be titrated to maintain WBC counts between 4,000 and 6,000/mm^3 (Evrard et al., 1990). Other side effects include alopecia, nausea, and vomiting, which occur more frequently with higher dosages (see Table 4.1).

CORTICOSTEROIDS (PREDNISONE, METHYLPREDNISOLONE, PREDNISOLONE)

Originally used in the 1960s, corticosteroids remain a consistent and controversial component of modern-day immunosuppressive strategies. Despite long-standing experience with these agents, clinicians continue to debate the role of corticosteroids in the continuum of immunotherapy (Hricik, 1998b). Corticosteroids are nonspecific anti-inflammatory agents that inhibit both humoral and cell-mediated immunity. Corticosteroids exert their immunosuppressive effects by several mechanisms:

- Inhibition of macrophage and T-cell cytokine production including IL-2, tumor necrosis factor, and interferon-gamma
- Inhibition of IL-1, IL-2, and IL-6 synthesis

As a result, T-cell activation is blocked. Given their nonselective immuno-suppressive properties, the use of corticosteroids has been successful in many facets of solid organ transplantation, including prevention and treatment of rejection.

Prednisone and methylprednisolone are the most commonly prescribed corticosteroids for transplant recipients. Both of these agents are metabolized into the active metabolite prednisolone. Despite a relatively short half-life (2 hours), the pharmacologic activity demonstrated by inhibition of lymphokines persists for 24 hours; thus, once daily dosing is adequate. Once daily dosing is preferentially used in most transplant centers.

Corticosteroids are administered in a variety of ways, including

- High-dose, short courses of intravenous methylprednisolone 250 to 1,000 mg for 3 days for acute rejection
- Oral pulse doses in cases of acute rejection (100 mg)
- Gradually tapered regimens where doses are decreased over an appropriate period of time and discontinued when possible
- Maintenance therapy at a standard low dose

Corticosteroids are metabolized via the cytochrome p450 (3A4) enzyme system. Agents that induce or inhibit this system can alter plasma concentrations of prednisolone, the circulating immunosuppressive active metabolite of prednisone and methylprednisolone. Corticosteroid dosage modifications may be empirically considered especially if used in concert with potent interacting agents including rifampin, phenytoin, phenobarbital, or ketoconazole. Dosage adjustments are generally not required with hepatic or renal dysfunction.

Glucocorticoid receptors are readily available throughout the body. As a result, corticosteroids exert far-reaching effects on the body. This is most notably reflected by the numerous side effects associated with chronic corticosteroid use. Similar to CSA, hyperlipidemia, glucose intolerance, and hypertension are common (Denton, Magee, & Sayegh, 1999). Additionally, cataracts, glaucoma, growth impairment, sodium and water retention, and Cushingoid syndrome may occur (Fryer et al., 1994) (see Table 4.1).

These adverse effects are associated with additional comorbidities, such as cardiovascular and other diseases (Veenstra, Best, Hornberger, Sullivan, & Hricik, 1999). Cardiovascular sequelae remain the leading cause of death in the renal transplant population. Given the multiple deleterious effects of corticosteroid therapy, many clinicians have begun to assess the effects of immunosuppressive regimens that avoid or withdraw corticosteroids. However, this strategy continues to be debated in the transplant community because of the potential risk of rejection and long-term deleterious effects on graft function associated with steroid-free regimens (Denton et al., 1999; Hricik, 1998a). The development of novel therapeutic regimens will allow further exploration of steroid-free regimens and their potential benefits and disadvantages.

ANTIBODY PREPARATIONS

Polyclonal and monoclonal antibody preparations continue to play an important role in transplantation. Currently, they are used in combination with other immunosuppressive medications as induction or sequential therapy or in the treatment of acute rejection episodes. Many centers have developed additional strategies to optimize the use of these agents. Increasingly, antibody preparations have been used successfully in patients with high immunologic risks, including patients with high pretransplant PRA levels, African American recipients, or in cases of delayed graft function or retransplantation.

POLYCLONAL ANTILYMPHOCYTE PREPARATIONS

Anti-thymocyte globulin (Atgam) is a polyclonal antilymphocyte globulin solution. It is prepared by innoculating horses with human thymocytes. Thymoglobulin, [Anti-thymocyte Globulin (Rabbit)] is a recently approved polyclonal antithymocyte agent derived from rabbits. The resulting gamma globulin solution is then purified to remove unnecessary materials yielding a solution specific for lymphocytes. Following administration of the agent, there is a profound depletion of peripheral blood lymphocytes (Hong & Kahan, 2000). The immunosuppressive effects of these preparations are thought to be mediated through several mechanisms: Cells coated with antibodies undergo complement-mediated cell lysis of lymphocytes or clearance by the reticuloendothelial system (Hong & Kahan, 2000). T-lymphocyte proliferation may also be affected by these agents.

Atgam and Thymoglobulin have extended half-lives of approximately 5.7 days and 30 days, respectively. However, there have been large variations reported between patients. The recommended dose for Atgam is approximately 10 to 20 mg/kg/day for up to 14 days. The first dose should be administered over a 6-hour infusion; subsequent doses may be administered over 4 hours. The initial dose of Thymoglobulin is also administered over a 6-hour infusion, with remaining doses given over a minimum of 4 hours. The recommended dose of Thymoglobulin is 1.5 mg/kg/day. However, a number of centers have modified their protocols to use either lower doses (e.g., 1.0 mg/kg/day) or alternate day therapy (e.g., 1.5 mg/kg/day every other day for a total of 4 doses over 7 days) rather than wait to adjust the dose because of leukopenia and thrombocytopenia. Both agents may be given for up to 14 days; however, many centers administer much shorter courses of therapy for induction regimens. Often patients are premedicated with acetaminophen, diphenhydramine, and methyl-prednisolone 1 hour prior to administration to ameliorate side effects.

Atgam and Thymoglobulin have similar side effects. Common side effects associated with Atgam include leukopenia (29%), fever (63%), chills (43%), nausea (28%), diarrhea (32%), arthralgias, and headache. Anaphylactic-type reactions have rarely occurred with these agents. Both agents are associated with leukopenia and thrombocytopenia, either of which may require dosage adjustment and/or discontinuation of the agent. However, Thymoglobulin has been associated with an increased incidence of leukopenia (approximately 57%). Patients should be monitored daily while on therapy. Dosages should be decreased by approximately 50% if the WBC count decreases to less than 3,000 cells/mL or if platelets fall between 50,000 and 100,000 cells/mL. Doses should be held if the WBC count drops below 2,000 cells/mL or platelets fall below 50,000 cells/mL. These agents are also associated with increased risk of malignancies as well as opportunistic bacterial, viral, and fungal infections. Appropriate anti-infective prophylaxis therapy is warranted while administering these agents.

MONOCLONAL ANTIBODY PREPARATIONS

Since its introduction, muromonab-CD3 (OKT3) has been successfully used in the treatment of severe acute rejection. In addition, muromonab-CD3 has been used as induction therapy or for steroid-resistant rejection (Kreis, Legendre, & Chatenoud, 1991). Muromonab-CD3, a murine mon-oclonal antibody preparation, causes depletion of circulating T lympho-cytes by binding CD3 receptor complex located on T cells (Miller, Maloney, McKillop, & Levy, 1981). As a result, T cells are rendered immunologi-cally incompetent and are unable to respond to foreign antigen stimuli. Muromonab-CD3 depletes virtually all circulating T cells within minutes to hours following intravenous administration. Throughout the course of muromonab-CD3 therapy, CD3 positive cells will remain depleted while T cells bearing CD2, CD4, and CD8 surface markers reappear. However, shortly following discontinuation of the agent (approximately 48 hours), T cells bearing CD3 as well as other surface markers begin to reappear. Therefore, immunosuppressants are required to be at therapeutic levels prior to discontinuation of the agent. Failure to decrease CD3 positive cells may be indicative of the production of human antimurine antibodies, which negate the action of muromonab-CD3 (Burk & Matuszewski, 1997). This may be more apparent in patients receiving a second course of therapy and may be monitored by measurement of CD3 cells. Additionally, some patients may exhibit an abnormally increased clearance rate of murine immunoglobilin, resulting in potential therapeutic failures. Patients receiving concomitant immunosuppressants typically have a lower incidence of murine antibody production (Schroeder, Hariharan, & First, 1993).

Muromonab-CD3 is associated with many significant adverse drug reactions. Generally, side effects are most notable following the administration of the initial dose of therapy or following an increase in dose. These side effects are largely due to cytokine release syndrome, which results in increased IL-1, IL-6, and tumor necrosis factor from muromonab-CD3-activated T cells and monocytes (Chatenoud et al., 1990). Some patients experience flulike symptoms that may range in severity. Occasionally, some patients experience rapidly developing pulmonary edema, hypotension, seizures, encephalopathy, renal dysfunction, or aseptic meningitis. Muromonab-CD3 has also been associated with rare instances of coagulopathies, manifested by thrombocytopenia, or graft thrombosis.

Generally, patients receive premedications such as steroids, acetaminophen, and diphenhydramine approximately 1 hour prior to muromonab-CD3 administration to reduce clinical symptoms associated with cytokine release syndrome (Todd & Brogden, 1989). Other agents such as indomethacin or anti-TNF antibodies have also been employed to minimize the severity of these side effects.

Patients may also be at higher risk of infections or lymphomas. The development of infection, most commonly manifested as cytomegalovirus (CMV) infection, is likely but also dependent on the overall amount of immunosuppression the patient receives. It is important to insure that patients receive the appropriate antiviral prophylaxis therapy with ganciclovir while receiving muromonab-CD3 or any potent immunosuppressive regimen. As with any immunosuppressive agent, muromonab-CD3 has been associated with an increased risk for the development of lymphoma (Swinnen et al., 1990).

IL-2 RECEPTOR ANTAGONISTS

Basiliximab (Simulect) and daclizumab (Zenapax) are the newest monoclonal antibody preparations introduced onto the market. Basiliximab is a chimeric murine-human monoclonal antibody preparation; it contains a larger proportion of murine antibody (25%) constituents (Onrust & Wiseman, 1999). Daclizumab is humanized monoclonal antibody containing a smaller percentage (approximately 10%) of murine antibody sequence (Wiseman & Faulds, 1999). These medications contain primarily human antibody components; therefore, they have demonstrated improved side effect profiles as well as low immunogenic potential when compared to muromonab-CD3. The IL-2 receptor antagonists bind specifically to the alpha-subunit, also known as the Tac subunit, of the interleukin-2 receptor, which is expressed on the surface of activated T lymphocytes. As a result, T-lymphocyte proliferation and differentiation are inhibited.

The IL-2 inhibitors yield a prolonged immunosuppressive action, resulting from half-lives exceeding 7 days. The half-life of basiliximab is approximately 13 days; the mean half-life of daclizumab has been estimated at approximately 20 days, with a range of approximately 11 to 38 days (Onrust & Wiseman 1999; Wiseman & Faulds 1999). The extended half-life allows the agents to be administered over long dosage intervals. Following administration of basiliximab and daclizumab, the alpha-subunit of IL-2 receptors are effectively saturated for approximately 30 days and 120 days, respectively, potentially contributing to their long-lasting immunosuppressive activity (Onrust & Wiseman, 1999; Wiseman & Faulds, 1999).

Basiliximab is administered intravenously as a 20 mg single daily dose on the day of transplant and on the fourth day posttransplantation. The recommended dose of daclizumab is 1 mg/kg/day within 24 hours of transplant surgery followed by equal doses administered every 14 days for 5 doses. However a number of centers have modified their protocols to 2 doses of daclizumab.

Both agents exert similar pharmacologic properties as well as side effect profiles. Unlike their predecessors, basiliximab and daclizumab have demonstrated a relatively mild side effect profile and do not seem to elicit cytokine release syndrome or first dose effects. In clinical trials, both daclizumab and basiliximab exhibited similar side effects to those associated with patients receiving placebo. Although these agents may be associated with an increased risk of infection and lymphoproliferative disorders, the overall incidence of infection as well as malignancy was similar to that experienced by patients receiving placebo (Nashan et al., 1997; Vincenti et al., 1998). Additionally, the IL-2 inhibitors have been used concomitantly with a large variety of immunosuppressive agents including CSA, tacrolimus, MMF, and corticosteroids. No significant drug interactions have been identified for basiliximab or daclizumab.

CONCLUSION

Immunosuppressive agents are potent medications with a wide variety of side effects and interactions with other drugs (prescription and over-the-counter), supplements, and herbal preparations. Health care providers are encouraged to contact the transplant center when prescribing or recommending other medications for transplant recipients. If a particular agent is contraindicated, the transplant center can recommend a safer alternative.

REFERENCES

Barone, G. W., Gurley, B. J., Ketel, B. L., Lightfoot, M. L., & Abul-Ezz, S. R. (2000). Drug interaction between St. John's Wort and cyclosporine. *The Annals of Pharmacotherapy, 34,* 1013–1016.

Brennan, D. C., Flavin, K., Lowell, J. A., Howard, T. K., Shenoy, S., Burgess, S., Dolan, S., Kano, J. M., Mahon, M., Schnitzler, M. A., Woodward, R., Irish, W., & Singer, G. G. (1999). A randomized, double-blinded comparison of Thymoglobulin versus Atgam for induction immunosuppressive therapy in adult renal transplant recipients. *Transplantation, 67*(7), 1011–1018.

Brooks R. J., Dorr, R. T., & Durie, B. G. (1982). Interaction of allopurinol with 6-mercaptopurine and azathioprine. *Biomedicine and Pharmacotherapy, 36*(4), 217–222.

Bullingham, R. E., Nicholls, A. J., & Kamm, B. R. (1998). Clinical pharmacokinetics of mycophenolate mofetil. *Clinical Pharmacokinetics, 34*(6), 429–455.

Bullingham R., Shah, J., Goldblum R., & Schiff, M. (1996). Effects of food and antacid on the pharmacokinetics of single doses of mycophenolate mofetil in rheumatoid arthritis patients. *British Journal of Clinical Pharmacology, 41*(6), 513–516.

Burk, M. L., & Matuszewski, K. A. (1997). Muromonab-CD3 and antithymocyte globulin in renal transplantation [Review]. *Annals of Pharmacotherapy, 31*(11), 1370–1377.

Canafax, D. M. (1995). Minimizing cyclosporine concentration variability to optimize transplant outcome. *Clinical Transplantation, 9*(1), 1–13.

Chan, G. L., Canafax, D. M., & Johnson, C. A. (1987). The therapeutic use of azathioprine in renal transplantation. *Pharmacotherapy, 7*(5), 165–177.

Chatenoud, L., Ferran, C., Legendre, C, Thouard, I., Merite, S., Reuter, A., Gevaert, Y., Kreis, H., Franchimont, P., & Bach, J. F. (1990). In vivo cell activation following OKT3 administration: Systemic cytokine release and modulation by corticosteroids. *Transplantation, 49*(4), 697–702.

Christians, U., First, M. R., & Benet, L. Z. (2000). Recommendations for bioequivalence testing of cyclosporine generics revisited. *Therapeutic Drug Monitoring, 22*(3), 330–345.

Christians, U., & Sewing, D. F. (1993). Cyclosporin metabolism in transplant patients. *Pharmacology & Therapeutics, 57*(2–3), 291–345.

Coffey, J. J., White, C. A., Lesk, A. B., Rogers, W. I., & Serpeck, A. A. (1972). Effect of allopurinol on the pharmacokinetics of 6-mercaptopurine (MSC 775) in cancer patients. *Cancer Research, 32*(6), 1283–1289.

Cunningham, D., Cummings, J., Blackie, R. B., McTaggart, L., Banham, S. W., Kaye, S. B., & Soukop, M. (1988). The pharmacokinetics of high dose cyclophosphamide and high dose etoposide. *Medical Oncology Tumor Pharmacotherapy, 5*(2), 117–123.

Denton, M. D., Magee, C. C., & Sayegh, M. H. (1999). Immunosuppressive strategies in transplantation. *Lancet, 353*(9158), 1083–1091.

Dumont, R. J., & Ensom, M. H. H. (2000). Methods for clinical monitoring of cyclosporin in transplant patients. *Clinical Pharmacokinetics, 38*(5), 427–447.

Dumont, R. J., Partovi, N., Levy, R. D., Fradet, G., Ensom M. H. H. (2001) A limited sampling strategy for cyclosporine area under the curve monitoring in lung transplant recipients. *Journal of Heart and Lung Transplantation, 20,* 897–900.

European Mycophenolate Mofetil Cooperative Study Group. (1995). Placebo-controlled study of mycophenolate mofetil combined with cyclosporine and corticosteroids for prevention of acute rejection. *Lancet, 345*(8961), 1321–1325.

Evrard, H. M., Miller, C., Schwartz, M., Thung, S. N., & Mayer, L. (1990). Resistant hepatic allograft rejection successfully treated with cyclophosphamide and plasmapheresis. *Transplantation, 50*(4), 702–704.

Food and Drug Administration Talk Paper. (2000, July 10). *Nationwide recall of Sangcya Oral Solution.* Retrieved March 14, 2001, from http://www.fda.gov/bbs/topics/ANSWERS/ANS01025.html

Fryer, J. P., Granger, D. K., Leventhal, J. R., Gillingham, K., Najarian, J. S., & Matas, A. J. (1994). Steroid-related complications in the cyclosporine era. *Clinical Transplantation, 8*(3, Pt. 1), 224–229.

Fugh-Burman, A. (2000). Herb-drug interactions. *Lancet, 355,* 134–138.

Fulton, B., & Markham, A., (1996). Mycophenolate mofetil: A review of its pharmacodynamic and pharmacokinetic properties and clinical efficacy in renal transplantation. *Drugs, 51*(2), 278–298.

Glanemann, M., Klupp, J., Langrehr, J. M., Schroer, G., Platz, K. P., Stange, B., Settmacher, U., Bechstein, W. O., & Neuhaus, P. (2000). Higher immunosuppressive efficacy of mycophenolate mofetil in combination with FK 506 than in combination with cyclosporine A. *Transplantation Proceedings, 32*(3), 522–523.

Hariharan, S., Tomlanovich, S. J., Filo, R. S., Dessiomz, M., Wisemandle, W., & Townsend, R. W. (2001, May). *Pharmacokinetics and tolerability of tacrolimus and sirolimus in stable renal transplant patients.* Paper presented at the meeting of the American Society of Transplantation, Chicago.

Hong, J. C., & Kahan, D. K. (2000). Immunosuppressive agents in organ transplantation: Past, present, and future. *Seminars in Nephrology, 20*(2), 108–125.

Hricik, D. E. (1998a). Steroid withdrawal in renal transplant recipients: Pro point of view [Review]. *Transplantation Proceedings, 30*(4), 1380–1382.

Hricik, D. E. (1998b). Withdrawal of immunosuppression: Implication for composite tissue allograft transplantation [Review]. *Transplantation Proceedings, 30*(6), 2721–2723.

Ingle, G. R., Sievers, T. M., & Holt, C. D. (2000). Sirolimus: Continuing the evolution of transplant immunosuppression. *Annals of Pharmacotherapy, 34,* 1044–1055.

Johnson, C., Ahsan, N., Gonwa, T., Halloran, P., Stegall, M., Hardy, M., Metzger, R., Shield, C., 3rd, Rocher, L., Scandling, J., Sorensen, J., Mulloy, L., Light, J., Corwin, C., Danovitch, G., Wachs, M., van Veldhuisen, P., Salm, K., Tolzman, D., & Fitzsimmons, W. E. (2000). Randomized trial of tacrolimus (Prograf) in combination with azathioprine or mycophenolate mofetil vs. cyclosporine (Neoral) with mycophenolate mofetil after kidney transplantation. *Transplantation, 69*(5), 834–841.

Kahan, B. D. (1989). Cyclosporine. *New England Journal of Medicine, 321*(25), 1725–1738.

Kahan, B. D. (2000). Efficacy of sirolimus compared with azathioprine for reduction of acute renal allograft rejection: A randomised multicentre study. The Rapamune US Study Group. *Lancet, 356*(9225), 194–202.

Kahan, B. D., Dunn, J., Fitts, C., Van Buren, D., Wombolt, D., Pollak, R., Carson, R., Alexander, J. W., Choc, M., & Wong, R., et al. (1995). Reduced inter- and intrasubject variability in cyclosporine pharmacokinetics in renal transplant recipients treated with the microemulsion formulation in conjunction with fasting, low-fat meals, or high-fat meals. *Transplantation, 59*(4), 505–511.

Kaplan, B., Meier-Kriesche, H. U., Friedman, G., Mulgaonkar, S., Gruber, S., Korecka, M., Brayman, K. L., & Shaw, L. M. (1999). The effect of renal insufficiency on mycophenolic acid protein binding. *Journal of Clinical Pharmacology, 39*(7), 715–720.

Kaplan, B., Meier-Kriesche, H. U., Napoli, K. L., & Kahan, B. D. (1998). The effects of relative timing of sirolimus and cyclosporine microemulsion formulation coadministration on the pharmacokinetics of each agent. *Clinical Pharmacology & Therapuetics, 63*(1), 48–53.

Kelly, P. A., Burckart, G. J., & Venkataramanan, R. (1995). Tacrolimus: A new immunosuppressive agent [Clinical Review]. *American Journal of Health-System Pharmacy, 52*(14), 1521–1535.

Kennedy, D. T., Hayney, M. S., & Lake, K. D. (1996). Azathioprine and allopurinol: The price of an avoidable drug interaction. *Annals of Pharmacotherapy, 30*(9), 951–954.

Klein, A. (1999). Tacrolimus rescue in liver transplant patients with refractory rejection or intolerance or malabsorption of cyclosporine. The US Multicenter FK506 Liver Study Group. *Liver Transplantation Surgery, 5*(6), 502–508.

Kreis, H., Legendre, C., & Chatenoud, L. (1991). OKT3 in organ transplantation. *Transplantation Reviews, 5,* 181–199.

Lake, K. D., & Canafax, D. M. (1995). Important interactions of drugs with immunosuppressive agents used in transplant recipients. *Journal of Antimicrobial Chemotherapy, 36*(Suppl. B), 11–22.

Lennard, L., Murphy, M. F., & Maddocks, J. L. (1984). Severe megaloblastic anemia associated with abnormal azathioprine metabolism. *British Journal of Clinical Pharmacology, 17*(2), 171–172.

Mathew, T. (1998). A blinded, long-term randomized multi-center study of mycophenolate mofetil in cadaveric renal transplantation. *Transplantation, 65,* 1450–1454.

Matsuda, S., & Koyasu, S. (2000). Mechanisms of action of cyclosporine. [Review]. *Immunopharmacology, 47*(2–3), 119–125.

Mele, T. S., & Halloran, P. F. (2000). The use of mycophenolate mofetil in transplant recipients [Review]. *Immunopharmacology, 47*(2–3), 215–245.

Mignat, C. (1997). Clinically significant drug interactions with new immunosuppressive agents. *Drugs, 16,* 267–278.

Miller, J., Mendez, R., Pirsch, J. D., & Jensik, S. C. (2000). Safety and efficacy of tacrolimus in combination with mycophenolate mofetil (MMF) in cadaveric renal transplant recipients. *Transplantation, 69*(5), 875–880.

Miller, R. A., Maloney, D. G., McKIllop, J., & Levy, R. (1981). In vivo effects of murine hybridoma monoclonal antibody in a patient with T-cell leukemia. *Blood, 58*(1), 78–86.

Morii, M., Ueno, K., Ogawa, A., Kato, R., Yoshimura, H., Wada, K., Hashimoto, H., Takada, M., Tanaka, K., Nakatani, T., & Shibakawa, M. (2000). Impairment of mycophenolate mofetil absorption by iron ion. *Clinical Pharmacology and Therapeutics, 68*(6), 613–616.

Nashan, B., Moore, R., Amlot, P., Schmide, G. G., Abeywichrama, K., & Soulillou, J. P. (1997). Randomised trial of basiliximab versus placebo for control of acute cellular rejection in renal allograft recipients. CHIB 201 International Study Group. *Lancet, 350*(9086), 1193–1198.

Onrust, S. V., & Wiseman, L. R. (1999). Basiliximab. *Drugs, 57*(2), 207–213.

Plosker, G. L., & Foster, R. H. (2000). Tacrolimus: A further update of its pharmacology and therapeutic use in the management of organ transplantation. *Drugs, 59*(2), 323–389.

Schroeder, T. J., Hariharan, S., & First, M. R. (1993). Antibody response to OKT3 and methods for monitoring. *Transplantation Proceedings, 25*(Suppl. 2), 77–80.

Shapiro, R. (1999). Tacrolimus in solid organ transplantation: An update. *Transplantation Proceedings, 31*(6), 2203–5.

Shapiro, R. (2000). Tacrolimus in renal transplantation—A review. *Graft, 3*(2), 64–80.

Shapiro, R., Jordan, M. L., Scantlebury, V. P., Vivas, C., McCauley, J., Johnston, J., Fung, J. J., & Starzl, T. E. (1998). Alopecia as a consequence of tacrolimus therapy [Letter; Comment]. *Transplantation, 65*(9),1284.

Sievers, T. M., Rossi, S. J., Rafik, M. G., Arriola, E., Nishimura, P., Kawano, M., & Holt, C. D. (1997). Mycophenolate mofetil. *Pharmacotherapy, 17*(6), 1178–1197.

Smak Gregoor, P. J. H., de Sévaux, R. G. L., Hené, R. J., Hesse, C. J., Hilbrands, L. B., Vos, P., van Gelder, T., Hoitsma, A. J., & Weimar, W. (1999). Effect of discontinuing cyclosporine on mycophenolic acid trough levels in kidney transplant recipients. *Transplantation, 68*(10), 1603–1606.

Sollinger, H. W. (1995). Mycophenolate mofetil for the prevention of acute rejection in primary cadaveric renal allograft recipients: U.S. Renal Transplant Mycophenolate Mofetil Study Group. *Transplantation, 60*(3), 225–32.

Starzl, T. E., Halgrimson, C. G., & Penn, I. (1971). Cyclophosphamide and human organ transplantation. *Lancet, 2,* 70–74.

Swinnen, L. J., Costanzo-Nordin, M. R., Fisher, S. G., O'Sullivan, E. J., Johnson, M. R., Heroux, A. L., Dizikes, G. J., Pifarre, R., & Fisher, R. I. (1990). Increased incidence of lymphoproliferative disorder after immunosuppression with the monoclonal antibody OKT3 in cardiac transplant. *New England Journal of Medicine, 323*(25), 1723–1728.

Taylor, D. O., Barr, M. L., Radovancevic, B., Renlund, D. G., Mentzer, R. M. Jr, Smart, F. W., Tolman, D. E., Frazier, O. H., Young, J. B., & VanVeldhuisen, P. (1999). A randomized, multicenter comparison of tacrolimus and cyclosporine immunosuppressive regimens in cardiac transplantation: Decreased hyperlipidemia and hypertension with tacrolimus. *Journal of Heart and Lung Transplantation, 18*(4), 336–345.

Taylor, D. O., Barr, M. L., Meiser, B. M., Pham, S. M., Mentzer, R. M., & Gass, A. L. (2001). Suggested guidelines for the use of tacrolimus in cardiac transplant recipients. *Journal of Heart and Lung Transplantation, 20*(7), 734–738.

Todd, P. A., & Brogden, R. N. (1989). Muromonab CD3: A review of its pharmacology and therapeutic potential. *Drugs, 37,* 871–899.

Tricontinental Mycophenolate Mofetil Renal Transplantation Study Group. (1996). A blinded, randomized clinical trial of mycophenolate mofetil for the prevention of acute rejection in cadaveric renal transplantation. *Transplantation, 61,* 1029–1037.

Ushigome, H., Yoshimura, N., Okamoto, M., Najima, H., Hamajima, T., Nakai, I., & Oka, T. (1999). Two cases of tacrolimus-induced alopecia following kidney transplantation. *Transplantation Proceedings, 31*(7), 2885–2886.

Van Gelder, T., Klupp, J., Barten, M., Christians, U., & Morris, R. E. (1999). Coadministration of tacrolimus (FK) and mycophenolate mofetil (MMF) does not increase mycophenolic acid (MPA) exposure, but coadministration of cyclosporine (CsA) and MMF inhibits the enterohepatic recirculation of MPA, thereby decreasing its exposure. *32nd Annual Meeting and 1999 Renal Week of the American Society of Nephrology. Journal of the American Society of Nephrology, 10* (Abstract No. A3622).

Veenstra, D. L., Best, J. H., Hornberger, L., Sullivan, S. D., & Hricik, D. E. (1999). Incidence and long-term cost of steroid-related side effects after renal transplantation. *American Journal of Kidney Diseases, 33*(5), 829–839.

Vincenti, F., Kirk man, R., Light, S., Baumgartner, G., Passivity, M., Halloran, P., Nylon, J., Wilkinson, A., Ember, H., Gaston, R., Backman, L., & Burdick, J. (1998). Interleukin-2-receptor blockade with Daclizumab to prevent acute rejection in renal transplantation. *New England Journal of Medicine, 338*(3), 161–165.

Wiseman, L. R., & Faulds, D. (1999). Daclizumab. A review of its use in the prevention of acute rejection in renal transplant recipients. *Drugs, 58*(6), 1029–1042.

Yatscoff, R. W. (1996). Pharmacokinetics of rapamycin. *Transplantation Proceedings, 28,* 985–986.

Zimmerman, J. J., & Kahan, B. D. (1997). Pharmacokinetics of sirolimus in stable renal transplant patients after multiple oral dose administration. *Journal of Clinical Pharmacology, 37,* 405–415.

5

Neurocognitive Issues in Transplantation

William Garmoe

Successful long-term outcome following organ transplant depends on many factors, not the least of which is inclusion of the patient as an active member of the medical team. The best efforts of the medical team will fail if the patient either will not or cannot comply with the treatment regimen prior to and following transplantation. At minimum, there will be complications and an increased likelihood of graft rejection episodes; in the worst case, the patient may not survive. Lack of compliance has been identified as a major risk factor for morbidity and mortality following transplantation (Dew, Roth, Thompson, Kormos, & Griffith, 1996).

It is critical for physicians and other health care professionals to be aware of factors that affect the capacity of patients to successfully manage the demands of transplantation. This chapter will focus on neurobehavioral factors that may interfere with the transplant process. Patients with impaired cognitive functioning may have difficulties remembering and following through on treatment plans. Because of problems with memory or executive functioning, they may fail to spontaneously report important information during medical visits. As a result, the risk of complications that compromise health and potentially contribute to graft rejection increases. Sensitivity to issues of cognitive functioning will help the entire medical team and the patient be more effective in achieving a higher level of treatment compliance and overall health.

Much has been written about psychosocial and psychiatric issues affecting transplant with respect to depression and anxiety (Dew et al.,1996; Fisher, Lake, Reutzel, & Emery, 1995), quality of life (Grady, Jalowiec, & White-Williams,1999; Ramsey, Patrick, Lewis, Albert, & Raghu, 1995) and psychosocial exclusion criteria for transplantation (Olbrisch & Levenson, 1991). These topics per se will not be the focus here except to the extent that such factors interact with neurobehavioral factors. Less has been written about the prevalence and potential impact of cognitive impairment in transplant candidates and recipients, though this clearly has been identified as an area of concern (Bornstein, Starling, Myerowitz, & Haas, 1995; Kramer et al., 1996; Putzke, Williams, Rayburn, Kirklin, & Boll, 1998; Schall, Petrucci, Brozena, Cavarocchi, & Jessup, 1989).

Group studies lack consensus on a number of issues such as the extent to which cognitive dysfunction is present among transplant patients, whether it is reversible following transplant, and how much it influences overall outcome. However, it is clear that many individuals present with significant cognitive impairment during both the pre- and posttransplant process, and this represents a potential threat to treatment adherence and outcome. This chapter will focus on the clinical aspects of cognitive functioning in transplant patients and discuss strategies for working with such individuals who present for medical care.

DEMANDS OF THE TRANSPLANT PROCESS

It should be noted that, irrespective of the integrity of brain functioning, the transplant process is very demanding on cognitive and psychological resources. Individuals begin the process only as a function of life-threatening and often chronic illness. They then must cope with a very uncertain future in which progressive decline in health is balanced against the hope for a replacement organ, which in many cases can happen only through the death of the donor. An added challenge is learning to negotiate a very complex medical system. Finally, despite the best efforts of transplant teams, many individuals retain the fantasy that once they have received a new organ, they will be free of medical problems, long lists of medications, and frequent physician visits. It should not be surprising, then, that even individuals with good cognition may at times have difficulty processing all of the complex information that they need to know. The principles discussed for individuals with cognitive impairment can also be used to enhance the effectiveness of information processing of those without such difficulties.

COGNITIVE FUNCTIONING IN PATIENTS
AWAITING TRANSPLANT

Cognitive deficits are commonly reported among individuals suffering major organ failure (Bremer, Wert, Durica, & Weaver, 1998; Farmer, 1994; Putzke et al., 1998; Schall et al., 1989). For example, Bremer and colleagues (1998) reported that individuals with end-stage renal disease (ESRD) were impaired relative to control subjects on tests of cognitive performance. Similarly, Kramer and colleagues (1996) reported that, compared to healthy controls, chronic hemodialysis patients awaiting transplant showed greater p300 latencies, and lower performance on two common cognitive functioning tasks (e.g., Mini-Mental State, Trail Making Test). ESRD results in a range of metabolic disturbances that can produce uremic encephalopathy. Ensuing neurobehavioral sequelae may include

- Cognitive changes such as poor concentration, slowed information processing speed, memory deficits, and decreased mental flexibility (Bornstein et al., 1995; Cummings & Benson, 1992)
- Changes in mood and perceptions
- Alterations in motor functioning

There is some evidence that neurobehavioral deficits related to uremic dysfunction may abate when clinically effective renal dialysis is provided. Umans and Pliskin (1998) and Pliskin, Yurk, Ho, and Umans (1996) found no differences in performance on neuropsychological tests between well-dialyzed patients and control subjects. They hypothesize that deficits reported in end-stage renal patients in many other studies may be related to either insufficiently treated uremia or methodological flaws.

Portosystemic (or hepatic) encephalopathy is a syndrome to be considered when evaluating patients for liver transplantation. This condition can develop in patients with end-stage liver disease when portal venous blood is shunted into the peripheral circulation by collateral blood vessels that have developed (Adams, Victor & Ropper, 1997). A progressive encephalopathy may develop that begins with dementia or confusion and progresses to coma. Arousal, attention, memory, and constructional abilities may be impaired. The patient may show changes in mood or thought processes. At times, bizarre behavior may emerge (Cummings & Benson, 1992). Physical/motor changes that may be seen include asterixis, hyper-reflexia, gait ataxia, and suck and grasp reflexes. Although progression to coma (and possibly death) is not uncommon, patients often do not progress beyond a mild dementia state that may be reversible (Adams et al., 1997). It is important to attempt to rule out portosystemic encephalopathy during the transplant assessment process, in order to differentiate a potentially reversible condition. Many of these patients will show improvement with treatment or transplantation.

Studies of cognitive functioning in individuals with chronic cardiac illness similarly report high rates of impairment. Bornstein and colleagues (1995) performed neuropsychological testing with a group of 62 patients being considered for cardiac transplantation and concluded that 58% fell in the impaired range on the test battery used. Highest rates of impairment were seen on tasks of reasoning and concept formation, attention, and psychomotor skills. The severity of impairment was mild in most patients, and was not accounted for by variables such as age and fatigue, though there was some relationship to depression. Schall and colleagues (1989) similarly reported a high frequency of cognitive impairment in their group of pretransplant patients, with deficits seen in the areas of memory, information processing, and motor speed. Impaired cognitive performance in cardiac transplant candidates has been associated with stroke volume and cardiac index (Bornstein et al., 1995; Putzke et al., 1998). Others have also reported that the etiology of cardiac disease did not differentially affect incidence of cognitive impairment (Schall et al., 1989).

> *Clinical Example:* The patient was a 60-year-old female with a 3-year history of cardiomyopathy who was listed for transplant. Her ongoing medical management was complicated by problems with generalized pain, depression and anxiety, and problems with cognitive functioning. Prior to the onset of her cardiac disease, the patient had been married for more than 20 years and was employed as an administrative assistant. She had no history of alcohol or other drug abuse or psychiatric illness prior to her cardiac disease. Transplant team members were concerned about the patient's inability to remember important information and generalize skills taught in the clinic. When seen for neuropsychological evaluation, the patient displayed impairments in the areas of attention/concentration, speed of processing, new learning and recent memory, and executive functions; there were subtle language deficits as well. These deficits appeared to represent an interaction of brain dysfunction with the effects of mood on attention and information processing.

COGNITIVE FUNCTIONING IN PATIENTS FOLLOWING TRANSPLANT

There is little consensus regarding whether cognition improves following transplant. It is clear that cognitive problems are common in the postoperative period and early months following transplantation, although estimates of prevalence vary considerably.

LUNG TRANSPLANT RECIPIENTS

Craven (1990) reported that more than 70% of patients studied experienced delirium during the first 2 weeks following lung transplantation. Goldstein and colleagues (1998) reported that as many as 26% of lung transplant recipients had symptoms of central nervous system events following transplantation, although confusional states, seizures, and stroke had a relatively low frequency.

CARDIAC TRANSPLANT RECIPIENTS

Bornstein and colleagues (1995) reported that cognitive functioning improved significantly following cardiac transplantation. Fifty-eight percent of their pretransplant sample was cognitively impaired based on a standardized neuropsychological evaluation. A subset of this group was reexamined following transplantation, and significant improvement in cognitive functioning was found. Patients who had not undergone transplantation showed limited improvement on some measures but deteriorated on many others. Improvement in patients who had undergone transplantation could not be explained on the basis of improved mood, as their depression scores had actually worsened. In contrast to these findings, Schall and colleagues (1989) reported that cognitive functioning did not improve following heart transplantation. Those who were impaired before transplantation continued to show deficits following transplantation even though physical functioning improved significantly. Cognitive deficits involved new learning and recent memory, higher cognitive functions, and motor speed. The pattern of impairment was most consistent with diffuse rather than focal brain dysfunction. A similar picture emerges when considering other types of organ transplantation (e.g., Kramer et al., 1996).

Overall there are very mixed findings about whether transplantation results in improved cognitive functioning. However, although reports vary about the frequency of impairment and whether cognition improves, it is clear that a significant percentage of individuals will have cognitive deficits following transplantation.

Clinical Example: The patient is a 57-year-old male with a history of hypertension and diabetes (type 2), who developed ESRD and was on hemodialysis for 1 year prior to receiving a kidney transplant. He was seen one year posttransplant because he could not remember treatment instructions regarding medications and warning signs of acute illness or graft rejection. His medical history was significant for loss of his right eye during childhood when he picked up an undetonated artillery shell that subsequently exploded. As an adult, he had a long history of alcohol abuse but quit drinking 3 years prior to his transplant as a result of a serious medical illness. He had no prior psychiatric history. Neuropsychological evaluation showed moderately severe cognitive impairment in the areas of memory, attention and mental speed, complex reasoning, and mental flexibility. He also showed evidence of focal right hemisphere deficits, pointing to a probable earlier unrecognized cerebral vascular event.

MEDIATING FACTORS AFFECTING PRE- AND POSTTRANSPLANT PATIENTS

Cognitive impairment can also stem from other mediating variables that are common in pre- and posttransplant patients. These comorbidities include

- Other forms of neurologic illness
- Psychiatric disorders
- Medication effects.

NEUROLOGICAL ILLNESS OR INJURY

Based on population demographics alone, a certain percentage of patients will have suffered a neurologic illness or injury such as traumatic brain injury or stroke, with possible residual effects on cognitive functioning. In addition, the etiologic processes that lead to organ failure can further increase the risk for neurologic illnesses such as cerebrovascular disease and dementia.

PSYCHIATRIC DISORDERS

Mood Disorders (Depression, Dysthmia, and Anxiety)

Psychiatric disorders represent a very important factor that may affect cognition both in pre- and posttransplant patients. It is a well-documented finding that depression often has a negative impact on cognitive functioning. The most frequent psychiatric problem affecting transplant patients is major depression and dysthymia.

- Dew and colleagues (1999) found a prevalence rate of 16% for major depression in the first year following cardiac transplantation. This prevalence exceeds estimates of the disorder in the general population based on epidemiological studies (Kaelber, Moul, & Farmer, 1995).
- These investigators also reported an increased prevalence of other psychiatric conditions such as posttraumatic stress disorder (16%) and adjustment disorder (9%). When patients were followed over 3 years, Dew and colleagues (1999) concluded that the prevalence of depression and other indices of psychiatric distress increased the risk of noncompliance and morbidity.

On a more general level, it is important to consider the impact of any form of chronic illness on adjustment. Studies examining the relationship of mood disorders to medical illness are both voluminous and highly variable in results reported. Rates of depression vary considerably across studies, but a recent review estimated that 12% to 36% of chronically ill medical outpatients suffer from depression (Stevens, Merikangas, & Merikangas, 1995). Stevens and colleagues (1995) also examined the relationship between depression and specific medical illnesses. Although results are highly variable, they can be briefly summarized by stating that mood disorders are considerably more common in patients with most forms of chronic medical illness than in normal control subjects. Similar conclusions can be drawn about anxiety disorders in medical patients. Additionally, it is difficult for many patients to distinguish symptoms of anxiety from depression when both are present (Maser, Weise, & Gwirtsman, 1995).

Substance Abuse Disorders

Substance abuse disorders represent an additional group of psychiatric conditions that may affect cognition. As with other disorders, the impact on cognition may be direct or indirect. Chronic alcohol abuse is strongly associated with cognitive impairment, although sustained abstinence may reverse many of the deficits seen (Adams et al., 1997). Chronic alcohol abuse may contribute to organ system failure, increase risk for brain trauma and stroke, and exacerbate other illnesses that may in turn affect cognition. Also, individuals whose alcohol abuse was severe enough to contribute to organ system failure may be those more likely to suffer lasting cognitive impairment even with sustained abstinence. Transplant programs screen for active alcohol and other substance abuse, but they do not typically exclude candidates who have achieved sustained abstinence.

EFFECTS OF MEDICATIONS

The potential impact of medication on cognition represents a third factor that must be considered with transplant patients. Of course, this is a general principle that is applicable across all forms of medical illness. Transplant patients additionally are maintained on immunosupressive therapy, with the most commonly used medication being cyclosporine. Cyclosporine has been associated with neurotoxicity and encephalopathy in a number of anecdotal or single-patient reports (Drachman, DeNofrio, Acker, Galetta, & Loh, 1996; Garcia-Escrig, Martinez, Fernandez-Ponsati, Diaz, & Soto, 1994). In addition, concern has been raised about the potential long-term effects of cyclosporine on brain functioning. Grimm and colleagues (1996) concluded that negative changes in brain functioning over a 2-year posttransplant period were related to cumulative cyclosporine effects. Finally, Cohen and Raps (1995) point out that patients who are immunocompromised may be more susceptible to neurologic illness as a function of opportunistic infection or underlying disease states.

EFFECTIVE ASSESSMENT AND TREATMENT OF IMPAIRED TRANSPLANT PATIENTS

Transplant patients with cognitive impairment most often present with deficits that reflect generalized brain dysfunction. These deficits often present in a subtle form that may not be immediately evident during office or clinic visits (Farmer, 1994). The point cannot be overemphasized that medical office visits are often so structured and brief that cognitive impairment may go undetected. Thus, a patient may appear reasonably intact during a structured office visit yet have significant cognitive and functional impairment in daily life.

Deficits in attention, memory, and executive functions are the most disabling with regard to the transplant process.

Patients with significant attention and memory impairment

- May be easily distracted and have difficulty focusing on information being told to them by the medical team
- Will have greater difficulty remembering important information, and, as a consequence, may be at risk for not following through on treatment plans
- May fail to inform health care providers about important symptoms or medications they are taking

Patients with impaired executive functioning may

- Have problems with complex reasoning, initiation, and judgment
- Fail to comprehend complicated or multistep instructions
- Fail to spontaneously report important information
- Fail to generalize knowledge to new settings
- Show deficient self-awareness about cognitive deficits
- Make poor decisions about health behavior

However, there are things the medical team can be sensitive to that may indicate the presence of brain dysfunction. One indication comes from thorough history taking and asking specifically about conditions such as prior brain injury, stroke, and periods of confusion. It is often the case that such conditions are not asked about or are overlooked during examinations. In addition, two or three direct questions about whether the person notices problems with daily memory, keeping track of appointments, or finances can provide a hint of possible cognitive problems. Furthermore, the patient's behavior can be observed during initial interviews. The clinician can observe how well the patient seems to be able to concentrate, maintain a continuous flow of thoughts, remember things discussed earlier in the interview, and comprehend the basic information being shared about the transplant process. The interview can also be structured to examine how well a patient remembers and follows through on instructions. Giving the patient an assignment or task that is to be completed prior to the next contact will help identify problems with remembering, initiating, and follow-through.

It is also recommended that routine neuropsychological screening of cognitive functioning be conducted with all candidates for transplantation. Screening of transplant candidates can identify preexisting cognitive deficits that might otherwise go undetected, and which would likely interfere with the transplant process. Knowing the patient's cognitive capabilities will help identify those patients with deficits who are in need of specific assistance or compensatory strategies in order to remember treatment regimens. Follow-up screening after transplantation is also recommended. Some patients will show significant change following surgery and impairment at this point can represent a significant threat to graft survival, because a patient who is unable to follow the posttransplant regimen is at great risk for rejection and other complications.

Neuropsychological screening of pre- and posttransplant patients can be accomplished through several means:

1. Routine screenings of pre- and posttransplant patients by a neuropsychologist. The neuropsychologist can provide an efficient screening and identify those patients who require a more detailed assessment battery. Screening by a neuropsychologist can also help identify other potential problems that may not be due to brain dysfunction but can affect compliance with the transplant process, such as poor reading skills, low general intellectual level, and psychiatric illnesses.

2. Use of a structured mental status exam such as the Mini-Mental Status Examination (MMSE) will give a global picture of cognitive functioning, although it may not be sensitive to the memory and executive deficits of many patients with mild impairment.

   • Other structured mental status examinations will likely be more sensitive (e.g., Cognistat, Repeatable Battery for the Assessment of Neuropsychological Status) but may not be tenable given time constraints of office medical visits.

3. Asking the patient and family members about the patient's cognitive functioning. This is particularly useful when there is insufficient time or resources to perform a detailed mental status examination and when problems are suspected even in the face of good performance on the MMSE or other brief screening.

   • Many patients are aware of their memory or other cognitive problems based on prior assessment or experience and can provide such information, but they may not do so if not explicitly asked. Particularly in the cases of impaired executive functioning, the patient may not initiate disclosure of such problems or may not have full self-awareness of the deficits.

   • Although it is always important to protect patient privacy and confidentiality, it may be necessary to ask specific questions of family members. Most transplant patients are accustomed to having family members involved with their care and will be open to having them provide information.

   • There are structured inventories that ask about specific cognitive and behavioral deficits; these inventories have the benefit of identifying symptoms that might not be spontaneously reported by patients and families. These can be incorporated as part of a screening assessment done by a neuropsychologist.

INTERVENTIONAL STRATEGIES

In summary, all of the factors discussed in the preceding sections lead to the conclusion that particular care must be taken to maximize the transplant patient's potential to follow through on treatment plans. Health care providers must be alert to the possibility of cognitive deficits and, when present, adapt treatment interventions to help the patient compensate for these deficits. A number of strategies will help facilitate a positive outcome with regard to treatment compliance:

1. Provide memory aids to help the patient remember treatment recommendations, new medications, and so on.
   - Focus on the most important information. Patients with cognitive impairment will be much more likely to retain and use information that is written down in a structured and organized way. Too much information can be just as difficult as too little information for someone with memory deficits, so it is important to include the essential things that the patient needs to remember and respond to.
   - Help the patient write a list of medications, doses, schedule, and so on, to enhance compliance with treatment. Although it may seem unrealistic to devote the time to helping the patient make organized lists or memory aids, doing so will help prevent future problems that threaten the patient's health and require more cost and resources to address.
   - Use multimodal cues and aids. For example, when developing a list of medications for a patient with memory deficits, include photos of the medications to facilitate learning and retention. One creative team member developed a set of color-coded reminder cards that could be carried in the patient's pocket as an easily accessed reference about potentially dangerous symptoms.
2. Follow up with patients to be sure they have followed through on treatment prescriptions and directions. This usually can be done with a very brief phone call by office staff, which, once again, represents a modest investment of time that helps reduce the possibility of future problems.
3. Patients with impaired planning and initiation may know they need to remember to do something but still fail to follow through. In such cases, it will be important to identify another person who can provide reminders and checks to be sure that important tasks are being completed and medications are being taken correctly.
4. Verify the effectiveness of any strategies developed. The most elegant strategy to help a patient with cognitive deficits is useless if the patient does not use it. Strategies need to be tailored to the individual's skills and preferences, and many a creative intervention has gone unused because the patient either could not or would not use

it. The most effective tool is one that is used by the patient.

5. Be sensitive to the possibility that patients who have undergone transplantation may, as a function of existing cognitive problems, be more vulnerable to the effects of certain medications on attention and memory.

6. At times the types of strategies discussed here may not be effective. In such cases, it may be helpful to seek consultation with a neuropsychologist, speech-language pathologist, or occupational therapist who is familiar with brain dysfunction. There are many other strategies used in rehabilitation that may be beneficial to transplant patients.

7. As has been noted above, good communication among all health care professionals involved in the patient's care is essential. This point need not be belabored here, but effective communication becomes even more critical when working with any patient who is compromised in his or her capacity to remember information, recognize and report important symptoms, or follow through on treatment recommendations.

Clinical assessment and intervention strategies must be done on an individual basis, and there are no "cookbook" strategies that can be applied in all cases. However, it may be useful to have suggested strategies that can be individualized to meet specific patients' needs. See Table 5.1 for additional strategies for specific cognitive deficits.

REFERENCES

Adams, R. D., Victor, M., & Ropper, A. H. (1997). *Principles of neurology* (6th ed.). New York: McGraw-Hill.

Bornstein, R. A., Starling, R. Co., Myerowitz, P. D., & Haas, G. J. (1995). Neuropsychological function in patients with end-stage heart failure before and after cardiac transplantation. *Acta Neurologica Scandanavica, 91*(4), 260–265.

Bremer, B. A., Wert, K. M., Durica, A. L., & Weaver, A. (1998). Neuropsychological, physical, and psychosocial functioning of individuals with end-stage renal disease. *Annals of Behavioral Medicine, 19*(4), 348–352.

Cohen, J. A., & Raps, E. C. (1995). Critical neurologic illness in the immunocompromised patient. *Neurology Clinics, 13*(3), 659–677.

Craven, J. L. (1990). Postoperative organic mental syndromes in lung transplant recipients. *Journal of Heart Transplantation, 9*(2), 129–132.

Cummings, J. L., & Benson, D. F. (1992). *Dementia: A clinical approach.* (2nd ed.). Boston: Butterworth-Heinemann.

Dew, M. A., Kormos, R. L., Roth, L. H., Murali, S., DiMartine, A., & Griffith, B. P.

TABLE 5.1 Common Strategies for Managing Cognitive Deficits in Transplant Patients

Problem	Strategy
Attention deficits	1. Review medications for possible agents that may impair alertness and attention. 2. Meet with patient in quiet, nondistracting settings. 3. Focus conversations and meetings on one task at a time, and write down important information discussed.
Memory deficits	1. Provide organized list of medications, appointments, etc., using multimodal cues. 2. Train patient to use a memory logbook that contains important information, so he or she learns to rely on it for daily functioning. 3. Break down information into smaller units or chunks, so that learning and memory do not become over-loaded. 4. Utilize frequent practice/rehearsal of important information to be learned 5. Use alarms to cue daily tasks such as taking medications. 6. Use pill dispensers and similar devices to simplify daily memory demands. 7. Use reminders for upcoming appointments and other tasks that are not part of the daily routine. Reminders can be in the form of phone calls, postcards, e-mail, etc. 8. Begin as much teaching as possible prior to transplantation, as patients often will not learn well during the early posttransplant period. 9. Involve family members or friends to help the patient.
Preexisting learning disabilities	1. Modify training and reading materials to fit the reading level of patients.

(1999). Early post-transplant medical compliance and mental health predict physical morbidity and mortality one to three years after heart transplantation. *Journal of Heart and Lung Transplantation, 18*(6), 549–562.

Dew, M. A., Roth, L. H., Schulberg, H. C, Simmons, R. G., Kormos, R. L., Trzepacz, P. T., & Griffith, B. P. (1996). Prevalence and predictors of depression and anxiety-related disorders during the first year after heart transplantation. *General*

Hospital Psychiatry, 18, 48S–61S.

Dew, M. A., Roth, L. H., Thompson, M. E., Kormos, R. L., & Griffith, B. P. (1996). Medical compliance and its predictors in the first year after heart transplantation. *Journal of Heart and Lung Transplantation, 15*(6), 631–645.

Drachman, B. M., DeNofrio, D., Acker, M. A., Galetta, S., & Loh, E. (1996). Cortical blindness secondary to cyclosporine after orthotopic heart transplantation: A case report and review of the literature. *Journal of Heart and Lung Transplantation, 15*(11), 1158–1164.

Farmer, M. E. (1994). Cognitive deficits related to major organ failure: The potential role of neuropsychological testing. *Neuropsychology Review, 4*(2), 117–160.

Fisher, D. C., Lake, K. D., Reutzel, T. J., & Emery, R. W. (1995) Changes in health-related quality of life and depression in heart transplant recipients. *Journal of Heart and Lung Transplantation, 14*(2), 373–381.

Garcia-Escrig, M., Martinez, J., Fernandez-Ponsati, J., Diaz, J., & Soto, O. (1994). Severe central nervous system toxicity after chronic treatment with cyclosporine. *Clinical Neuropharmacology, 17*(3), 298–302.

Goldstein, L. S., Haug, M. T., Perl, J., Perl., M. K., Maurer, J. R., Arroliga, A. C., Mehta, A. C., Kirby, T., Higgins, B., & Stillwell, P. C. (1998). Central nervous system complications after lung transplantation. *Journal of Heart and Lung Transplantation, 17*(2), 185–191.

Grady, K. L, Jalowiec, A., & White-Williams, C. (1999). Predictors of quality of life in patients at one year after heart transplantation. *Journal of Heart and Lung Transplantation, 18*(3), 202–210.

Grimm, M., Yeganehfar, W., Laufer, G., Madl, C., Kramer, L., Eisenhuber, E., Simon, P., Kupilik, N., Schreiner, W., Pacher, R., Bunzel, B., Wolner, E., & Grimm, G. (1996). Cyclosporine may affect improvement of cognitive brain function after successful cardiac transplantation. *Circulation, 94*(6), 1339–1345.

Kaelber, C. T., Moul, D. E., & Farmer, M. E. (1995). Epidemiology of depression. In E. E. Beckham & W. R. Leber (Eds.), *Handbook of depression* (2nd ed., pp. 3–35). New York: The Guilford Press.

Kramer, L., Madl, C., Stockenhuber, F., Yeganehfar, W., Eisenhuber, E., Derfler, K., Lenz, K., Schneider, B., & Grimm, G., (1996). Beneficial effect of renal transplantation on cognitive brain function. *Kidney International, 49*(3), 833–838.

Maser, J. D., Weise, R., & Gwirtsman, H. (1995). Depression and its boundaries with selected Axis I disorders. In E. E. Beckham & W. R. Leber (Eds.), *Handbook of depression* (2nd ed., pp. 86–106). New York: The Guilford Press.

Olbrisch, M. E., & Levenson, J. L. (1991). Psychosocial evaluation of heart transplant candidates: An international survey of process, criteria, and outcomes. *Journal of Heart and Lung Transplantation, 10*(6), 948–955.

Pliskin, N. H., Yurk, H. M., Ho, L. T., & Umans, J. G. (1996). Neurocognitive function in chronic hemodialysis patients. *Kidney International, 49,* 1435–1440.

Putzke, J. D., Williams, M. A., Rayburn, B. K., Kirklin, J. K., & Boll, T. J. (1998). The relationship between cardiac function and neuropsychological status among heart transplant candidates. *Journal of Cardiac Failure, 4*(4), 295–303.

Ramsey, S. D., Patrick, D. L., Lewis, S., Albert, R. K., & Raghu, G. (1995). Improvement in quality of life after lung transplantation: A preliminary study.

Journal of Heart and Lung Transplantation, 14(5), 870–877.

Schall, R. R., Petrucci, R. J., Brozena, S. C., Cavarocchi, N. C., & Jessup, M. (1989). Cognitive function in patients with symptomatic dilated cardiomyopathy before and after transplantation. *Journal of the American College of Cardiology, 14*(7), 1666–1672.

Stevens, D. E., Merikangas, K. R., & Merikangas, J. R. (1995). Comorbidity of depression and other medical conditions. In E. E. Beckham & W. R. Leber (Eds.), *Handbook of depression* (2nd ed., pp. 147–199). New York: The Guilford Press.

Umans, J. G., & Pliskin, N. H. (1998). Attention and mental processing speed in hemodialysis patients. *American Journal of Kidney Disease, 32*(5), 749–751.

6

Heart Transplantation

Sandra A. Cupples,
Steven W. Boyce, and
Sotiris C. Stamou

What began as a highly experimental procedure in 1967 now has become an effective treatment modality for end-stage heart disease (ESHD). Current 1- and 3-year heart transplant patient survival rates are 85.6% and 79.5%, respectively (Hosenpud, Bennett, Keck, Boucek, & Novick, 2000). Current 1- and 3-year graft survival rates are 84.4% and 76.6%, respectively.

RATIONALE FOR EXTENSIVE EVALUATION PROCESS

Despite the success of heart transplantation, there remains a shortage of donor organs. As of December 2001, there were 4,137 patients on the national heart transplant waiting list (United Network for Organ Sharing [UNOS], 2001). Over the last 10 years, the number of heart donors has remained relatively constant (Frantz & Olson, 1997). Each month, approximately 200 more candidates are added to the waiting list than there are available donor organs. This imbalance between supply and demand has resulted in prolonged waiting times. At present, the average waiting time for a donor heart exceeds 300 days (Miller, 1998). The mortality rate for patients on the heart transplant waiting list ranges between 10% and 30%

(Frantz & Olson, 1997; Miller, 1998). These sobering statistics mandate that heart transplant programs carefully evaluate potential candidates so that only those patients who have the greatest need for and who will obtain the greatest benefit from transplantation are actually placed on the waiting list.

TYPES OF PATIENTS REFERRED FOR HEART TRANSPLANTATION

Patients referred for heart transplant evaluation have one of the following diagnoses:

- Ischemic cardiomyopathy (CDM) (45% of referrals)
- Nonischemic CDM (44% of referrals): peripartum, inflammatory, familial, toxic, or idiopathic CDM
- Miscellaneous (11% of referrals): congenital abnormalities, refractory ventricular arrhythmias, valvular disease, or retransplantation (Costanza, 1996; Grady, 1996; Hosenpud et al., 2000).

INDICATIONS FOR HEART TRANSPLANTATION

Before the actual transplant evaluation process begins, the transplant team must first determine if there are any other viable treatment options that will confer similar or better long-term survival (Achuff, 1990). Patients with ischemic CDM undergo extensive testing to determine if there is any reversible ischemia that may be amenable to either surgery or catheter intervention (Miller, 1998). Patients with nonischemic CDM are typically given a trial of optimal medical therapy that may include vasodilators, diuretics, digoxin, angiotensin-converting enzyme (ACE) inhibitors, and beta-blocking agents designed to reduce preload and afterload (Conte 1998; Cross & Stevenson, 1998).

Accepted indications for heart transplantation include

- Maximal oxygen consumption (VO_2) < 10 mL/kg/min with achievement of anaerobic metabolism
- Severe, limiting ischemia not amenable to surgical or catheter intervention
- Recurrent, refractory ventricular arrhythmias

Probable indications for heart transplantation include

- Maximal VO_2 < 14 mL/kg/min with major limitation of daily activity
- Recurrent unstable ischemia not amenable to surgical or catheter intervention
- Instability of fluid balance and renal function not associated with patient noncompliance (Mudge et al., 1993).

EVALUATION PROCESS

The purpose of the heart transplant evaluation process is to determine

- The likelihood that the patient will be able to resume an active and relatively normal lifestyle after transplantation
- The patient's potential to comply with a strict posttransplant medical regimen that involves daily medications and frequent follow-up visits (Achuff, 1990)

Therefore, the patient selection process includes a review of both physiological and psychosocial criteria. This evaluation process is typically conducted by a multidisciplinary team that includes the surgeon, cardiologist, nurse coordinator, social worker, psychologist or psychiatrist, and dietitian. Other specialists are consulted as needed.

PHYSIOLOGICAL CRITERIA

Severity and Prognosis

The first step is to evaluate the severity of the patient's functional impairment and prognosis by determining New York Heart Association classification, hemodynamic status, and exercise tolerance level (Cupples & Spruill, 2000). The metabolic exercise test is the most accurate predictor of survival; therefore, it is the gold standard by which patients are stratified (Miller, 1998). This test is typically performed after the ambulatory patient has been on optimal medical therapy for at least 2 weeks (Frantz & Olson, 1997; Miller, 1998).

Contraindications and Comorbidities

Once it has been established that disease severity and prognosis warrant transplantation, the patient is evaluated for any contraindications to transplantation. A contraindication is defined as "any condition that would place a recipient at excessive risk of morbidity due to transplant-related interventions such as immunosuppression, or limit survival independent of transplantation" (Kao, Winkel, & Costanzo, 1995, p. 164). Table 6.1 lists the generally accepted physiological contraindications to heart transplantation.

Although septuagenarians have successfully undergone transplantation (Conte, 1998; Cross & Stevenson, 1998), age remains a controversial issue. Most transplant programs consider physiological as well as chronological age, although some programs exclude patients older than 60 to 65 years (Achuff, 1990). Comorbidity typically increases with age; therefore, older patients must meet more stringent selection criteria (Miller et al., 1995). A few transplant centers offer an alternative waiting list. Older candidates who are placed on this list agree to accept hearts from older, marginal donors. Several of these programs have achieved excellent short- and midterm results (Laks et al., 1997).

Screening Tests

Patients who have no obvious contraindications to transplantation then undergo a rigorous screening process. This evaluation is tailored to the individual patient. Some tests are standard for all patients; additional tests may be added based on the patient's medical history and/or test results. Table 6.2 lists the studies and consultations that are routinely obtained.

PSYCHOSOCIAL CRITERIA

Given the multiple stressors and lifestyle changes associated with the transplant experience, most transplant centers consider psychosocial criteria during the evaluation process. Psychosocial factors that are assessed include

- Tangible and emotional support systems
- Compliance history
- Substance abuse history
- Neurocognitive status
- Emotional stability
- Commitment to the transplantation process.

TABLE 6.1 Physiological Contraindications to Heart Transplantation

General
- Advanced age (typically > 60 to 65)
- Morbid obesity ($\geq$ 30% of ideal body weight)
- Severe cachexia

Systemic
- Active infection
- Acquired immunodeficiency disorder
- Sarcoidosis
- Amyloidosis
- Coexisting systemic disease likely to limit survival and/or rehabilitation
- Insulin-dependent diabetes mellitus with end-organ damage

Pulmonary
- Irreversible pulmonary hypertension (> 4–8 Wood units)
- Irreversible pulmonary parenchymal disease
- Recent unresolved pulmonary infarction
- Severe obstructive/restrictive pulmonary disease (forced expiratory volume in 1 second < 50% of predicted or ratio of forced expiratory volume in 1 second to forced vital capacity < 40% to 50% of predicted)
- Severe chronic bronchitis

Renal
- Irreversible renal disease with serum creatinine > 2.0–2.5 mg/dL or creatinine clearance < 50 mL/min)

Hepatic
- Irreversible hepatic disease (total bilirubin > 2.5 mg/dL)

Cardiovascular
- Significant, uncorrectable peripheral vascular disease
- Cerebrovascular disease
- Myocardial infiltrative and inflammatory disease

Gastrointestinal
- Active peptic ulcer disease
- Current or recent diverticulitis

Skeletal
- Severe osteoporosis

Other
- Recent or active neoplasm

Source: Achuff, 1990; Blum & Aravot, 1996; Costanzo, 1996; Costanzo et al., 1995; Frantz & Olson, 1997; Mudge et al., 1993; Olivari, 1996

TABLE 6.2 Evaluation Process: Routine Studies and Consultations

Comprehensive history and physical examination

Cardiovascular
- ECG
- Right heart catheterization
- Left heart catheterization
- Metabolic exercise test
- Echocardiogram (M-mode and two-dimensional; Doppler)
- 24-hour Holter monitoring*
- Endomyocardial biopsy*
- Radionuclide ventriculography*
- Multigated blood panel imaging scan*
- Carotid and peripheral Doppler flow studies*

Pulmonary
- Chest radiograph
- Pulmonary function tests
- Tuberculin purified protein derivative
- Skin test anergy battery
- Lung ventilation–perfusion scanning*

Renal
- Urinalysis
- 24-hour urine for creatinine clearance and protein excretion

Gastrointestinal
- Stool guaiac (three tests)
- Abdominal ultrasound
- Colonoscopy*
- Sigmoidoscopy*

Immunological
- Blood type and antibody screen
- Panel reactive antibody
- Human leukocyte antigen typing

Infectious disease
- History (travel, exposure, risk factors)
- Vaccinations
- Tuberculin skin test; anergy panel
- Stool culture
- Stool for ova and parasites

Laboratory studies
- Blood chemistries
- Renal and liver function panels
- Lipid profile
- Complete blood count with differential leukocytic count
- Prothrombin time, partial thromboplastin time, fibrinogen
- Carcinoembryonic antigen
- Glycosylated hemoglobin*
- Hemoglobin A_{1c}*
- Toxicology screen*

Serology
- Human immunodeficiency virus
- Hepatitis profile
- Herpes group virus
- Cytomegalovirus IgG and IgM antibodies
- Epstein-Barr IgG and IgM antibodies
- Rapid plasma reagin test
- Varicella titers
- *Toxoplasma gondii* IgG and IgM antibodies
- Fungal antibody screen
- Lyme titers*

Gender-specific
- Mammography
- Papanicolaou's smear
- Prostate specific antigen
- Prostate: digital rectal examination
- Beta human chorionic gonadotropin*

Consultations
- Dental
- Social work
- Nutrition
- Gynecological
- Psychiatry*
- Neuropsychology*
- Ophthalmology*
- Endocrinology*

* If indicated
Source: Grady, 1996; Mudge et al., 1993

Typically, patients who are currently using tobacco, drugs, or alcohol are asked to enroll in formal smoking cessation and/or rehabilitation programs and to demonstrate abstinence for a given period of time (e.g., 6 months) before being placed on the waiting list (Cupples & Spruill, 2000). The major psychosocial contraindications to transplantation are listed in Table 6.3.

LISTING THE PATIENT

Adult patients who are accepted as candidates for heart transplantation are initially placed on the list in one of three categories (Table 6.4). However, certain patients may move back and forth among these statuses over the course of the waiting period.

CARE OF THE HEART TRANSPLANT CANDIDATE

Pretransplant care is often provided in collaboration with local clinicians. Key points regarding the primary care of the transplant candidate are listed in Table 6.5.

PERIODIC TESTING

Due to the dynamic nature of ESHD, transplant candidates typically undergo frequent reassessment by the transplant team that may include

TABLE 6.3 Psychosocial Contraindications to Heart Transplantation

- Current substance abuse (drugs, tobacco, alcohol)
- Psychosocial instability
- Behavior pattern likely to preclude compliance
- Unmanaged mental illness (active psychosis or schizophrenia; severe personality disorder)
- Dementia
- Severe mental retardation
- Suicidal behavior or ideation

Source: Miller et al., 1993; Miller, 1998; Olbrisch & Levenson, 1991

TABLE 6.4 Heart Transplant: United Network for Organ Sharing Statuses

Status	Requirements
1A	Mechanical circulatory support for acute hemodynamic decompensation that includes at least one of the following: • Left and/or right ventricular assist device implanted for ≤ 30 days • Total artificial heart • Intra-aortic balloon pump; or • Extracorporeal membrane oxygenator Mechanical circulatory support for > 30 days with objective medical evidence of significant device-related complications such as • Thromboembolism • Device infection (VAD, pocket, or driveline) • Mechanical failure and/or • Life-threatening ventricular arrhythmia Mechanical ventilation Continuous infusion of a single high-dose intravenous inotrope (e.g., dobutamine ≥ 7.5 mcg/kg/min, or milrinone ≥ 0.5 mcg/kg/min, or multiple intravenous inotropes in addition to continuous hemodynamic monitoring of left ventricular filling pressures A patient who does not meet any of the criteria specified above may be listed as status 1A if the patient is admitted to the listing transplant center hospital and has a life expectancy without a heart transplant of < 7 days.
1B	Left and/or right ventricular assist device implanted for > 30 days and/or Continuous infusion of intravenous inotropes (hospitalized or at home)
2	Patient is waiting at home on oral medications

VAD = ventricular assist device

TABLE 6.5 Key Points: Primary Care of the Transplant Candidate

- Frequently monitor renal and hepatic function and serum electrolytes, particularly potassium and magnesium levels
- For patients on oral anticoagulant therapy, check prothrombin time and international normalized ratio levels frequently
- Perform routine cancer screening according to American Cancer Society guidelines
- Monitor for infection, allergic reactions, weight changes; report these to transplant center
- If blood products are required, administer either leukocyte-depleted blood or use leukocyte-removing filter
- For candidates who are CMV seronegative, administer only CMV-negative blood products
- Report administration of any blood products to transplant center so that PRA levels can be rechecked
- Keep all immunizations current
- Report following clinical conditions to transplant center:
    Significant azotemia
    Refractory fluid retention
    Persistent hypotension
    Altered mental status
    Unexplained GI symptoms
    Nonorthostatic presyncopal episodes
    Any other signs/symptoms of low cardiac output

CMV = cytomegalovirus
PRA = panel-reactive antibody
Source: Frantz & Olson, 1997; Tolman et al., 1995

- Echocardiograms or nuclear scans to evaluate ejection fraction
- Right heart catheterizations to determine current pulmonary vascular resistance
- Periodic metabolic exercise tests; in some situations, left ventricular (LV) function improves, thereby precluding or deferring the need for transplantation (Mudge et al., 1993; Tolman, Taylor, Olsen, Karwande, & Renlund, 1995)

PROGRAMABLE PACER-CARDIOVERTER-DEFIBRILLATORS

Patients with severe CDM are at increased risk for ventricular tachyarrhythmias. The incidence of sudden death in patients with ESHD ranges from 10% to 50%. Factors associated with sudden cardiac death include prior cardiac arrest, recurrent syncope, ventricular tachycardia, and ejection fraction less than 20%. For these patients, programable pacer-cardioverter-defibrillators may be implanted prophylactically (Hauser & Kallinen, 1996).

LEFT VENTRICULAR ASSIST DEVICES

Given the imbalance between the supply and demand for donor organs, the median waiting time for heart transplant candidates has increased substantially. As a result, approximately 25% of heart transplant candidates die while on the waiting list (Blum & Aravot, 1996), and many more patients are at increased risk of multisystem organ failure (MSOF) during the waiting period. Candidates with life-threatening heart failure may require left ventricular assist devices (LVADs) as a bridge to transplantation.

Several types of implantable LVADs are currently available. Regardless of specific type, LVADs confer physiological benefits by

- Reducing the workload of the heart by decreasing preload and myocardial oxygen consumption
- Improving systemic circulation by providing a stable and adequate cardiac output
- Improving tissue perfusion, thereby reversing premorbid MSOF (Duke & Perna, 1999)

Although LVADs confer life-saving benefits, infection is a common complication. Patients are at increased risk of infection due to their deteriorated medical status prior to LVAD implantation. In addition, prolonged stimulation of the immune system by the LVAD itself predisposes patients to immune deficiencies (Morales et al., 2000). Device-related infections have been reported in 30% to 50% of LVAD patients (Piccione, 2000). These infections can be located in the LVAD driveline, pocket, sternum, substernal space, or within the pump itself. Device-related septicemia mimics prosthetic-valve endocarditis. Even though relatively minor, driveline infections can lead to major pocket infections or mediastinitis (Dyke, Pagani, & Aaronson, 2000). See Table 6.6 for care of the LVAD patient at home.

ORGAN SELECTION AND PROCUREMENT

The suitability of a donor organ for a given recipient is based on blood type compatibility and a height and weight ratio match. In most instances,

TABLE 6.6 Key Points: Care of the Patient with a Left Ventricular Assist Device

- Monitor patient for device-related and other types of infection
- Signs and symptoms of device-related infections:

Systemic: Fever, elevated white blood cell count, signs/symptoms of prosthetic valve endocarditis

Local: Erythema, swelling, drainage, purulent exudate, warmth, tenderness, or induration at the driveline exit site

- Notify transplant center of any suspected infection
- Provide antibiotic prophylaxis according to American Heart Association guidelines for high-risk patients

---

human leucocyte antigen (HLA) matching is done retrospectively. However, if the candidate's panel-reactive antibody (PRA) levels exceed 10%, a prospective donor-specific lymphocytotoxic cross-match is performed (Lavee et al., 1991).

Criteria used to determine the suitability of the donor organ typically include the following:

- Age less than 45 to 50 years
- Negative serologies (human immunodeficiency virus, hepatitis B surface antigen, hepatitis C)
- Arterial saturation greater than 80% on ventilatory support
- No active systemic infections, significant ventricular dysrhythmias, extracranial malignancies, history of intravenous drug use, or significant cardiac disease, abnormalities, or trauma (Tolman et al., 1995).

Coronary angiography is typically performed for male and female donors over the age of 45 and 50 years, respectively, or for any donor who has risk factors for coronary artery disease (CAD). The final decision to accept the donor heart is made by the transplant surgeon after visual inspection of the organ.

PREPARATION OF THE RECIPIENT

Once a potentially suitable donor organ has been located, preoperative preparations begin. In addition to obtaining routine preoperative tests, transplantation typically involves

- Assessing the patient for any concurrent infection
- Administering prophylactic antibiotics and immunosuppressants
- Discontinuing and reversing anticoagulation
- Treating any elevated pulmonary vascular resistance with sodium nitroprusside, nitroglycerine, or prostaglandin E_1 (Rourke, Droogan, & Ohler, 1999: Tolman et al., 1995).

Occasionally, the candidate arrives in the preoperative holding area, only to be informed that the donor heart is not suitable. In this circumstance, both the patient and family members require emotional support to cope with their disappointment.

TYPES OF HEART TRANSPLANTATION PROCEDURES

There are two types of heart transplantation procedures: orthotopic and heterotopic. With orthotopic transplantation, the recipient's native heart is excised and replaced with a donor heart. Most heart transplantation procedures today involve the orthotopic technique. Heterotopic transplantation involves the "piggyback" placement of a donor heart into the recipient's right chest cavity. Although heterotopic transplantation is rarely performed, this procedure may be done, for example, if the recipient has high pulmonary vascular resistance and a normal-size donor heart alone would not be capable of maintaining right ventricular function. In this situation, the heterotopically implanted donor heart serves as an auxiliary pump to the recipient's own native heart (Augustine & Masiello-Miller, 1995; Baumgartner, 1990).

SURGICAL PROCEDURE—ORTHOTOPIC TRANSPLANTATION

Heart transplantation mandates careful orchestration of the explantation and implantation procedures so as to minimize ischemic time and optimize outcomes.

PROCUREMENT OF THE DONOR HEART

Once the donor organ has been visually inspected and found to be suitable for transplantation in accordance with the preoperative echocardiogram and, if indicated, cardiac catheterization, the surgical procedure begins with cross-clamping the donor aorta and arresting the heart with cold hyperkalemic cardioplegic solution. The inferior vena cava is divided following ligation of the superior vena cava, and the heart is vented via the left inferior pulmonary vein. Following infusion of the cardioplegic solution, the heart is excised by dividing the pulmonary veins within the pericardial sac. The pulmonary artery is divided at the bifurcation, and the aorta is transected at the level of the innominate artery. The heart is removed, placed in cold saline solution surrounded by ice slush, and transported to the recipient's hospital.

PREPARATION OF THE DONOR HEART

The right atrium is incised in an oblique line from the junction of the inferior vena cava toward the right atrial appendage. This technique protects the donor sinoatrial node from incorporation in the suture (Barnard, 1968) and preserves two of the major internodal pathways. The foramen ovale is closed, if patent, to prevent postoperative hypoxemia from right to left shunting. The pulmonary artery and aorta are appropriately trimmed, and the left atrium is opened through the four pulmonary veins to form a left atrial cuff.

RECIPIENT OPERATION

The timing of the operation in the recipient is coordinated with the activity at the donor's hospital. Once the donor heart is determined to be acceptable, the recipient's procedure begins in standard fashion with a median sternotomy. The patient is cannulated via the ascending aorta and with venous cannulas in the superior and inferior vena cava. Once the donor organ has arrived at the recipient's hospital, the diseased heart is excised following cross-clamping of the aorta. The aorta and pulmonary artery are both transected at the level of their respective valves. Either a cuff of the left and right atrium is preserved, or the operation is modified to perform bicaval anastomoses with the superior and inferior vena cava.

IMPLANTATION OF THE DONOR HEART

Implantation of the donor heart in the traditional manner begins with a suture line anastomosing the donor left atrium to the recipient's left atrial cuff. The donor right atrium is then anastomosed to the recipient's right atrium, and the donor and the recipient aortae and pulmonary arteries are joined by end-to-end anastomosis. The heart is then allowed to fill with blood, and air is displaced as the aortic suture line is completed. Following removal of the aortic cross-clamp, most hearts begin beating spontaneously; however, defibrillation may be required. Cardiopulmonary bypass (CPB) is discontinued with the aid of chronotropic and inotropic support, which is usually continued for several days.

IMMEDIATE POSTOPERATIVE CARE

In many respects, the immediate postoperative care of the transplant recipient is similar to that of any patient who undergoes cardiac surgery. However, the transplant recipient is at risk for several unique problems due to denervation of the transplanted heart and global ischemia during explantation, transportation, and implantation of the allograft (e.g., decreased diastolic compliance, impaired contractility, depressed systolic function) (Tolman et al., 1995) (see Table 6.7). The primary goals in the immediate postoperative period are to

- Achieve adequate gas exchange and hemodynamic stability
- Promote systemic and peripheral perfusion
- Prevent or treat potential problems associated with heart transplantation (see Table 6.7) (Rourke et al., 1999)

IMMUNOSUPPRESSIVE THERAPY

Immunosuppressive therapy may be categorized according to when and why it is administered: early prophylaxis, maintenance prophylaxis in the absence of rejection, and treatment of documented rejection. There is wide variation among transplant programs with respect to immunosuppressant protocols, (see Table 6.8).

The goal of long-term maintenance therapy is to prevent rejection while avoiding the potential side effects of immunosuppressant agents (e.g., nephrotoxicity, hypertension, infection, and neoplasms). This is achieved by carefully monitoring the patient's drug levels, white blood cell count, endomyocardial biopsy results, and clinical signs and symptoms. Immunosuppressant doses are titrated accordingly (Blum & Aravot, 1996).

TABLE 6.7 Immediate Postoperative Period: Major Potential Problems, Precipitating Factors, and Potential Treatment Options

Potential problem	Precipitating factors	Potential treatment options
Compromised fluid status		
Hemorrhage	Preoperative anticoagulants Prior cardiac surgery Coagulopathy Prolonged CPB time Enlarged pericardial space	Blood products (whole blood, packed red blood cells, fresh frozen plasma, platelets) Protamine sulfate or Aprotinin Surgical reexploration
Hypovolemia	3rd spacing of fluids ↑ in intravascular space during rewarming Failure to maintain adequate preload	Optimize preload fluid volume Maintain higher filling pressures
Hypervolemia	Preoperative heart failure CPB High-dose steroids Preoperative renal dysfunction Nephrotoxic immunosuppressants	Diuretics Renal dose dopamine
Myocardial dysfunction Right ventricular failure	Pulmonary hypertension Undersized allograft Prolonged ischemia (> 5 hours) Reactive pulmonary vasoconstriction due to CPB and/or protamine administration	Vasodilators Pulmonary vasodilators (isoproterenol, prostaglandin E_1, prostacyclin, nitroglycerin, sodium nitroprusside, amrinone) Minimal use of vasopressors Mechanical right ventricular support

TABLE 6.7 *(continued)*

Potential problem	Precipitating factors	Potential treatment options
Left ventricular failure	Prolonged ischemia	Inotropic agents (dopamine, dobutamine, epinephrine, ephedrine) Intra-aortic balloon pump Extracorporeal membrane oxygenation Left ventricular assist device Retransplantation
Dysrhythmias (junctional rhythms, atrioventricular blocks, bradyarrhythmias)	Inadequate myocardial preservation Prolonged ischemia Sinus node dysfunction secondary to surgical trauma Pulmonary hypertension Cardiac edema Rejection Pretransplant amiodarone	Atrial ventricular pacing Isoproterenol Terbutaline Theophylline
Hypertension	Cyclosporine and steroid therapy	Antihypertensive agents (diltiazem, nifedipine, enalapril)

CPB = cardiopulmonary bypass
Source: Augustine & Masiello-Miller, 1995; Miller, Wolford, & Donohue, 1996; Ohler, Morris, McCauley, & DiSanto, 1994; Rourke et al., 1999; Tolman et al., 1995

REJECTION

Rejection is the process by which the immune system attempts to destroy alloantigenic tissue. The Bethesda Conference Task Force has defined rejection as "any clinical event, usually, but not always, accompanied by abnormal endomyocardial biopsy findings, that is treated with significant augmentation of immunosuppression" (Miller, Schlant, Kobashigawa, Kubo, & Renlund, 1993, p. 42). All transplant recipients are at risk for rejection. The risk of rejection is highest during the first 6 months after transplantation. In addition, an increased risk of rejection is associated with

TABLE 6.8 Immunosuppression Regimens

Category	Time Frame	Examples
Early prophylaxis	Immediately preoperatively, intraoperatively, and during the first several weeks after transplantation	Cyclospsorine (Sandimmune), or cyclosporine USP [MODIFIED] (Neoral, Gengraf) Azathioprine (Imuran) Methylprednisolone (SoluMedrol) Triple therapy regimens include combinations of • Cyclospsorine • Prednisone (Deltazone, Orazone) • Azathioprine • Mycophenolate mofetil (CellCept) • Tacrolimus (Prograf)
	Induction therapy consists of intravenous agents that are given 7 to 14 days postoperatively to reduce the risk of rejection	Murine monoclonal CD3 antibody Antithymocyte globulin Antilymphocyte globulin Antilymphocyte serum
Maintenance prophylaxis	For the remainder of the patient's life. Note: Given the morbidity associated with corticosteroid administration, some transplant programs taper and withdraw steroid therapy.	Dual therapy: • Cyclosporine and azathioprine Triple therapy: • Cyclosporine, corticosteroids, azathioprine • Cyclosporine, corticosteroids, mycophenolate • Cyclosporine, corticosteroids, tacrolimus Quadruple therapy: • Triple combination therapy plus one of following for 7–10 days: • Antithymocyte globulin (ATGAM) • Antilymphocyte globulin • Antilymphocyte serum • Murine monoclonal CD3 antibody

TABLE 6.8 *(continued)*

Category	Time Frame	Examples
		Cyclophosphamide (Cytoxan) or Methotrexate may be substituted for one of the above drugs
Rejection therapy	Immediately upon diagnosis of rejection	Oral or intravenous bolus of corticosteroids such as • Prednisone 50 mg BID × 3 days • SoluMedrol 500–1,000 mg IV qd × 3 days Intravenous antithymocyte or antilymphocyte agents Monoclonal antibodies Total lymphoid irradiation or photochemotherapy may be used for refractory rejection

Source: Tolman et al., 1995; Wagoner, 1997

- Age < 55
- Female gender (especially multiparous women)
- Increased preoperative PRA levels
- Preoperative myocarditis
- Positive retrospective donor-specific cross-match

TYPES OF REJECTION

Rejection may be mediated by cellular or humoral factors. In cellular rejection, T cells infiltrate the allograft. Humoral (vascular) rejection is mediated by antibodies. Cell-mediated rejection is more common than humoral rejection. There are three types of rejection: hyperacute, acute, and chronic (see Table 6.9).

TABLE 6.9 Types of Rejection

Type	*Typically occurs*	*Description*
Hyperacute (rare)	In the operating room or immediately after transplantation	Mediated by antibodies (humoral rejection) Characterized by rapid tissue necrosis and allograft failure Usually fatal Only treatment is retransplantation
Acute	During the first few months after transplantation; incidence decreases thereafter, but can occur anytime after the transplant procedure	Delayed hypersensitivity reaction Characterized by interstitial and perivascular mononuclear cell infiltrates
Chronic	After 6 months	Characterized by intimal thickening and vascular fibrosis Associated with cell-mediated and humoral injury to the endothelium

DIAGNOSIS OF REJECTION

Endomyocardial Biopsy

Endomyocardial biopsy is the gold standard for diagnosing rejection. This brief (10 to 15 minutes) outpatient procedure typically involves a right internal jugular vein approach. Fluoroscopy or echocardiography may be used to guide a bioptome through the right atrium and tricupsid valve and into the right ventricle. Biopsy specimens are obtained from the septum. The International Society for Heart and Lung Transplantation (ISHLT) has established a standardized cardiac biopsy grading system (Table 6.10).

TABLE 6.10 ISHLT Endomyocardial Grading System

0 =	no rejection
1A =	mild rejection, focal infiltrate without necrosis
1B =	mild rejection, diffuse infiltrate without necrosis
2 =	moderate rejection, one focus only, with aggressive infiltration or focal myocyte damage
3A =	moderate rejection, multifocal aggressive infiltrates or myocyte damage
3B =	severe rejection, diffuse inflammatory process with necrosis
4 =	severe rejection, diffuse aggressive polymorphous infiltrate, edema, hemorrhage, vasculitis, and necrosis

Source: Billingham et al., 1990

Endomyocardial biopsy is associated with a relatively low morbidity (Billingham, 1981); nevertheless, potential complications include the following:

- Pneumothorax
- Hematoma
- Atrial or ventricular dysrhythmias
- Vasovagal reaction
- Myocardial perforation (tamponade)
- Hemothorax
- Perforation of carotid artery
- Bleeding (Ohler et al., 1994)

Clinical Manifestations

Rejection may be associated with vague signs and symptoms such as malaise, shortness of breath, low-grade fever, or mood changes (Augustine & Masiello-Miller, 1995; Rourke et al., 1999). However, there may be no clinical signs or symptoms of rejection unless it is severe. Typical clinical manifestations may include the following:

- New onset peripheral edema
- Weight gain
- Decreased exercise tolerance

- New S_3 or S_4 heart sounds
- Hypotension
- Jugular venous distention
- Pulmonary crackles
- Pericardial friction rub
- Enlarged cardiac silhouette
- Electrocardiogram findings: bradyarrhythmias, decreased voltage or atrial fibrillation or flutter
- Echocardiography findings: decreased systolic function, change in LV mass and wall thickness, increase in pericardial effusion, shortening of isovolumic relaxation time, or increase in early transmittal filling velocity (Wagoner, 1997).

TREATMENT OF REJECTION

Factors Considered

Specific treatment protocols depend on a number of factors including the

- Histologic grade of rejection
- Type of rejection (e.g., acute vs. chronic)
- Time elapsed since transplantation
- Effectiveness of previous rejection treatment strategies
- Patient's current hemodynamic status
- Patient's prior rejection pattern
- Patient's current immunosuppression regimen (Blum & Aravot, 1996; Wagoner, 1997)

Treatment Options

Asymptomatic patients with mild rejection may not be treated; however, these patients are closely observed because 18% to 33% of low-grade rejection episodes may escalate to higher grades of rejection (Lloveras et al., 1992).

- Higher grades of rejection may be treated with either an oral or an intravenous bolus of corticosteroids.
- Outpatients with hemodynamic instability are always readmitted to the transplant center.
- Refractory or severe rejection warrants more aggressive therapy such as intravenous antithymocyte or antilymphocyte agents or monoclonal antibodies. Failure of these therapies may necessitate total lymphoid irradiation or photochemotherapy (Blum & Aravot, 1996; Wagoner, 1997).

LONG-TERM CARE

ROUTINE FOLLOW-UP

At the time of their regularly scheduled endomyocardial biopsies, transplant recipients have laboratory tests that typically include a complete blood cell count, chemistry profile, and electrolyte, blood urea nitrogen, creatinine, glucose, magnesium, and trough immunosuppression levels (cyclosporine or tacrolimus). Chest radiographs and lipid profiles may be done every 6 to 12 months. Echocardiograms, electrocardiograms, coronary angiography, and extensive infection screening tests are typically included in the annual checkup at the transplant center.

Routine follow-up by both primary care providers and the transplant center involves careful monitoring for and treatment of the following potential posttransplant complications: infection, vasculopathy, hypertension, metabolic disorders, renal insufficiency, malignancy, gastrointestinal disorders, and reduced exercise tolerance (Mills, 1994; Wagoner, 1997).

INFECTION

Infection is the primary cause of posttransplant morbidity and mortality (Miller et al., 1993) and a leading cause of death during the first year after heart transplantation (Smart et al., 1996). It is estimated that two thirds of all heart transplant recipients will have at least one significant infection (Thaler & Rubin, 1996). Recent data from the ISHLT/UNOS Thoracic Registry morbidity study indicated that 22% of heart transplant recipients who survived 1 year were rehospitalized for infection during the first posttransplant year (Brann, Bennett, Keck, & Hosenpud, 1998). (See Chapter 2.)

CARDIAC ALLOGRAFT VASCULOPATHY

Cardiac allograft vasculopathy (CAV), an accelerated form of coronary artery disease, is the major impediment to long-term survival following heart transplantation (Conraads et al., 1998). First noted among the original heart transplant recipients at Stanford in the late 1960s, the incidence of CAV has not decreased despite the introduction of newer immunosuppressants (Miller, Donohue, & Wolford, 1996). The majority of allograft failures after the first year are due to CAV (Dong et al., 1996). CAV remains the most common reason for retransplantation (Anderson, 1999).

Prevalence

- CAV significantly affects over 40% of heart transplant recipients who survive more than 4 years (Dong et al., 1996).
- The prevalence of CAV at 1 and 5 years posttransplant is 8% and 22%, respectively (Hosenpud et al., 2000)

Characteristics

CAV is an unusual form of CAD that affects both epicardial and myocardial vessels. It differs from CAD in the following respects (Parameshwar, 1996; Weis & von Scheidt, 1997):

Natural CAD	*Transplant CAV*
Asymmetrical lesions	Concentric intimal lesions
Involves focal lesions	Diffuse process; affects entire length of vessel
Affects small branches	Typically does not affect small branches
Internal elastic lamina disrupted	Internal elastic lamina intact
Does not affect intramyocardial vessels	Affects intramyocardial vessels
Calcification common	Calcification rare
Develops slowly over years	Develops rapidly (may develop over months)
Development of collaterals common	Development of collaterals rare
Children typically not affected	Children affected

Interestingly, CAV stops at the junction between recipient and donor tissue.

Etiology

Both immunological and nonimmunological processes play a role in the development of CAV (Anderson, 1999; Conraads et al., 1998). Etiological factors of note include the folowing:

Immunological factors	Nonimmunological factors
HLA mismatching	Donor characteristics: age, sex, ischemic time, preexisting CAD
Suboptimal immunotherapy	Recipient characteristics: age, sex obesity, hypertension, hyperlipidemia, diabetes mellitus (DM), cytomegalovirus (CMV) infection, smoking, oxidative injury
Acute and chronic rejection	

Clinical Manifestations

Unlike classic CAD, angina is rarely associated with CAV because the allograft is denervated. Clinical manifestations of CAV may include

- Increasing exertional dyspnea, fatigue
- Elevated left ventricular filling pressures
- Arrhythmias, sudden death (Conraads et al., 1998; Mills, 1994).

Diagnostic Tests

- Noninvasive tests such as exercise electrocardiography and myocardial nuclear imaging generally lack sufficient sensitivity to be reliable screening tools (Conraads et al., 1998).
- CAV causes diffuse, concentric narrowing of arteries; focal stenoses are rare. Therefore, conventional coronary angiography also lacks sensitivity and underestimates the presence of this disease.
- More recently, intravascular ultrasound (IVUS) has been shown to be an effective imaging modality. IVUS permits delineation of the actual lumen diameter, assessment of vessel wall morphology, and quantification of stenosis (Conraads et al., 1998).

Treatment

- Revascularization procedures such as percutaneous transluminal coronary angioplasty (PTCA) or coronary artery bypass graft (CABG) surgery are limited treatment options because of the diffuse, concentric nature of CAV (Conraads et al., 1998).
- For those recipients with focal lesions in epicardial vessels, PTCA has been somewhat successful; however, follow-up angiography has demonstrated that restenosis occurs in 50% to 60% of these patients within 6 months.
- The only definitive treatment for CAV is retransplantation. Given the current shortage of donor organs, many centers do not offer this option.

HYPERTENSION

Hypertension is a significant problem among heart transplant recipients. It frequently develops within the first few weeks after transplantation.

Prevalence

- Hypertension requiring drug therapy is the most common first-year morbidity complication, occurring in 61% of survivors (Brann et al., 1998).
- The prevalence of hypertension increases over time (Singer & Jenkins, 1996); it has been reported in 50% to 90% of all heart transplant recipients (Parameshwar, 1996).
- Posttransplant hypertension is more common in
  - Males
  - Older recipients
  - Recipients with pretransplant hypertension
  - Recipients with a family history of hypertension, myocardial infarction, or stroke
  - Recipients with preceding ischemic CDM

Characteristics

In the general population, blood pressure (BP) typically falls 20% during sleep. In heart transplant recipients, however, this nocturnal decline in BP is blunted and may disappear entirely. As a result of this abnormal circadian BP rhythm, the total daily BP load in transplant recipients is actually greater for any given clinic pressure than in patients with essential hypertension. Therefore, BP-related complications in heart transplant recipients may be greater than expected from their clinic readings. Potential causes of this abnormal 24-hour BP profile include impaired afferent and efferent baroreceptor reflexes secondary to denervation and failure to decrease heart rate (HR) and vasodilate in response to supine posture-induced increases in central volume and filling pressure (Singer & Jenkins, 1996).

Etiology

The etiology of posttransplant hypertension is multifactorial. Major contributing factors include:

- Abnormal regulation of sodium balance associated with cyclosporine, cardiac denervation, and renal impairment
- Structural changes in resistance arteries (increase in wall:lumen ratio)
- Immunosuppressive therapy (Singer & Jenkins, 1996)

Treatment

- Nonpharmacological measures:
  - Cyclosporine-associated hypertension is salt-sensitive; therefore, reduction of dietary salt intake is useful.
  - Other conventional measures include weight loss, regular exercise, and reversing other cardiovascular risk factors, for example, smoking and hyperlipidemia (Singer & Jenkins, 1996).
- Pharmacological measures:
  - Hypertension exacerbates cyclosporine-induced nephrotoxicity; therefore, aggressive pharmacological therapy is essential.
  - Pharmacological options include calcium antagonists, ACE inhibitors, beta-adrenergic blockers, and diuretics.
  - These agents may exacerbate renal dysfunction and alter cyclosporine and lipid metabolism. Therefore, it is important to monitor cyclosporine levels, renal function, serum electrolytes, and lipid profiles (Parameshwar, 1996; Singer & Jenkins, 1996).

METABOLIC DISORDERS

Hyperlipidemia, obesity, osteoporosis, and DM are common problems following heart transplantation.

Hyperlipidemia

Prevalence of hyperlipidemia

- Hyperlipidemia occurs in 60% to 83% of heart transplant recipients receiving triple-drug immunosuppressant therapy (Lake, 1996).
- Cholesterol levels increase as early as 3 weeks after transplantation.
- Patients who develop hypercholesterolemia typically do so within 6 to 18 months following surgery.
- Total cholesterol levels generally increase 30 to 80 mg/dL over pre-transplant levels. If untreated, however, much higher cholesterol levels are observed (Miller et al., 1993).

Etiology of hyperlipidemia

Factors associated with the development of posttransplant hyperlipidemia include

- History of pretransplant hyperlipidemia and/or CAD
- Obesity
- Male gender
- Diabetes
- Age
- Renal dysfunction
- Proteinuria
- Antihypertensive medications
- Cyclosporine and prednisone dosage (Augustine, Baumgartner, & Kasper, 1998; Kubo et al., 1992; Lake, 1996).

Treatment of hyperlipidemia

Hyperlipidemia in transplant recipients is usually treated (Johnson, 1995). Posttransplant hyperlipidemia and obesity are multifactorial problems; therefore, a multifaceted, individualized treatment strategy is imperative.
   Nonpharmacologic strategies include

- Weight loss, exercise, and smoking cessation
- National Cholesterol Education Program Step 2 diet (often necessary for many patients) (Lake, 1996)

Pharmacologic interventions:

- Indications for initiation of drug therapy vary among transplant centers
- Given the survival benefits observed with statins, some centers prescribe statins for all recipients, even those with normal lipid profiles (Yamani & Starling, 2000).

Drug therapy is typically instituted if

- Total or LDL cholesterol levels are elevated, or
- Nonpharmacological interventions have failed after a 3 to 6-month trial, or
- Pretransplant compliance with diet therapy has been ineffective, or
- Immunosuppressant medications have been reduced to a maintenance level and lipid levels remain elevated (Lake, 1996).

Typically, dosing is titrated to achieve low-density lipoprotein (LDL) < 100 mg/dL and a total cholesterol level < 200 mg/dL. 3-hydroxy-3-methylglutaryl coenzyme A (HMG-CoA) reductase inhibitors are the treatment of choice for mixed hyperlipidemias because they decrease LDL and triglycerides and increase high-density lipoprotein (HDL) (Lake, 1996). Drug-specific precautions are listed in Table 6.11.

Regardless of when drug therapy begins, the patient must understand that this therapy is in conjunction with, and not in place of, diet and exercise (Lake, 1996).

Obesity

Prevalence of obesity

- Approximates that of hyperlipidemia
- During the first posttransplant year, most recipients gain between 5 and 10 kilograms
- Patients who gain 5 or more kilograms in the year following transplantation are more likely to have total serum cholesterol levels that exceed 240 mg/dL (Lake, 1996).

Etiology of obesity

Factors contributing to posttransplant weight gain include

- Chronic immunosuppression with cyclosporine and prednisone
- Lack of compliance with a low-fat diet
- Lack of exercise
- A sense of well-being associated with normal heart function—a newly found joie de vivre that may be associated with the feeling that life is to be lived to the fullest (Augustine et al., 1998; Grady, Costanzo-Nordin, Herold, Sriniavasan, & Pifarre, 1991).

Treatment of obesity

Aggressive weight management strategies are necessary for patients who are at or above 120% of their ideal body weight (Lake, 1996).

Osteoporosis

Prior to transplantation, transplant candidates' vertebral bone density is approximately 20% lower than that of age- and gender-matched controls. This decrease is attributed to cigarette smoking, physical inactivity, cardiac cachexia, and administration of heparin and loop diuretics (Wagoner, 1997).

TABLE 6.11 Key Points: Lipid-Lowering Therapy

Bile acid sequestrants
  • May interfere with the absorption of cyclosporine
  • Side effects may preclude long-term compliance
  • May transiently increase triglycerides
  • Cyclosporine and other medications should not be taken 1 hour
    before or 4 to 6 hours after this medication is taken

Nicotinic acid
  • For patients on cyclosporine: May increase LFTs and uric acid
    level; monitor patient for hepatotoxicity and/or gout
  • Can cause hyperglycemia; not recommended for diabetic patients
  • Increased incidence of hepatotoxicity and decreased efficacy
    reported with sustained-released formulation
  • Concurrent use of niacin with cyclosporine, lovastatin, and/or
    gemfibrozil may cause myositis and rhabdomyolysis
  • Concurrent use with prednisone may increase risk of peptic ulcer
    disease

Fibric acid derivatives
  • Have only a moderate effect on LDL
  • Most effective for elevated triglycerides
  • May cause gallstones (transplant recipients already at increased
    risk for cholelithiasis)
  • Concurrent use with lovastatin and cyclosporine can cause rhab-
    domyolysis
  • May potentiate the effects of warfarin
  • Use with caution in diabetic patients; interacts with insulin and
    sulfonylureas

HMG-CoA Reductase Inhibitors
  • Can increase creatine kinase level and cause myositis and rhab-
    domyolysis, especially in patients taking other medications that are
    metabolized by the cytochrome p450 system
  • Cyclosporine inhibits the metabolism of lovastatin

All Agents
  • Monitor LFTs, particularly when patient begins medication and
    any time dose is increased

HMG CoA = 3-hydroxy-3-methylglutaryl coenzyme A
LDL = low-density lipoproteins
LFT = liver function tests
Source: Blum & Aravot, 1996; Lake, 1996

Prevalence of osteoporosis

- Significant bone loss occurs in almost 100% of heart transplant recipients and can be severe during the first 6 to 12 months (Brann et al., 1998).
- The rate of bone loss can approach 20% during the first posttransplant year. Both lumbar and hip regions are involved.
- The prevalence rate for vertebral fractures ranges from 18% to 50% (Epstein, Shane, & Bilezikian, 1995).
- Osteoporosis has been reported in up to 50% of heart transplant recipients on long-term steroid therapy (Wagoner, 1997).

Etiology of osteoporosis

- Immunosuppressant therapy, particularly with glucocorticoids, cyclosporine, or tacrolimus, is the main factor that is associated with the development of osteoporosis
- Steroid therapy affects both bone resorption and formation (Epstein et al., 1995).
- Other contributing factors include older age, renal failure, and postmenopausal status in women (Wagoner, 1997).

Clinical manifestations of osteoporosis

Common clinical manifestations include

- Back pain
- Vertebral compression fractures
- Avascular necrosis of weight-bearing joints

Diagnostic tests

Tests to diagnose posttransplant osteoporosis typically include

- Bone mineral density measurements (baseline, then every 6 months for first 18 months, then annually)
- Radiograph of spine
- Blood tests (calcium, phosphate, vitamin D metabolites, intact parathyroid hormone, free or total testosterone [males], osteocalcin)
- Urine tests (calcium, collagen breakdown products: D-pyridinoline and N-telopeptides) (Epstein et al., 1995).

Prevention and treatment

Preventive therapy should begin immediately after transplantation and should continue for at least 1 year (Shane et al., 1997). It is important to diagnose and treat any underlying disorders that may also affect bone and mineral metabolism. Many transplant programs will reduce or discontinue steroid therapy provided that the recipient does not experience rejection. Other therapies include

- Weight-bearing exercise
- Smoking cessation
- Supplemental calcium (1 to 2 grams per day)
- Vitamin D supplements (400–800 IU daily; monitor patient for hypercalciuria and hypercalcemia)
- Substitution of hydrochlorothiazide for loop diuretics
- Antiresorptive agents (calcitonin, biphosphonates, estrogens [if not contraindicated])
- Agents to increase bone formation (sodium fluoride, parathyroid hormone)
- Testosterone (Epstein et al., 1995)

Diabetes Mellitus

Prevalence of DM

- Recent data indicate that posttransplant DM occurs in 20% and 16% of heart transplant recipients at 1- and 5-year follow-up, respectively (Hosenpud et al., 2000).

Etiology of DM

The development of DM results from a reduction in the action and secretion of insulin.

- Glucocorticoids increase insulin resistance.
- Cyclosporine is also known to be toxic to beta cells and can decrease insulin production. However, this effect may only be clinically manifested in patients with prior decreased beta cell reserve or increased insulin resistance.
- Unlike glucocorticoids, cyclosporine-induced DM is not dose dependent (Depczynski, Daly, Campbell, Chisholm, & Keogh, 2000).
- Newer immunosuppressive agents, such as tacrolimus, may also be diabetogenic.

Management of DM

Insulin-dependent transplant candidates may require a three- to fourfold increase in insulin following transplantation. Hyperinsulinemia is a contributing factor to the development of CAV; therefore, strict control of posttransplant DM is essential.

Renal Insufficiency

Nephrotoxicity is a common side effect of cyclosporine and tacrolimus therapy.

Prevalence of renal insufficiency

- Recent data on 55,359 heart transplant recipients indicate that 12% and 13% of these patients had renal dysfunction at 1- and 5-year follow-up, respectively.
- Serum creatinine levels above 2.5 mg/dL occurred in 7.5% and 8.5% of recipients at 1- and 5-year follow-up, respectively.
- Approximately 1% of these patients were on chronic dialysis at 1 year posttransplant.
- Two percent were on dialysis at 5 years posttransplant (Hosenpud et al, 2000).

Etiology of renal insufficiency

As with many posttransplant morbidities, the pathogenesis of renal insufficiency is multifactorial and not completely understood.

- Cyclosporine causes renal vasoconstriction of the afferent arterioles; this vasoconstriction subsequently leads to increased renal vascular resistance, decreased renal plasma flow and glomerular filtration rate, and chronic ischemia—all of which result in renal fibrosis.
- The direct tubular toxicity of cyclosporine is a secondary pathogenic mechanism (Richenbacher & Hunt, 1996).

Clinical manifestations of renal insufficiency

- The development of renal insufficiency often follows a biphasic pattern:
- During the first 6 months, renal function declines rapidly. This rapid decline is followed by a gradual improvement and eventual stabi-

lization of serum creatinine levels. This plateau is associated with a reduction in cyclosporine dose over time.
- With long-term follow-up, a second, more gradual and progressive decline in renal function has been noted in recipients who are 7 to 8 years posttransplant (Sehgal, Radhakrishnan, Appel, Valeri, & Cohen, 1995).

In addition to elevated serum creatinine levels, other clinical manifestations of renal dysfunction include

- Reduced creatinine clearance
- Disproportionate azotemia
- Hyperkalemia
- Increased serum uric acid levels
- Proteinuria
- Decreased sodium excretion
- Hypertension
- Fluid retention (Miller et al., 1993; Rickenbacher & Hunt, 1996)

Management of renal insufficiency

Strategies to limit the progressive decline in renal function include the following:

- Monitor and adjust trough cyclosporine or tacrolimus levels carefully to keep them within a therapeutic but not toxic range.
- Avoid drugs that alter cyclosporine levels and/or potentiate nephrotoxicity, for example, aminoglycosides, erythromycin, ketoconazole, and nonsteroidal anti-inflammatory drugs (see Chapter 4).
- If drugs with additive nephrotoxicity cannot be avoided, monitor cyclosporine or tacrolimus levels and renal function before, during, and after these drugs are administered; call transplant center for adjustments in cyclosporine dose (Parameshwar, 1996; Richenbacher & Hunt, 1996).

Malignancy

Prolonged immunosuppressive therapy after transplantation is associated with an increased risk of malignancy. The overall risk of de novo malignant tumors among heart transplant recipients ranges from 3% to 9% (mean: 6%) (Penn, 1993a). This risk is 100 times higher than in a matched general population (Pham et al., 1995). Malignancy is among the common causes of mortality after the first posttransplant year (other causes of mortality include cardiac allograft vasculopathy, nonspecific graft failure, and infection) (Hosenpud et al., 2000).

According to the Cincinnati Transplant Tumor Registry (CTTR) data, the most frequently occurring types of malignancies in heart transplant recipients (in descending order) are lymphomas, skin and lip, lung, Karposi's sarcoma, head/neck, colon/rectum, kidney, prostate, and hepatobiliary tumors (Penn, 1993a).

Prevalence of malignancy

- Recent data indicate that the incidence of malignancy among heart transplant recipients at 1- and 5-year follow-up is 4% and 10%, respectively.
- Skin cancer occurred in 35% and 52% of recipients at 1 and 5 years, respectively.
- Lymphomas occurred in 28% and 15% of recipients at 1 and 5 years, respectively (Hosenpud et al., 2000).
- Neoplasms that are most common in the general population, such as tumors of the lung, breast, and colon, do not occur more frequently in heart transplant recipients (Blum & Aravot, 1996).

Diagnosis of malignancy

- Transplant recipients should obtain regular screening tests as recommended by the American Cancer Society.
- Carcinoembryonic antigen markers are useful for detecting lung and colon cancer (Nagele, Bahlo, Klapdor, & Rodiger, 1999).
- Many transplant centers recommend yearly chest radiographs. However, lung tumors often have rapid doubling times, and this routine surveillance may not be adequate for the early diagnosis of lung cancer. Lung lesions may not be immediately obvious and radiographic abnormalities in this population may be initially attributed to an infectious process rather than a neoplastic process. Requisitions for chest radiographs should include the patient's transplant history, smoking history, and current smoking status (Goldstein et al., 1996).

Posttransplant Lymphoproliferative Disease

Primary infection with EBV is a significant risk factor for posttransplant lymphoproliferative disease (PTLD) (Wagoner, 1997). The incidence of PTLD is approximately 10% among heart transplant recipients who have received antilymphocyte antirejection therapy while on triple immuno-suppressants (Rubin, 1994). PTLD typically develops 8 to 18 months post-transplant; it occurs most frequently within the abdomen (including bowel involvement). Diffuse involvement of nodal and extranodal tissue is common. It less frequently involves the CNS (Wagoner, 1997).

Clinical manifestations of PTLD may include

- Fever of unknown origin
- Mononucleosis-like syndrome of fever, malaise, and lymphadenopathy (with or without tonsillitis or pharyngitis)
- GI symptoms: bleeding, abdominal pain, diarrhea, obstruction, perforation
- Weight loss
- Night sweats
- Upper respiratory infection
- Hepatocellular dysfunction
- CNS dysfunction: seizures, focal neurologic disease, change in state of consciousness.
- Infiltration of cardiac allograft (Penn, 1993b; Rubin, 1994).

Management of PTLD

Management of PTLD remains controversial. Treatment options include reduction in immunotherapy coupled with more frequent biopsies, high-dose acylovir or ganciclovir, anti-B-cell monoclonal antibody, interferon-alpha with intravenous IgG, or chemotherapy. Radiotherapy or surgery may be indicated for localized disease (Rubin, 1994).

Cutaneous Neoplasms

Cutaneous malignancy is associated with the use of azathioprine, possibly because its metabolite, nitromidazole, enhances photosensitivity. Azathioprine is also associated with more metastatic disease (Miller et al., 1993). Cutaneous neoplasms in transplant recipients differ from those in the general population in the following respects:

- Squamous cell carcinomas (SCCs) outnumber basal cell carcinomas by almost 2:1 (possibly related to an immunosuppression-mediated change in papillovirus-induced warts)
- Skin cancer in transplant recipients occurs at a much younger age.
- The incidence of multiple skin cancers is significantly higher.
- SCCs are more aggressive and metastatic in transplant recipients (Penn, 1993a, 1993b).

Management of skin neoplasms includes surgical excision, cryosurgery, and radiotherapy. Prevention of skin cancer is extremely important. Heart transplant recipients are advised to

- Avoid undue exposure to sunlight.
- Avoid tanning beds.
- Wear wide-brimmed hats, sun visors, and protective clothing.
- Use a sunscreen that filters out ultraviolet-B rays.
- Have a yearly checkup with a dermatologist.
- Obtain prompt treatment of any premalignant or malignant skin lesions.

GASTROINTESTINAL DISORDERS

Common posttransplant gastrointestinal (GI) complications include upper GI lesions (gastritis, esophagitis, duodenitis), biliary tract disease, and pancreatitis (Table 6.12). Administration of glucocorticoid therapy is associated with GI irritation and hemorrhage. Antisecretory compounds and H_2 histamine receptor antagonists are frequently prescribed for the first 6 to 12 months posttransplant.

Biliary Tract Disease

Prevalence

- Biliary tract disease is the most common posttransplant GI problem, with an incidence that ranges between 1% and 17% (Begos et al., 1995).

TABLE 6.12 Key Points: GI Complications

- Steroid therapy may mask clinical manifestations such as leukocytosis, abdominal guarding, and rebound.

- Subtle symptoms may belie the actual severity of the disease.

- An attack of acute cholecystitis that rapidly progresses to a septic crisis may be the first manifestation of gallstone disease.

- Cyclosporine cholestasis is associated mainly with an elevated serum bilirubin level.

- Aggressive management of GI complications is essential.

Source: Begos et al., 1995; Lord et al., 1998; Miller et al., 1993

Predisposing factors

- The most important predisposing factor is the effect of cyclosporine on bile metabolism.
- Other contributing factors include DM, older age, female gender, use of cholelithogenic antihyperlipidemic agents, steroid-induced obesity, perioperative ischemia, and gallbladder dysmotility due to vagotomy (Miller et al., 1993; Vega, Pina, & Krevsky, 1996; Wagoner, 1997).

Cholelithiasis that involves the common bile duct has higher morbidity and mortality than gallbladder cholelithiasis alone (Begos et al., 1995). Both minilaparotomy and laparoscopy have been safely used to treat gallstone disease in heart transplant recipients. Higher morbidity and mortality are associated with urgent rather than elective cholecystectomy (Lord, Ho, Coleman, & Spratt, 1998; Wagoner, 1997).

Pancreatitis

Pancreatitis occurs in 2% to 18% of heart transplant recipients. Major contributing factors include perioperative hypoperfusion, preexisting disease, and the use of azathioprine (Wagoner, 1997).

REDUCED EXERCISE TOLERANCE

The physiology of the transplanted heart differs from that of the innervated heart. Explantation of the native heart results in severance of sympathetic and parasympathetic fibers; however, beta-adrenergic receptors are intact. Lack of parasympathetic innervation causes a higher resting HR (approximately 100 beats per minute). Increases in HR, conduction, and contractility are mediated by circulating catecholamines, rather than reflex tachycardia (Augustine & Masiello-Miller, 1995; Ohler et al., 1994).

Some heart transplant recipients can achieve extremely high levels of exercise activity. However, when compared to age-, gender-, and body habitus–matched controls, many recipients may have impaired maximal exercise tolerance (Mills, 1994). Mean VO_{2max} for heart transplant recipients is typically 55% to 60% of predicted VO_{2max} values (Braith, 1998). Proposed mechanisms associated with this phenomenon include pretransplant deconditioning, chronotropic incompetence, diastolic dysfunction, glucocorticoid-induced myopathy, abnormalities in peripheral oxygen uptake or use, and arterial desaturation caused by elevated left heart filling pressures that interfere with ventilation (Braith, 1998; Johnson, 1995; Mills, 1994).

Important considerations relative to exercise include the following:

- Beta-blockers should be used cautiously because they can increase exercise intolerance.
- Transplant recipients require prolonged warm-up and cool-down periods.
- Formal outpatient cardiac rehabilitation programs can help heart transplant recipients improve peripheral oxygen use and increase their exercise tolerance.
- Exercise training should be temporarily suspended if rejection episodes require enhanced glucocorticoid therapy (Johnson, 1995; Braith, 1998).

WHEN TO CALL TRANSPLANT CENTER

As a consequence of managed care, primary care providers (PCPs) are becoming increasingly more involved with the management of the heart transplant recipient (Wagoner, 1997). The transplant center will continue to routinely see the patient for surveillance endomyocardial biopsies and laboratory tests, but problems such as hypertension, simple infections, hyperlipidemia, and osteoporosis are frequently managed by the PCP and/or consultants. Although this team approach can be successful, there are certain indications for which the transplant center should be consulted:

- Requirement for medications that may interact with immunosuppressive agents
- Suspected allograft rejection
- Allograft dysfunction
- New onset or exacerbation of renal failure
- Fever of unknown origin
- Complicated infections, especially CMV and fungal infections
- Recurrent simple infections
- Cardiac events: myocardial infarction, syncope, arrhythmias, sudden death
- Suspected major abdominal disease
- Malignancy other than cutaneous carcinoma
- Anticipated (e.g., perioperative) intolerance of oral medications and substitution of intravenous immunosuppressants
- Noncompliance (Wagoner, 1997)

Transplant centers usually prefer to manage the recipient's immuno-suppressants. Because of third-party payer constraints, however, cyclosporine levels may have to be drawn at contract laboratories that use different assays to measure drug levels (whole blood vs. serum; fluorescent poly-clonal immunoassay vs. high-performance liquid chromatography). When possible, the transplant team may request that blood samples be sent to the transplant center so that a consistent assay methodology is used.

Over the course of the oftentimes lengthy pretransplant waiting period and during the posttransplant recovery period, transplant center personnel develop close relationships with their patients. Transplant teams are most willing to answer questions regarding the care of their patients and to collaborate with community providers to achieve optimal outcomes.

REFERENCES

Achuff, S. C. (1990). Clinical evaluation of potential heart transplant recipients. In W. A. Baumgartner, B. A. Reitz, & S. C. Achuff (Eds.), *Heart and heart–lung transplantation* (pp. 51–57). Philadelphia: W. B. Saunders.

Anderson, H. O. (1999). Heart allograft vascular disease: An obliterative vascular disease in transplanted hearts. *Atherosclerosis, 142,* 243–263.

Augustine, S. M., Baumgartner, W. A., & Kasper, E. K. (1998). Obesity and hyper-cholesterolemia following heart transplantation. *Journal of Transplant Coordination, 8*(3), 164–169.

Augustine, S. M., & Masiello-Miller, M. M. (1995). Heart transplantation. In M. T. Nolan & S. M. Augustine (Eds.), *Transplantation nursing: Acute and long-term management* (pp. 109–140). Norwalk, CT: Appleton & Lange.

Barnard, C. N. (1968). What have we learned about heart transplantation? *Journal of Thoracic and Cardiovascular Surgery, 56*(4), 457–468.

Baumgartner, W. A. (1990). Operative techniques utilized in heart transplantation. In W. A. Baumgartner, B. A. Reitz, & S. C. Achuff (Eds.), *Heart and heart-lung transplantation* (pp. 113–133). Philadelphia: W. B. Saunders.

Begos, D. G., Franco, K. L., Baldwin, J. C., Lee, F. A., Revkin, J. H., & Modlin, I. M. (1995). Optimal timing and indications for cholecystectomy in cardiac transplant patients. *World Journal of Surgery, 19,* 661–667.

Billingham, M. E. (1981). Diagnosis of cardiac rejection by endomyocardial biopsy. *Heart Transplantation, 1*(1), 25–30.

Billingham, M. E., Cary, N. R., Hammond, M. E., Kemnitz, J., Marobe, C., McCallister, H. A., Snovar, D. C., Winters, G. L. & Zerbe, A. (1990). A working formulation for the standardization of nomenclature in the diagnosis of heart and lung rejection: Heart rejection study group. *Journal of Heart and Lung Transplantation, 9,* 587–593.

Blum, A., & Aravot, D. (1996). Heart transplantation: An update. *Clinical Cardiology, 19,* 930–938.

Braith, R. W. (1998). Exercise training in patients with CHF and heart transplant recipients. *Medicine and Science in Sports & Exercise, 30*(10), S367–S378.

Brann, W. M., Bennett, L. E., Keck, B. M., & Hosenpud, J. D. (1998). Morbidity, functional status, and immunosuppressive therapy after heart transplantation: An analysis of the Joint International Society for Heart and Lung Transplantation/United Network for Organ Sharing Thoracic Registry. *Journal of Heart and Lung Transplantation, 17*(4), 374–382.

Conraads, V., LaHaye, I., Rademakers, F, Heuten, H., Rodrigus, I., Vrints, C., & Moulijn, A. (1998). Cardiac graft vasculopathy: Aetiologic factors and therapeutic approaches. *Acta Cardiologia, 1,* 37–43.

Conte, J. V. (1998). Thoracic transplantation in 1998. *Maryland Medical Journal, 47,* 235–240.

Costanza, M. R. (1996). Selection and treatment of candidates for heart transplantation. *Seminars in Thoracic and Cardiovascular Surgery, 8,* 113–125.

Costanza, M. R., Augustine, S., Bourge, R., Bristow, M., O'Connell, J. B., Driscoll, D., & Rose, E. (1995). Selection and treatment of candidates for heart transplantation: A statement for health professionals from the Committee on Heart Failure and Cardiac Transplantation of the Council on Clinical Cardiology, American Heart Association. *Circulation, 92,* 3593–3612.

Cross, A. M., & Stevenson, L. W. (1998). Pre-transplant evaluation of the recipient. In D. J. Norman & W. N. Suki (Eds.), *Primer on transplantation* (pp. 409–417). Thorofare, NJ: American Society of Transplant Physicians.

Cupples, S. A., & Spruill, L. C. (2000). Evaluation criteria for the pretransplant patient. *Critical Care Nursing Clinics of North America, 12*(1), 35–47.

Depczynski, B., Daly, B., Campbell, L. V., Chisholm, J., & Keogh, A. (2000). Predicting the occurrence of diabetes mellitus in recipients of heart transplants. *Diabetic Medicine, 17,* 15–19.

Dong, C., Redenbach, D., Wood, S., Battistini, B., Wilson, J. E., & McManus, B. M. (1996). The pathogenesis of cardiac allograft vasculopathy. *Current Opinion in Cardiology, 11,* 183–190.

Duke, S. A., & Perna, J. (1999). The ventricular assist device as a bridge to cardiac transplantation. *AACN Clinical Issues, 10*(2), 2217–2228.

Dyke, D. B. S., Pagani, F. D., & Aaronson, K. D. (2000). Circulatory assist devices 2000: An update. *Congestive Heart Failure, 6,* 259–271.

Epstein, S., Shane, E., & Bilezikian, J. P. (1995). Organ transplantation and osteoporosis. *Current Opinion in Rheumatology, 7*(3), 255–261.

Frantz, R. P., & Olson L. J. (1997). Recipient selection and management before cardiac transplantation. *American Journal of the Medical Sciences, 314,* 139–152.

Goldstein, D. J., Austin, J. H., Zuech, N., Williams, D. L., Stoopler, M. B., Michler, R. E., & Schulman, L. L. (1996). Carcinoma of the lung after heart transplantation. *Transplantation, 62*(6), 772–775.

Grady, K. L. (1996). When to transplant: Recipient selection for heart transplantation. *Journal of Cardiovascular Nursing, 10,* 58–70.

Grady, K. L., Costanzo-Nordin, M. R., Herold, L. S., Sriniavasan, S., & Pifarre, R. (1991). Obesity and hyperlipidemia after heart transplantation. *Journal of Heart and Lung Transplantation, 10*(3), 449–454.

Hauser, R. G., & Kallinen, L. M. (1996). Implantable cardioverter defibrillator as a bridge to transplantation. In R. W. Emery & L. W. Miller (Eds.), *Handbook of cardiac transplantation* (pp. 11–16). Philadelphia: Hanley & Belfus.

Hosenpud, J. D., Bennett, L. E., Keck, B. M., Boucek, M. M., & Novick, R. H. (2000). The registry of the International Society for Heart and Lung Transplantation: Seventeenth official report—2000. *Journal of Heart and Lung Transplantation, 19*(10), 909–931.

Johnson, M. R. (1995). Clinical follow-up of the heart transplant recipient. *Current Opinion in Cardiology, 10,* 180–192.

Kao, W., Winkel, E., & Costanzo, M. R. (1995). Candidate evaluation and selection for heart transplantation. *Current Opinion in Cardiology, 10,* 159–168.

Kubo, S. H., Peters, J. A., Knutson, K. R., Hertz, M. I., Olivari, M. T., Bolman, R. M., & Hunninghake, D. B. (1992). Factors influencing the development of hypercholesterolemia after cardiac transplantation. *American Journal of Cardiology, 70,* 520–526.

Lake, K. L. (1996). Management of posttransplant obesity and hyperlipidemia. In R. W. Emery & L. W. Miller (Eds.), *Handbook of cardiac transplantation* (pp.147–164). Philadelphia: Hanley & Belfus.

Laks, H., Scholl, F. G., Drinkwater, D. C., Blitz, A., Hamilton, M., Moriguchi, J., Fonarow, G., & Kobashigawa, J. (1997). The alternative recipient list for heart transplantation: Does it work? *Journal of Heart and Lung Transplantation, 16*(7), 735–742.

Lavee, J., Kormos, R. L., Duquesnoy, R. J., Zerbe, T. R., Armitage, J. M., Vanek, M., Hardesty, R. L., & Griffith, B. P. (1991). Influence of panel-reactive antibody and lymphocytotoxic crossmatch on survival after heart transplantation. *Journal of Heart and Lung Transplantation, 10,* 921–928.

Lloveras, J. J., Escourrou, G., Delisle, M. B., Fournial, G., Cerene, A., Bassanetti, I., & Durand, D. (1992). Evolution of untreated mild rejection in heart transplant recipients. *Journal of Heart and Lung Transplantation, 11*(4, Pt. 1), 751–756.

Lord, R. V. N., Ho, S., Coleman, M. J., & Spratt, P. M. (1998). Cholecystectomy in cardiothoracic organ transplant recipients. *Archives of Surgery, 133,* 73–79.

Miller, L. W. (1998). Listing criteria for cardiac transplantation. *Transplantation, 66,* 947–951.

Miller, L. W., Donohue, T., & Wolford, T. L. (1996). Allograft coronary disease. In R. W. Emery & L. W. Miller (Eds.), *Handbook of cardiac transplantation* (pp. 135–139). Philadelphia: Hanley & Belfus.

Miller, L. W., Kubo, S. H., Young, J. B., Stevenson, L. W., Loh, E., & Costanzo, M. R. (1995). Medical management of heart and lung failure and candidate selection: Report of the Consensus Conference on Candidate Selection for Heart Transplantation—1993. *Journal of Heart and Lung Transplantation, 14*(3), 562–571.

Miller, L. W., Schlant, R. C., Kobashigawa, J., Kubo, S., & Renlund, D. G. (1993). 24th Bethesda conference on cardiac transplantation: Task Force 5—complications. *Journal of the American College of Cardiology, 22,* 41–54.

Miller, L. W., Wolford, T. L., & Donohue, T. (1996). Nonspecific graft dysfunction in cardiac transplantation. In R. W. Emery & L. W. Miller (Eds.), *Handbook of cardiac transplantation* (pp. 129–133). Philadelphia: Hanley & Belfus.

Mills, R. M., Jr. (1994). Transplantation and problems afterward including coronary vasculopathy. *Clinical Cardiology, 17,* 287–290.

Morales, D. L. S., Catanese, K. A., Helman, D. N., Williams, M. R., Weinberg, A., Goldstein, D. J., Rose, E. A., & Oz, M. C. (2000). Six-year experience of caring for forty-four patients with a left ventricular assist device at home: Safe, economical, necessary. *Journal of Thoracic and Cardiovascular Surgery, 119,* 251–259.

Mudge, G. H., Goldstein, S., Addonizio, L. J., Caplan, A., Mancini, D., Levine, T. B., Ritsch, M. E., & Stevenson, L. W. (1993). 24th Bethesda conference on cardiac transplantation: Task Force 3—recipient guidelines. *Journal of the American College of Cardiology, 22,* 21–30.

Nagele, H., Bahlo, M., Klapdor, R., & Rodiger, W. (1999). Tumor marker determination after heart transplantation. *Journal of Heart and Lung Transplantation, 18,* 957–962.

Ohler, L., Morris, K. H., McCauley, M. F., & DiSanto, P. (1994). Cardiac transplantation: A review for critical care nurses. *Journal of Intensive Care Medicine, 9,* 211–226.

Olbrisch, M. E., & Levenson, J. L. (1991). Psychosocial evaluation of heart transplant candidates: An international survey of process, criteria and outcomes. *Journal of Heart and Lung Transplantation, 10,* 948–955.

Olivari, M. T. (1996). Cardiac transplantation: Current indications, short- and long-term results, economic implications, and future developments. *Journal of Cardiac Failure, 2,* 141–152.

Parameshwar, J. (1996). Follow-up after cardiac transplantation. *British Journal of Hospital Medicine, 56*(7), 350–354.

Penn, I. (1993a). Incidence and treatment of neoplasia after transplantation. *Journal of Heart and Lung Transplantation, 12,* S328–S336.

Penn, I. (1993b). Tumors after renal and cardiac transplantation. *Hematology/Oncology Clinics of North America, 7*(2), 431–445.

Pham S. M., Kormos, R. L., Landreneau, R. J., Kawai, A., Gonzalez-Cancel, I., Hardesty, R. L., Hattler, B. G., & Griffith, B. P. (1995). Solid tumors after heart transplantation: Lethality of lung cancer. *Annals of Thoracic Surgery, 60,* 1623–1626.

Piccione, W., Jr. (2000). Left ventricular assist device implantation: Short- and long-term surgical complications. *Journal of Heart and Lung Transplantation, 19,* S89–S94.

Rickenbacher, P. R., & Hunt, S. A. (1996). Long-term complications of transplantation. In R. W. Emery & L. W. Miller (Eds.), *Handbook of cardiac transplantation* (pp. 201–216). Philadelphia: Hanley & Belfus.

Rourke, T. K., Droogan, M. T., & Ohler, L. (1999). Heart transplantation: State of the art. *AACN Clinical Issues, 10*(2), 185–201.

Rubin, R. H. (1994). Infection in the organ transplant recipient. In R. H. Rubin & L. S. Young (Eds.), *Clinical approach to infection in the compromised host* (3rd ed., pp. 629–705). New York: Plenum.

Sehgal, V., Radhakrishnan, J., Appel, G. B., Valeri, A., & Cohen, D. J. (1995). Progressive renal insufficiency following cardiac transplantation: Cyclosporine, lipids, and hypertension. *American Journal of Kidney Diseases, 26*(1), 193–201.

Shane, E., Rivas, M., McMahon, D. J., Staron, R. B., Silverberg, S. J., Seibel, M. J., Mancini, D., Michler, R. E., Aaronson, K., Addesso, V., & Lo, S. H., (1997). Bone loss and turnover after cardiac transplantation. *Journal of Clinical Endocrinology and Metabolism, 82,* 1497–1506.

Singer, D. R. J., & Jenkins, G. H. (1996). Hypertension in transplant recipients. *Journal of Human Hypertension, 10,* 395–402.

Smart, F. W., Naftel, D. C., Costanzo, M. R., Levine, T. B., Pelletier, G. B., Yancy, C. W., Hobbs, R. E., Kirklin, J. K., & Bourge, R. C. (1996). Risk factors for early, cumulative, and fatal infections after heart transplantation: A multiinstitutional study. *Journal of Heart and Lung Transplantation, 15*(4), 329–341.

Thaler, S. J., & Rubin, R. H. (1996). Opportunistic infections in the cardiac transplant patient. *Current Opinion in Cardiology, 11,* 191–203.

Tolman, D. E., Taylor, D. O., Olsen, S. L., Karwande, S. V., & Renlund, D. G. (1995). Heart transplantation. In L. Makowa & L. Sher (Eds.). *Handbook of organ transplantation* (pp. 107–131). Austin, TX: Landes.

United Network for Organ Sharing. (2001). *Critical data: Waiting list.* Retrieved January 19, 2002, from http:// www.unos.org/Newsroom/critdata_wait.htm

Vega, K. J., Pina, I., & Krevsky, B. (1996). Heart transplantation is associated with an increased risk for pancreaticobiliary disease. *Annals of Internal Medicine, 124*(11), 980–983.

Wagoner, L. E. (1997). Management of the cardiac transplant recipient: Roles of the transplant cardiologist and primary care physician. *American Journal of the Medical Sciences, 314*(3), 173–184.

Weis, M., & von Scheidt, W. (1997). Cardiac allograft vasculopathy: A review. *Circulation, 96,* 2069–2077.

Yamani, M. H., & Starling, R. C. (2000). Long-term medical complications of heart transplantation: Information for the primary care physician. *Cleveland Clinic Journal of Medicine, 67*(9), 673–680.

7

Kidney Transplantation

Marilyn Rossman Bartucci
and Donald E. Hricik

As recently as the late 1960s, little hope was available for patients with end-stage renal disease (ESRD). Only a few kidney transplants were performed and a small number of patients were being maintained on chronic dialysis. In the early 1970s, Medicare entitlement legislation provided equal access to dialysis and transplantation for all patients in the Social Security system and led to a rapid expansion of ESRD care in the United States.

Despite increased knowledge and skill in the management of ESRD, the most efficient hemodialysis techniques used today provide only 10% to 12% of the small solute removal of two normal kidneys and considerably less removal of larger solutes. Patients on dialysis often have impaired quality of life, dependence on others, poor rehabilitation, and depressed sexual function, which contribute to physical and emotional disabilities that may persist even in well-dialyzed patients with ESRD.

Despite ever-improving health care and new advances in medical technology, the number of Americans with ESRD continues to increase. Although there is some debate about when a patient with renal insufficiency should be referred to nephrology, studies have shown the earlier the referral, the better the outcome. Diabetes remains the leading cause of new cases (42%), followed by hypertension (26%) and glomerulonephritis (11%). There are currently more than 233,000 patients who require dialysis in the United States (United States Renal Data System, [USRDS], 1998).

ESRD TREATMENT OPTIONS

The three treatment options for ESRD are hemodialysis, peritoneal dialysis, and transplantation.

HEMODIALYSIS

- Hemodialysis can be performed in medical facilities specifically designed for this purpose or in the patient's home.
- It requires the creation of a permanent vascular access.
- Treatments range from 2 to 5 hours, 3 times a week.
- During dialysis, solutes are removed by diffusion across a semipermeable membrane.
- Fluid removal is achieved by adjusting the transmembrane pressure across the dialyzer usually by generating negative pressure in the dialysate compartment. Modern hemodialysis machines contain volumetrically controlled ultrafiltration systems that ensure accurate, programmable fluid removal during the treatment.
- Intermittent systemic heparinization is required to prevent clotting in the extracorporeal circuit.
- Dialysis is generally well tolerated, although ultrafiltration is at times associated with
  - Hypotension
  - Nausea
  - Muscle cramps
  - Postdialysis fatigue and malaise (due to the intermittent nature of this therapy)
  - Vascular access failure from clotting and decreased blood flow

PERITONEAL DIALYSIS

- Peritoneal dialysis depends on the fluid and solute transport characteristics of the peritoneal membrane. It can be performed as either continuous ambulatory peritoneal dialysis (CAPD) or continuous cycling peritoneal dialysis (CCPD).

- Access to the peritoneal cavity is achieved by the surgical placement of a Tenckhoff catheter through the abdominal wall.
- The dialysis procedure consists of instilling 1,500 to 3,000 mL of dialysate into the abdomen by gravity, letting the fluid dwell, then draining and discarding it.
- During the dwell period, solute removal and fluid ultrafiltration take place.
- The advantages of peritoneal dialysis include
  - Maintenance of steady-state blood chemistries
  - Higher hematocrit levels
  - Better blood pressure control
  - More liberal diet
  - Greater patient independence
  - No systemic anticoagulation requirement
- The major complication of peritoneal dialysis is peritonitis.

KIDNEY TRANSPLANTATION

Kidney transplantation offers the greatest potential for the full return of a healthy, productive life. In addition, recent analyses of registry data indicate that transplantation offers a distinct advantage over dialysis-based renal replacement therapies (Wolfe et al., 1999). The first human-to-human kidney transplant was performed in 1936. It was unsuccessful because rejection and the role of immunosuppression were not clearly understood. Major advances have been made in kidney transplantation since the first successful operation was performed in 1954 in Boston between identical twins. The advances made in organ procurement and preservation, surgical technique, tissue typing and matching, understanding the immune system, and preventing and treating rejection have led to 1-year patient and graft survival rates of 96% and 90%, respectively (UNOS, 2000).

With success comes greater demand. The number of patients waiting for kidneys has continued to increase, whereas the number of kidney transplants performed each year has remained fairly constant. At the end of December 2000, there were 44,824 patients awaiting kidneys for transplantation. In 1999, there were 12,518 kidney transplants performed in the United States (UNOS, 2000). Because the waiting list is so long, minimum listing criteria have been implemented. Any patient undergoing renal replacement therapy may be listed providing they are medically suitable for transplantation. Patients not receiving renal replacement therapy may not be listed for cadaveric kidney transplant until the creatinine clearance is ≤ 20 mL/minute.

EVALUATION OF THE POTENTIAL KIDNEY TRANSPLANT CANDIDATE

The purpose of the pretransplant evaluation process is to identify and treat all coexisting medical problems that may increase the morbidity and mortality rates and adversely impact the posttransplant course. The physiologic and psychosocial parameters considered in the evaluation of the potential kidney transplant candidate are listed in Table 7.1. Contraindications to kidney transplantation are listed in Table 7.2.

AGE

- The upper age limit beyond which patients are no longer accepted for transplantation is arbitrary.
- Older patients are not at a significantly increased risk of posttransplant morbidity as long as they do not have significant cardiovascular disease and their general medical evaluation is unremarkable.
- Most transplant centers, however, are reluctant to transplant patients over the age of 70 in the absence of superb extrarenal health.

OBESITY

- Most studies suggest that severe obesity is an independent risk factor for decreased long-term renal allograft survival (Pirsch et al., 1995).
- Obese patients are at greater risk for postoperative wound complications and pulmonary infections.
- The long-term risks of cardiovascular disease secondary to hyperlipidemia and hypertension are compounded by obesity.
- Many transplant centers will recommend specific weight reduction parameters before the patient can be listed for transplantation.

CARE OF THE RENAL TRANSPLANT CANDIDATE

- Waiting time: In general, candidates with blood types A and AB typically have a 1- to 2-year wait for a cadaveric kidney. Those with blood types B and O have a 3- to 5-year wait. However, there is marked geographic variability in these average waiting times.
- Periodic reassessment: Because of the long waiting time, candidates should be reevaluated on an annual basis to make certain they are

TABLE 7.1 (*continued*)

Assessment	Rationale
Hepatobiliary tests • Liver function tests with coagulation profile • Hepatitis B and C serologies • Ultrasonography of gallbladder*	Hepatobiliary complications • Hepatitis B and C are the most common etiologic agents in long-term dialysis patients, especially if the patient has received multiple blood transfusions • Most patients with Hepatitis B or C are asymptomatic • Most ESRD patients with serologic evidence of hepatitis C have normal liver function tests (Rosen, Friedman, & Martin, 1996) • Drug toxicity and alcohol abuse may contribute to liver dysfunction and may present in combination with viral hepatitis • Hepatomegaly does not necessarily indicate primary liver disease, but may reflect chronic, passive liver congestion associated with fluid overload or cardiac disease
Genitourinary tests • Urinalysis, urine culture (if patient is still making urine) • Voiding cystourethrogram* • Cystometrics* • Gynecologic examination, including • Papanicolaou's smear, for females who are sexually active or over 18 years of age • Prostate examination and prostate specific antigen test for males over 50 years of age • Mammogram*	Genitourinary complications • The lower urinary tract should be sterile and continent without urinary retention before transplantation • Pretransplant native nephrectomies are indicated for patients with ureteral reflux resulting in hydronephrosis or infection, polycystic kidney disease with grossly enlarged kidneys or frequently infected cysts, or severe uncontrolled hypertension

continued

TABLE 7.1 (*continued*)

Rationale	Assessment
Neurological complications • Patients with seizure disorders on anticonvulsant agents have an increased rate of metabolism of calcineurin inhibitors (cyclosporine and tacrolimus) • Pretransplant neurology consult is useful in determining whether anticonvulsant therapy is mandatory	Neurology consultation*
Immunologic data • All potential kidney transplant recipients are tissue typed to determine human leukocyte antigen (HLA) class 1 and class 2 loci; six HLA antigens are identified • Kidney donors are also HLA typed; the degree of incompatibility between donor and recipient is defined by the number of antigens that are mismatched at each HLA loci; there is mandatory sharing across the United States for all 6 antigen/0 mismatch kidneys • Lymphocytotoxic antibodies obtained from multiparous females or from recipients of multiple blood transfusions are used to determine the presence of preformed antibodies to HLA antigens; Results range from 0% to 100% and reflect the percentage of antigens on the test panel against which the potential recipient has preformed antibodies; the higher the panel reactive antibody (PRA) level, the more difficult it will be to find a donor to whom the potential recipient would have a negative T-cell cross-match	Immunologic tests • History of autoimmune disease, previous transplants, blood transfusions, pregnancy (in females) • Blood type • Human leukocyte antigen testing • Cytotoxic screening or panel reactive antibody testing • Lymphocyte cross-match with potential donor

continued

TABLE 7.1 (*continued*)

Rationale	Assessment
Immunization status • Because of their increased susceptibility to infection posttransplant, transplant candidates should have current immunizations	**Immunization status** • All immunizations current, including pneumonia vaccination (Pneumovax)® and Hepatitis B vaccination (Heptavax)®
Psychosocial assessment • Organic mental syndromes, psychosis, and severe mental retardation may seriously impair the patient's capacity to understand the entire transplant process and related complications • Patients addicted to alcohol or any other drug should enter and successfully complete a rehabilitation program before being placed on the waiting list • Chemical dependency counselor must clear patient for placement on the waiting list • There is a relationship between pretransplant noncompliance and posttransplant outcomes; When	**Psychosocial assessment** (history and emotional stability) • Patient and family's ability to cope with illness • Adjustment to and understanding of present illness • Support system (family, friends, significant others) • Preillness lifestyle • Work history • Education • Previous transplant experience (if any) • Expectations of transplantation

continued

TABLE 7.1 (*continued*)

Rationale	Assessment

compared with compliant recipients, noncompliant recipients have an increased mortality rate, more late acute rejection episodes, and lower graft survival rates (DeGeest et al., 1995; Douglas, Blixen, & Bartucci, 1996)
• Immunosuppressive agents and other medications can cost up to $20,000 per year. Although Medicare is often the primary payer for the kidney transplant procedure and related hospitalization, it only covers 80% of the cost of immunosuppressive medications for 44 months from the day of hospital discharge, unless the recipient remains disabled. After 44 months, the recipient is personally responsible for the entire cost of medications, unless he or she has a supplemental insurance policy that specifically covers prescriptions
• Financial counselors and social workers help patients develop a plan to ensure that medications can be obtained after transplantation
	• Chemical dependency (if any)
	  • Periodic random toxicology screening tests to assure that patients with prior chemical dependency remain alcohol/drug free
	• Noncompliance
	  • Some programs require a period of acceptable compliance with specific, measurable criteria as a condition for placement on the waiting list.
	• Financial/insurance status

* As indicated
CBC = complete blood count
ESRD = end-stage renal disease
INR = international normalized ratio
PA = posterior/anterior
PT = prothrombin time
PTT = partial thromboplastin time

TABLE 7.2 Relative Contraindications to Kidney Transplantation

- Reversible renal disease
- Recent malignancy
- Active infection
- Active systemic inflammatory disease (e.g., systemic lupus erythematosus)
- Uncorrectable cardiovascular disease
- Life expectancy < 1 year
- Sensitization to donor tissue
- Current psychosocial disorders that preclude compliance (e.g., substance abuse)

still medically suitable for transplantation. If medical problems occurred during the year, additional testing may be required. For those patients with a history of heart disease, noninvasive testing may be repeated at yearly intervals until transplantation.
- Communication with dialysis center: The dialysis center must be informed when a patient is listed for transplantation so monthly blood samples for cytotoxic antibody screening can be sent to the tissue typing laboratory.
- Communication with transplant center: Any change in the patient's health status must be reported to the transplant center by the patient, physician, or dialysis staff so suitability for transplantation can be reevaluated if necessary. A time-limited condition may require placing the patient in an inactive status on the list until the condition resolves.

TYPES OF DONORS

LIVING DONORS

Related donors may include a parent, sibling, child, grandparent, aunt, uncle, or cousin. Unrelated donors may include a spouse, in-law, adoptive parent or child, friend, significant other, anonymous, or "good Samaritan" donor.

Compared to cadaveric donors, the use of live donors

- Provides better patient and graft survival
- Permits transplantation to be performed electively at a time when the recipient is in optimal condition

- Reduces the complications of organ procurement and preservation thereby reducing the incidence of delayed graft function and nephrotoxicity from cyclosporine or tacrolimus
- Permits immunologic conditioning and initiation of immunosuppression before surgery
- Reduces the waiting period for transplantation
- Perhaps improves rehabilitation (Rosenthal & Danovitch, 1996)

In 1999, 4,487 live-donor kidney transplants were performed in the United States, accounting for approximately 36% of the total volume. Of these, 329 (16%) were from unrelated donors. From 1993 through 1999, kidney donation from biologically unrelated donors increased annually by 54% (UNOS, 2000). Ethical concerns about the use of living donors for kidney transplantation include the following:

- Subjecting a healthy person to the potential complications of an operation
- Loss of income if the donor is the primary wage earner in the family
- Unknown outcome for the recipient
- Guilt felt by the donor if the recipient dies (Caplan, 1993; Spital, 1997).

These implications for the donor must be weighed by the donor against the hope that living donation offers to the person with ESRD who is supported by long-term dialysis therapy. Respect for patient autonomy permits the donor to assume some risk if there is reasonable certainty that the donor's decision is informed, free from coercion, and truly autonomous. A psychosocial evaluation by a social worker, psychologist, or psychiatrist is an essential component of the live donor evaluation.

Exclusion criteria for living donors are listed in Table 7.3. Tests included in the medical assessment of the living donor are listed in Table 7.4.

CADAVERIC DONORS

Cadaveric kidney donors are previously healthy people who have had irreversible brain injury. The most common causes of injury are

- Cerebral trauma from motor vehicle accidents or gunshot wounds
- Intracerebral or subarachnoid hemorrhage
- Anoxic brain damage resulting from a drug overdose or cardiac arrest.

TABLE 7.3 Living Donors: Exclusion Criteria

- Age < 18 years or > 65 years of age
- Blood type incompatibility
- Positive T-cell cross-match with potential recipient
- Hypertension (> 140/90 or use of antihypertensive medications)
- Diabetes (abnormal glucose tolerance test or glycohemoglobin)
- Proteinuria (> 250 mg/24 hrs)
- History of kidney stones
- Abnormal glomerular filtration rate (creatinine clearance < 80 mL/min)
- Microscopic hematuria
- Urologic abnormalities in donor kidneys
- Significant medical illness (e.g., chronic lung disease, recent malignancy)
- Infectious disease (e.g. hepatitis B or C, HIV, syphilis)
- Obesity (30% above ideal weight)
- History of thrombosis or thromboembolism
- Psychosocial contraindication (e.g., substance abuse)

HIV = human immunodeficiency virus

Other important points:

- The donor in whom brain death has been declared must have effective cardiovascular function and must be supported on a ventilator to preserve organ viability.
- The age range of most suitable kidney donors is 2 to 70 years.
- The donor must be free of intravenous drug abuse, malignant disease, sepsis, and communicable diseases including human immunodeficiency virus, hepatitis B and C viruses, syphilis, and tuberculosis (Rosenthal & Danovitch, 1996).
- In some centers, hepatitis C virus (HCV) seropositive donor kidneys are used in recipients greater than 60 years (with the recipient's consent) or in recipients who are also HCV seropositive.

Patients who have been declared dead by traditional cardiopulmonary criteria (nonbeating heart) are another source of kidneys acceptable for transplantation. Recently, two methods for recovering kidneys from non-heart-beating donors have been implemented:

TABLE 7.4 Medical Assessment of Living Donors

- Blood type and histocompatibility testing to determine that the recipient has no preformed antibodies against the donor HLA antigens
- Thorough history and physical examination
- Chest X ray with PA and lateral views
- Electrocardiogram
- Complete blood count, chemistry panel, rapid plasma reagin, serologic studies for cytomegalovirus, human immunodeficiency virus, and hepatitis B and C
- 24-hour urine for total protein and creatinine clearance, urinalysis, and culture
- Pregnancy test in females
- Intravenous pyelogram or computed tomography to document the anatomy of the kidneys, ureters, and bladder
- Renal arteriogram or magnetic resonance angiography to outline the anatomy of the renal vasculature

PA = Posterior/Anterior

- In situ organ preservation after uncontrolled cardiopulmonary arrest
- Controlled procurement from patients whose death has been declared based on cardiopulmonary criteria after they have chosen to forgo life-sustaining treatment

ORGAN ALLOCATION AND DISTRIBUTION

Kidneys are distributed by UNOS using an objective computerized point system. The distribution of kidneys is based on blood type compatibility and points assigned for the quality of the human leukocyte antigen (HLA) match, waiting time, the presence of preformed antibodies, and pediatric status. The kidneys are transplanted locally unless there is a potential recipient with a perfect HLA match somewhere in the country.

SURGICAL PROCEDURES

PROCUREMENT OF DONOR KIDNEYS—LIVE DONORS

Open Nephrectomy

A flank incision above the 12th rib with an extrapleural, extraperitoneal approach is usually performed. Careful dissection and preservation of the renal artery, vein, and ureter is required. Donors are hydrated during the procedure, and mannitol is administered to ensure a brisk diuresis.

Laparoscopic Nephrectomy

With the patient in the lateral position, three operating ports are arranged in an arc equidistant from the target organ, and one extraction port is placed in the lower midline. Medial visceral rotation of the colon, adrenal and superior renal pole dissection, renal vascular dissection, ureteral dissection, and division of lateral attachments to the diaphragm and iliosoas muscle are the essential steps of the procedure. Extraction of the kidney is performed using an endoscopic retrieval bag placed through the lower abdominal midline incision or through a hand-port or endoscopic sleeve device. As in the open nephrectomy, donors are hydrated during the procedure and mannitol is administered intraoperatively to ensure a brisk diuresis (Farney et al., 2000). Advantages that have been attributed to this procedure compared to the standard open nephrectomy include decreased length of stay, decreased pain medication requirements, more rapid return to normal activity and work, and decreased risk of major and minor complications (Jacobs, Cho, & Dunkin, 2000).

PROCUREMENT OF DONOR KIDNEYS—CADAVERIC DONORS

- The kidneys are removed en bloc (remaining attached to the aorta and vena cava), flushed with a sterile, cold preservation solution, and preserved either in the iced solution or on a pulsatile perfusion machine that continuously pumps the preservation solution through the kidneys.
- Kidneys can be preserved for up to 72 hours, but most surgeons prefer to transplant kidneys before preservation time reaches 24 hours. Experience has shown that longer preservation time is associated with delayed graft function from acute tubular necrosis (ATN).

TRANSPLANTATION PROCEDURE

- The kidney transplant procedure takes approximately 3 hours.
- A hockey stick–shaped incision is made extending from the iliac crest to the symphysis pubis.
- The peritoneum is left intact and retracted upward while the common iliac, external iliac, hypogastric arteries, and common iliac veins are dissected.
- Any divided lymphatic vessels are ligated or cauterized to prevent future lymphocele formation.
- Intraperitoneal placement may be indicated in certain circumstances, such as in children in whom the transplanted kidney is too large to fit in the extraperitoneal space or in adults who have received previous transplants or have inadequate extraperitoneal vascular access.
- The kidney is positioned in the iliac fossa and revascularized. The kidney should be firm and pink.
- Urine often begins to flow from the ureter immediately. Diuretics may be administered intravenously to promote diuresis.
- The donor ureter is tunneled through the bladder submucosa before entering the bladder cavity and is sutured in place in a procedure called ureteroneocystostomy. This allows the bladder to clamp down on the ureter as it contracts for micturition, thereby preventing reflux of urine up the ureter into the kidney.
- After closing, a drain is inserted adjacent to the incision to facilitate removal of excess blood and serum from the operative site.

IMMEDIATE POSTOPERATIVE PERIOD

Common problems in the immediate postoperative period include hemodynamic instability, hypertension, electrolyte and acid-base imbalance, and renal dysfunction. The etiology, assessment parameters, and treatment options for each of these complications are summarized in Table 7.5.

IMMUNOSUPPRESSION REGIMENS

Immunosuppression regimens may be classified as induction therapy, maintenance regimens, and withdrawal and conversion regimens.

TABLE 7.5 Etiology and Treatment of Complications in the Immediate Postoperative Period

Complication	Etiology	Assessment	Treatment options
Hemodynamic instability	Ischemia due to organ procurement and/or denervation of allograft	Signs of volume depletion or volume overload Comparison of pre- and postoperative weights CVP monitoring Pulse oximetry or arterial blood gases	Maintenance of euvolemia by treating volume depletion with the administration of isotonic fluids to normalize blood pressure, heart rate, and CVP Treating volume overload with IV diuretics or dialysis, depending on urine flow
Hypertension	Inability to take or reliably absorb antihypertensive medications	Blood pressure	IV medications such as nitroprusside, labetolol, hydralazine, enalapril
Electrolyte imbalance	Preexisting electrolyte or acid-base abnormalities	Serial assessment of serum electrolytes	
Hyperkalemia	Effects of surgical tissue destruction; impaired renal function		Dietary potassium restriction Cation exchange resins (e.g., sodium polysytrene sulfonate [Kayexalate]®) Diuretics Dialysis
Hyponatremia	Excessive administration of hypotonic fluids in the presence of renal impairment		Water restriction Conversion to isotonic fluids

continued

TABLE 7.5 (*continued*)

Complication	Etiology	Assessment	Treatment options
Hypomagnesemia	May be a manifestation of "high-output" ATN; exacerbated by calcineurin inhibitors		IV magnesium sulfate for severe hypomagnesemia
Hypophosphatemia	Common when GFR suddenly normalizes in patients with preexisting hyperparathyroidism		Increased intake of dairy products
Metabolic acidosis	Impaired renal hydrogen ion excretion	Serial assessment of pH	Bicarbonate replacement generally warranted when the serum bicarbonate is <15 mEq/L
Anuria (urine output < 50 mL/24 hours)	Most commonly due to ATN; may be due to urine leak, ureteral obstruction, or vascular thromboses	Serial measurements of urine output and serum creatinine concentration	Trial of intravenous diuretics warranted to promote urine flow
Oliguria (urine output < 400 mL/24 hours)		Doppler ultrasonography or renal scans to determine structural abnormalities	Role of low-dose dopamine is controversial

continued

TABLE 7.5 (continued)

Complication	Etiology	Assessment	Treatment options
Polyuria	Most commonly observed after living-donor transplantation, reflecting an osmotic diuresis in the face of rapidly normalizing glomerular filtration Some patients with ATN develop a renal concentrating defect and may excrete relatively large amounts of urine despite persistent azotemia	Serial measurements of urine output	Matching urine output with replacement intravenous fluids is critical to avoiding severe volume depletion in first 12 to 24 hours posttransplant
DGF: the need for dialysis during the first week posttransplant	Ischemic ATN (incidence varies from 10%–40%) Immunologic mechanisms (Note: DGF is a risk factor for acute rejection; the combination of DGF and acute rejection portends a poor long-term prognosis for the allograft [Weir & Fink, 1999])	Serial measurements of urine output and serum creatinine concentration	Dialysis Fluid restriction

continued

TABLE 7.5 *(continued)*

Complication	Etiology	Assessment	Treatment options
Acute renal failure that develops after initial graft function has been established	Volume depletion Acute rejection (including "delayed hyperacute rejection") Arterial or venous thrombosis (more common in patients with hypercoagulable states and recipients of pediatric kidneys) Urine leak Ureteral obstruction Anastamotic stricture Obstruction by perinephric fluid (e.g., hematoma, lymphocele) Drug-induced nephrotoxicity Allergic interstitial nephritis Hemolytic uremic syndrome	Serial measurements of urine output and serum creatinine concentration Comparison of daily weights Percutaneous kidney biopsy to diagnose rejection Doppler ultrasonography to determine vascular or structural abnormalities	Fluid administration Treatment of rejection Correction of vascular abnormalities Correction of structural abnormalities Drainage of hematoma or lymphocele Dose adjustment—nephrotoxic drugs Plasmapheresis

ATN = acute tubular necrosis
CVP = central venous pressure
DGF = delayed graft function
GFR = glomerular filtration rate
IV = intravenous

INDUCTION ANTIBODY THERAPY

The benefits, risks, and costs associated with the routine use of antilymphocyte antibodies during the immediate posttransplant period is controversial (Norman, 1993). Administration of these agents may decrease the subsequent risk of acute allograft rejection or at least delay the onset of first rejection episodes.

Some centers reserve antibody induction therapy for patients deemed to be at high risk for rejection (e.g., African Americans, second transplant recipients, and patients with high pretransplant panel-reactive antibody [PRA] levels). Other transplant centers use induction therapy for patients with delayed graft function to delay the initiation of treatment with nephrotoxic calcineurin inhibitors.

Currently available choices include

- Polyclonal antibodies (e.g., horse or rabbit antithymocyte globulin)
- Monoclonal antibodies such as muromonab-CD3 (OKT3) or anti-CD25 (anti-IL2-receptor) antibodies

MAINTENANCE REGIMENS

Most centers administer a combination of two or three maintenance immunosuppressive drugs during the first posttransplant year (Hong & Kahan, 2000). Outside of the context of experimental protocols, corticosteroids generally are given for the first several months after transplantation.

The most common regimens are

- Double therapy: corticosteroids + calcineurin inhibitor (cyclosporine or tacrolimus)
- Triple therapy: corticosteroids + calcineurin inhibitor + purine antagonist (azathioprine or mycophenolate mofetil) or corticosteroids + calcineurin inhibitor + mTOR (mammalian target of rapamycin) inhibitor (i.e., sirolimus)

WITHDRAWAL AND CONVERSION REGIMENS

Because the use of newer immunosuppressants has been associated with lower rates of acute rejection, attention has focused increasingly on long-term minimization of immunosuppression to reduce drug toxicities in patients who are free of rejection during the early posttransplant period. Steroid- and calcineurin inhibitor–sparing protocols are examples of these types of regimens. With the availability of newer and more potent maintenance drugs, many centers convert recipients to a new maintenance regimen if acute rejection occurs while the patient is receiving another combination of drugs. An underlying concern that the calcineurin inhibitors may contribute to interstitial fibrosis and chronic graft dysfunction forms the basis for conversion protocols in which a new, non-nephrotoxic drug (most often either mycophenolate mofetil or sirolimus) is added to facilitate minimization or withdrawal of the calcineurin inhibitor in patients with established chronic allograft nephropathy (Gauthier & Helderman, 2000).

REJECTION

SURVEILLANCE

Acute renal allograft rejection can occur at any time following renal transplantation. However, the risk of acute rejection is highest in the first 6 months. Therefore, monitoring is performed frequently (usually once or twice weekly) early on and less frequently (two to four times yearly) in patients who are stable several years after the transplant. Chronic rejection (i.e., chronic allograft nephropathy) generally occurs beyond the sixth posttransplant month. Thus, renal function must be monitored for the life of the allograft.

Estimates of glomerular filtration rate (GFR) remain the most practical way to monitor kidney transplant recipients for acute and chronic rejection. The serum creatinine concentration only crudely estimates GFR and varies with muscle mass. Moreover, renal tubular secretion of creatinine may yield a deceivingly stable serum concentration in the face of a decreasing GFR (Ross, Wilkinson, Hawkins, & Danovitch, 1987). Nevertheless, in the absence of wide variations in muscle mass, the serum creatinine concentration remains the most widely employed means of monitoring transplant renal function. Some centers supplement measurement of serum creatinine with periodic measurements of either creatinine clearance or other estimates of GFR (e.g., iothalamate clearance).

It is now recognized that histologic evidence of acute allograft rejection can occur in the absence of a rise in serum creatinine concentration (Rush et al., 1999). Whether such subclinical episodes of rejection are predictive of long-term outcome remains a subject of active investigation In the absence of laboratory tests, which can reliably serve as surrogates for subclinical rejection, periodic "protocol" biopsies are the only satisfactory means for diagnosing subclinical rejection.

DIAGNOSIS OF REJECTION

Clinical Signs and Symptoms

Hyperacute rejection is mediated by preformed antibodies and may occur immediately following the vascular anastamosis or several days later (delayed hyperacute rejection). Necrosis of the renal parenchyma in this setting is often accompanied by a toxic state, including evidence of disseminated intravascular coagulation.

Acute rejection is characterized by an abrupt deterioration in renal function, usually manifested by a rise in serum creatinine concentration. Fever, general malaise, graft tenderness, and oliguria are characteristic of severe acute rejection, but are rarely observed in the modern era.

Chronic allograft nephropathy is characterized by a slow deterioration in GFR manifested by a slow rise in serum creatinine concentration, often accompanied by proteinuria, and new or worsening hypertension. One third of patients develop heavy proteinuria and frank nephrotic syndrome (edema, hypoalbuminemia, and hyperlipidemia) (Massy, Guijarro, Wiederkehr, Ma, & Kasiske, 1996; Matas, 1994).

Biopsy

Percutaneous biopsy remains the gold standard for diagnosis of acute and chronic rejection. The Banff classification (Table 7.6) was developed in an effort to provide a consistent approach for grading structural lesions in the transplanted kidney.

In patients with acute rejection, the Banff grade can be predictive of recurrent rejection and subsequent graft failure. In addition, many centers choose treatment strategies based on the grade of rejection as discussed below.

TREATMENT OF ACUTE REJECTION

Pulse Steroid Therapy

Administration of high doses of corticosteroids for 3 to 5 days is the first-line therapy for acute rejection in most centers and can reverse approximately 60% of rejection episodes. Some centers treat the patient empirically

TABLE 7.6 Simplified Banff Classification for Acute Renal Transplant Rejection

Grade	Criteria
"Borderline"	Patchy interstitial inflammation, mild tubulitis
1 (mild)	Interstitial inflammation involving > 25% of the renal parenchyma. Tubulitis with > 4 lymphocytes invading tubular basement membrane per tubular cross section
2 (moderate)	
2A	Interstitial inflammation as above. Tubulitis with > 10 lymphocytes invading tubular basement membrane per tubular cross section
2B	Same as 2A, but with mild intimal arteritis
3 (severe)	Severe intimal arteritis and/or transmural arteritis with necrosis and infarction

with steroids for clinical signs of rejection. Others prefer to perform a biopsy first and to use steroids only for patients with borderline or grade 1 acute rejection. Higher grades are treated with antilymphocyte antibodies (Kamath et al., 1998).

Antilymphocyte Antibodies

These agents are most often used in patients who fail to respond to pulse steroids, or as first-line therapy in patients with clinically or histologically severe episodes of rejection. The most commonly used agents are muromonab-CD3 (Orthoclone OKT3) and rabbit antithymocyte globulin.

Plasmapheresis and Intravenous Gamma Globulin

These interventions may be effective in removing and suppressing formation of the antibodies that mediate hyperacute rejection.

TREATMENT OF CHRONIC ALLOGRAFT NEPHROPATHY

Curative therapy is lacking. To date, none of the available immunosuppressants has proven to be effective in treating established chronic allograft nephropathy. Aggressive treatment of hyperlipidemia and systemic hypertension, including the use of the putatively renal protective angiotensin inhibitors (angiotensin converting enzyme inhibitors and angiotensin receptor blockers) is warranted, but the impact of these strategies on retarding the rate of renal functional deterioration remains to be proven.

LONG-TERM CARE

Long-term care of the renal transplant recipient involves management of infection, cardiovascular disease (hypertension and hyperlipidemia), post-transplant diabetes mellitus, malignancy, skeletal disorders, hemopoietic abnormalities, and recurrent renal disease.

INFECTIOUS COMPLICATIONS

Infections are frequent complications of systemic immunosuppression after transplantation. The principles of infectious disease management include

- Identification of the organism
- Identification of the organism's sensitivities to antimicrobials
- Localization of the site(s) of infections.

Different types of infections occur at three time periods after transplantation (Kubak, Pegues, & Holt, 2000).

FIRST MONTH

The most frequent infections occurring in this time period are related to surgical and nosocomial complications:

- Bacterial and fungal wound infections
- Urinary tract infections
- Nosocomial pneumonitis
- Line-associated bacteremias and fungemias

Urinary tract infections (UTIs) are the most frequent bacterial infection in kidney transplantation. Predisposing factors for UTIs include

- Renal insufficiency
- Decreased urine flow through the urinary epithelium
- Prolonged bladder catheterization
- Underlying diseases (e.g., diabetes and polycystic kidney disease)

Causative organisms are the same as the general population: Gram-negative enteric bacilli, enterococci, staphylococci, and *Pseudomonas aeruginosa.*

SECOND TO SIX MONTHS

During this time, the level of immunosuppression is the most intense. Patients are at risk for developing opportunistic infections including cytomegalovirus (CMV) disease, *Pneumocystis carinii* pneumonia (PCP), invasive aspergillosis, disseminated toxoplasmosis, disseminated varicella zoster infection, and certain bacterial infections such as listeriosis. CMV is the most common viral infection occurring in this time period. Other preexisting infections that can reactivate are tuberculosis and the endemic mycoses.

BEYOND SIX MONTHS

Patients who have not had acute rejection episodes requiring increased immunosuppression are at risk for the usual community acquired infections. Certain diseases can still occur during this time period: tuberculosis, cryptococcal disease, reactivation of hepatitis B and C infections, nocardiosis, and herpes zoster infection.

CARDIOVASCULAR DISEASE

Cardiovascular disease, including myocardial infarction, stroke, and complications of peripheral vascular disease, is now the most common cause of death in renal transplant recipients. The increasing frequency of cardiovascular death reflects a declining incidence of death due to infection, increasing age of the transplant population, and high prevalence of traditional cardiovascular risk factors such as hypertension, hyperlipidemia, and glucose intolerance.

HYPERTENSION

Hypertension occurs in 60% to 80% of recipients. The etiology is usually multifactorial and includes

- Effects of retained native kidneys
- Parenchymal disease of the transplanted kidney (mediated by rejection or recurrent disease)
- Hypertensive effects of immunosuppressants such as corticosteroids, cyclosporine, and tacrolimus
- Narrowing of the renal artery (renal artery stenosis) (First, Neylan, Rocher, & Tejani, 1994)

There is no consensus about optimal therapy, but calcium channel blockers are used as first-line agents in many centers. Hypertension may accelerate loss of allograft function, especially in African American patients (Cosio, Dillon, & Falkenheim, 1995).

HYPERLIPIDEMIA

Hyperlipidemia affects approximately 70% of patients at some time during the posttransplant course. Although many clinical factors are associated with posttransplant hyperlipidemia, immunosuppressants play a predominant pathophysiologic role (Hricik, 2000).

- Corticosteroids increase hepatic formation of lipoproteins.
- Cyclosporine impairs bile acid synthesis and cholesterol excretion.

The incidence and severity of hyperlipidemia are greater in transplant recipients receiving sirolimus (Rapamune).

The management of hyperlipidemia includes the folowing:

- 3-hydroxy-3-methylglutaryl coenzyme A (HMG-CoA) reductase inhibitors have proven to be the most effective agents for treating posttransplant hypercholesterolemia.
- Fibric acid derivatives or nicotinic acid may be used adjunctively and are sometimes required for management of isolated hypertriglyceridemia.

POSTTRANSPLANT DIABETES MELLITUS (PTDM)

PTDM occurs in 10% to 15% of patients and clearly reflects the effects of corticosteroids and calcineurin inhibitors on insulin and glucose metabolism in genetically susceptible individuals (Weir & Fink, 1999). Tacrolimus is more diabetogenic than cyclosporine.

Risk factors for PTDM include

- African American ethnicity
- Family history of diabetes
- Advanced age
- Posttransplant weight gain

Approximately two thirds of patients with PTDM require treatment with insulin, although the requirement for insulin may be eliminated with weight loss or minimization/withdrawal of steroids or calcineurin inhibitors.

MALIGNANCY

The mean incidence of malignancies of all types ranges between 1% and 18%. There is substantial geographic variation in the incidence of malignancy following renal transplantation. Carcinomas of the lung, prostate, colon, and breast do not occur with increased frequency in transplant recipients. Neoplasms that occur with increased frequency are posttransplant lymphoproliferative disease, skin cancer, Kaposi's sarcoma, and genital neoplasia.

POSTTRANSPLANT LYMPHOPROLIFERATIVE DISEASE (PTLD)

The overall incidence of PTLD is 1% to 3%. The unusual features of PTLD, compared to lymphomas in the general population, include

- The majority (96%) of cases are non-Hodgkin's lymphomas.
- Extranodal involvement (central nervous system, intestines, liver, transplanted organs) is common.
- There is a high rate of association with EBV infection. Seronegative recipients of organs from seropositive donors are at highest risk.
- The PTLD mortality rate is 50-fold higher than that of lymphomas in the general population.
- PTLD may respond to withdrawal or minimization of immunosuppression.

Treatment includes chemotherapy. Treatment with anti-CD20 antibodies holds some promise (Kuo, Dafoe, Alfrey, Sibley, & Scandling, 1995).

SKIN CANCER

The incidence of skin cancer is 20 times higher in transplant recipients than in the general population. Unusual features compared to the general population include

- Squamous cell carcinoma is more common than basal cell carcinoma
- Multiple skin cancers are often present at initial diagnosis
- Squamous cell carcinomas are more aggressive and metastasize more frequently

KAPOSI'S SARCOMA

In most series, up to 10% of all posttransplant malignancies are Kaposi's. The most common sites of involvement are

- Skin
- Oropharyngeal membranes
- Conjunctiva

Kaposi's presents as reddish blue macules and plaques. Treatment includes decreasing immunosuppression, chemotherapy, and radiotherapy.

GENITAL NEOPLASIA

Compared to the general population, renal transplant recipients have a 40-fold increase in vulvar and vaginal carcinoma and a 15-fold increase in cervical neoplasia.

SKELETAL DISORDERS

OSTEOPENIA

Bone density is often decreased in patients with ESRD and decreases further after transplantation with a rapid loss of density in the first 6 months

(Julian, Quarles, & Niemann, 1992). Corticosteroids play a preeminent role in the early loss of bone mineral. Beyond 6 months, cyclosporine may contribute to a state of low bone turnover. The severity of osteopenia is influenced by the degree of underlying renal osteodystrophy and by other common factors known to affect bone metabolism. Postmenopausal women and patients with diabetes mellitus are at particular risk for fractures related to posttransplant osteopenia.

Treatment options include calcium supplements, vitamin D, and biphosphonates, but their value remains to be proven.

OSTEONECROSIS

The incidence varies widely, but up to 15% of patients are affected in the first 3 years after transplantation. The femoral head is the most common site of involvement. The pathophysiology is uncertain, but corticosteroids are implicated as the major contributing factor. Treatments include core decompression and total arthroplasty.

HEMATOPOIETIC ABNORMALITIES

POSTTRANSPLANT ERYTHROCYTOSIS

The incidence of posttransplant erythrocytosis is about 10% to 20% (Danovitch et. al., 1995). Pathophysiologic mechanisms are uncertain, but are probably related to abnormal feedback regulation of erythropoietin metabolism. Treatment includes phlebotomy or angiotensin inhibitors.

PANCYTOPENIA

Pancytopenia is most often related to myelosuppressive immunosuppressants (azathioprine, mycophenolate mofetil, sirolimus). Anemia may be related to renal insufficiency.

RECURRENT RENAL DISEASE

The types of renal disease that may recur in the transplant recipient include

- Recurrent genetic and metabolic diseases
- Diabetic nephropathy

- Fabry's disease
- Primary oxalosis
- Sickle-cell nephropathy
- Amyloidosis
- Patients with Alport's syndrome may develop antiglomerular basement membrane antibody-mediated glomerulonephritis
- Recurrent forms of glomerulonephritis (see Table 7.7) (Ramos & Tisher, 1994)

WHEN TO CALL THE TRANSPLANT CENTER

- Rise in serum creatinine (30% or more) above baseline
- Requirement for medications that may interact with immunosuppression
- Fever of unknown origin
- Serious infections (life-threatening or requiring hospital admission)
- Unexplained weight loss
- Presence of enlarged lymph nodes
- Malignancy
- Noncompliance

TABLE 7.7 Rates of Recurrent Glomerulonephritis after Kidney Transplantation

Type of glomerulonephritis	*Frequency of recurrence (%)*
Membranoproliferative type 1	90–100
Membranoproliferative type 2	20–30
Focal glomerulosclerosis	25–45
IgA nephropathy	35–50
Henoch-Schönlein purpura	75–85
Membranous	5–10
Anti-GBM (globular basement membrane)	5–10
Hemolytic uremic syndrome	15–25
Lupus nephritis	< 2

CONCLUSION

Kidney transplantation is the treatment option for ESRD that offers the greatest potential for the full return to a healthy, productive life. Careful evaluation of the potential candidate and management of coexisting medical problems during the waiting period will decrease morbidity and mortality after transplantation. Management of infection, cardiovascular disease, diabetes mellitus, malignancy, skeletal disorders, hemopoietic abnormalities, and recurrent renal disease is key to long-term patient and graft survival. Successful outcomes depend on collaboration between the transplant team and the patient's primary health care providers.

REFERENCES

Caplan, A. (1993). Must I be my brother's keeper? Ethical issues in the use of living donors as sources of livers and other solid organs. *Transplantation Proceedings, 25,* 1997–2000.

Cosio, F. G., Dillon, J. J., & Falkenheim, M. E. (1995). Racial differences in renal allograft survival: The role of systemic hypertension. *Kidney International, 47*(4), 1136–1141.

Danovitch, G. M., Jamgotchian, N. J., Eggena, P. H., Paul, W., Barrett, J. D., Wilkinson, A., & Lee, D. B. (1995). Angiotensin-converting enzyme inhibition in the treatment of renal transplant erythrocytosis: Clinical experience and observation of mechanism. *Transplantation, 60,* 132–135.

DeGeest, S., Borgermane, L., & Gemoets, H., et al. (1995). Incidence, determinants, and consequences of subclinical noncompliance with immunosuppressive therapy in renal transplant recipients. *Transplantation, 59,* 340–347.

Douglas, S., Blixen, C., & Bartucci, M. R. (1996). Relationship between pretransplant noncompliance and posttransplant outcomes in renal transplant recipients. *Journal of Transplant Coordination, 6,* 53–58.

Farney, A. C., Cho, E., Schweitzer, E. J., Dunkin, B., Philosophe, B., Colonna, J., Jacobs, S., Jarrell, B., Flowers, J. L., & Bartlett, S. T. (2000). Simultaneous cadaver pancreas living-donor kidney transplantation: A new approach for the Type 1 diabetic uremic patient. *Annals of Surgery, 232*(5), 696–703.

First, M. R., Neylan, J. F., Rocher, L., & Tejani, A. (1994). Hypertension after renal transplantation. *Journal of the American Society of Nephrology, 4*(8, Suppl.), S30–S36.

Gauthier, P., & Helderman, J. H. (2000). Cyclosporine avoidance. *Journal of the American Society of Nephrology, 11,* 1933–1936.

Hong, J. C., & Kahan, B. D. (2000). Immunosuppressive agents in organ transplantation: Past, present, and future. *Seminars in Nephrology, 20,* 108–125.

Hricik, D. E. (2000). Hyperlipidemia in renal transplant recipients. *Graft, 4,* 11–19.

Jacobs, S., Cho, E., & Dunkin, B. (2000). Laparoscopic donor nephrectomy: Current role in renal allograft procurement. *Urology, 55*(6), 807–811.

Julian, B. A., Quarles, D., & Niemann, K. M. (1992). Musculoskeletal complications after renal transplantation: Pathogenesis and treatment. *American Journal of Kidney Diseases, 19,* 99–120.

Kamath, S., Dean, D., Peddi, V. R., Schroeder, T. J., Alexander, J. W., Cavallo, T., & First, M. R. (1998). Primary therapy with OKT3 for biopsy-proven acute renal allograft rejection. *Transplantation Proceedings, 30*(4), 1178–1180.

Kaufman, D. B. (1999). Kidney transplantation. In F. P. Stuart, M. M. Abecassis, & D. B. Kaufman (Eds.). *Organ transplantation* (pp. 105–144). Georgetown, TX: Vademecum Landes Bioscience.

Kubak, B. M., Pegues, D. A., & Holt, C. D. (2000). Infectious complications of kidney transplantation and their management. In G. M. Danovitch (Ed.). *Handbook of kidney transplantation,* 3rd ed. (pp. 221–262). Philadelphia: Lippincott, Williams, & Wilkins.

Kuo, P. C., Dafoe, D. C., Alfrey, E. J., Sibley, R. K., & Scandling, J. D. (1995). Posttransplant lymphoproliferative disorders and Epstein-Barr virus prophylaxis. *Transplantation, 59*(1), 135–138.

Massy, Z. A., Guijarro, C., Wiederkehr, M. R., Ma, J. Z., & Kasiske, B. L. (1996). Chronic renal allograft rejection: Immunologic and nonimmunologic risk factors. *Kidney International, 49*(2), 518–524.

Matas, A. (1994). Chronic rejection in renal transplant recipients—risk factors and correlates. *Clinical Transplantation, 8*(3, Pt. 2), 332–335.

Norman, D. J. (1993). Rationale for OKT3 monoclonal antibody treatment in transplant patients. *Transplantation Proceedings, 25*(2, Suppl. 1), 1–3.

Pirsch. J. D., Armbrust, M. J., Knechtle, S. J., D'Alessandro, A. M., Sollinger. H. W., Heisey, D. M., & Belzer, F. O. (1995). Obesity as a risk factor following renal transplantation. *Transplantation, 69*(4), 631–633.

Ramos, E. L., & Tisher, C. C. (1994). Recurrent diseases in the kidney transplant. *American Journal of Kidney Diseases, 24*(1), 142–154.

Rosenthal, J. T., & Danovitch, G. M. (1996). Live-related and cadaveric kidney donation. In G. M. Danovitch (Ed.). *Handbook of kidney transplantation* (pp. 95–108). Boston: Little, Brown.

Ross, E. A., Wilkinson, A., Hawkins, R. A., & Danovitch, G. M. (1987). The plasma creatinine is not an accurate reflection of the glomerular filtration rate in stable renal transplant patients receiving cyclosporine. *American Journal of Kidney Diseases, 10*(2), 113–117.

Rush, D. N., Karpinski, M. E., Nickerson, P, Dancea, S., Birk, P., & Jeffery, J. R. (1999). Does subclinical rejection contribute to chronic rejection in renal transplant patients? *Clinical Transplantation, 13*(6), 441–446.

Spital, A. (1997). Ethical and policy issues in altruistic living and cadaveric organ donation. *Clinical Transplantation, 11,* 77–87.

United Network for Organ Sharing. (2000). *1999 transplant statistics.* Richmond, VA: Author.

United States Renal Data System. (1998). Excerpts from the United States Renal Data System 1998 annual data report: Incidence and.prevalence of ESRD. *American Journal of Kidney Disease, 32,* S38–S49.

Weir, M. R., & Fink, J. C. (1999). Risk for posttransplant diabetes mellitus with current immunosuppressive medications. *American Journal of Kidney Diseases, 34*(1), 1–13.

Wolfe, R. A., Ashby, V. B., Milford, E. L., Ojo, A. O., Ettenger, R. E., Agodoa, L. Y., Held, P. J., & Port, F. K. (1999). Comparison of mortality in all patients on dialysis, patients on dialysis awaiting transplantation, and recipients of a first cadaveric transplant. *New England Journal of Medicine, 341*(23), 1725–1730.

8

Simultaneous Kidney–Pancreas Transplantation

Barbara Dimercurio, Leonard Henry and Allan D. Kirk

Approximately 1.4 million adults have type 1 diabetes mellitus (T1DM) in the United States (Libman, Songer, & LaPorte, 1993). Tight control over glucose metabolism has been shown to greatly improve the morbidity and mortality of T1DM, but it is difficult achieve (Diabetes Control and Complications Trial Research Group, 1993). To date, pancreas transplantation is the single most physiological method of controlling glucose metabolism and is the treatment of choice for those patients with T1DM who meet the criteria for the procedure. Nationally, the number of simultaneous kidney-pancreas (SPK) transplants performed has increased from 459 in 1990 to 946 in 1999 (U.S. Department of Health and Human Services, 2000). The outcome following SKP transplantation has improved over the last decade as a result of the advances in immunosuppression and surgical technique (Gruessner & Sutherland, 1999). Current kidney graft 1- and 3-year survival rates are 91% and 82%, respectively. Current pancreas graft 1- and 3-year survival rates are 83% and 75%, respectively. One- and 3-year SKP patient survival rates are 94% and 90%, respectively (United Network for Organ Sharing, *Transplant Patient DataSource*, 2001). As of January 2002, there were 2,452 patients on the SKP waiting list, (United Network for Organ Sharing, *Critical Data*, 2002). Median waiting times in 1999 were 550 days for females and 411 days for males (U.S. Department of Health and Human Services, 2000).

INDICATIONS FOR KIDNEY-PANCREAS TRANSPLANTATION

The indications for kidney–pancreas transplantation include (Freise, Narumi, Stock, & Melzer 1999):

- Insulin-dependent diabetes mellitus (Typically, this is predominantly T1DM, although select patients with type 2 diabetes mellitus [T2DM] may be considered.)
- Diabetic nephropathy

Because there are fewer than 5,000 pancreas donors per year, pancreas transplantation will never be a cure for most patients with diabetes. Thus, judicious patient selection is critical.

The complications of insulin-dependent diabetes mellitus that support the recommendation for SKP transplantation include (Freise et al., 1999):

- Retinopathy
- Neuropathy
- Gastroparesis

EVALUATION OF THE POTENTIAL SKP TRANSPLANTATION CANDIDATE

Individuals can be a self-referral or physician referral. Once referred, a multidisciplinary team conducts the evaluation process. This team typically includes an endocrinologist, nephrologist, surgeon, transplant coordinator, social worker, dietitian, and cardiologist. The comprehensive evaluation for SKP outlined in Table 8.1 is the standard protocol used at the National Institutes of Health. Additional diagnostic testing may be recommended by the endocrinologist, nephrologist, transplant surgeon, or other consultants.

The intent of a meticulous pretransplant evaluation is to identify surgical, medical, and psychosocial risk factors that may adversely affect patient and long-term graft survival. A patient's candidacy is established by multidisciplinary consensus. Particular attention is given to evidence of advanced diabetic vasculopathy.

TABLE 8.1 Comprehensive Simultaneous Pancreas–Kidney Evaluation

Professional consultations

- Endocrinologist: Confirms diagnosis of T1DM; determines the extent of diabetic complications; makes recommendations regarding improvements in control of diabetes while patient is on waiting list
- Nephrologist: Carefully evaluates all organ systems to determine any underlying comorbidities; focuses on the treatment of hypertensive complications and general health maintenance
- Transplant surgeon: Focuses primarily on identifying any reconstructable surgical comorbidities, particularly vascular disease
- Transplant coordinator: Establishes lines of communication and methods of transportation at time of transplantation; initiates pretransplant patient/family education
- Social worker: Evaluates the psychosocial needs of the patient and family; assesses patient's ability to comply with the immunosuppression regimen and other postoperative care requirements; identifies need for formal psychological evaluation
- Dietitian: Evaluates patient's nutritional status; guides the patient's fluid and dietary allowances

Basic laboratory studies
- Complete blood count, platelet count, prothrombin time, partial thromboplastin time, complete chemistry panel (electrolytes and minerals), aspartate aminotransferase, alanine aminotransferase, alkaline phosphate, lactic dehydrogenase, cholesterol panel, albumin, total protein, amylase, lipase, beta-2 microglobulin, thyroid panel

Diabetic laboratory studies
- C-peptide, hemoglobin A1C, anti-glutamate decarboxylase, arginine stimulation test

Urine laboratory studies
- 24-hour urine for creatinine and protein clearance, urinalysis, urine for microalbuminuria

Virology studies
- Cytomegalovirus IgG and IgM, Epstein-Barr Virus IgG and IgM, hepatitis B, hepatitis C, human immunodeficiency virus, herpes simplex virus, varicella zoster virus, Venereal Disease Research Laboratories test, rapid plasma reagent test

continued

TABLE 8.1 *(continued)*

Immunology studies
- Blood type and screen, human leukocyte antigen typing, panel-reactive antibody

Urologic studies
- Ultrasound of bilateral kidneys and gallbladder, voiding cystourethrogram if anuric ≥ 1 year

Gender-specific studies
- Prostate-specific antigen if ≥ 50 years old
- Gynecologic examination, Papanicolaou's smear, mammography if ≥ 35 years old

Cardiology evaluation
- Electrocardiogram, echocardiogram, chest radiograph, stress thallium test, cardiaccatheterization (for patients with a borderline or positive thallium)

Gastrointestinal evaluationv
- Flexible sigmoidoscopy, colonoscopy (for females ≥ 50 and males ≥ 45)

Ophthalmology evaluation
- Nondilated ophthalmoscopy (evaluation for retinal microaneurysm, neovascularization, and other changes consistent with diabetic retinopathy)

T1DM = type 1 diabetes mellitus

CONTRAINDICATIONS TO SKP TRANSPLANTATION

Absolute contraindications to SKP transplantation include the following (Freise et al., 1999):
- Active noncutaneous malignancy
- Active unconfined bacterial or fungal infection; ongoing osteomyelitis in a diabetic patient
- Active infection with any of the following viruses: human immunodeficiency virus (HIV), hepatitis C virus (HCV), or hepatitis B virus (HBV)
- Peripheral vascular disease precluding arterial anastomoses or threatening an extremity
- Irreversible large vessel cardiovascular disease (essentially, all patients with T1DM and diabetic nephropathy have some degree of microvascular vasculopathy that should be anticipated)

- Positive T-cell cross-match
- ABO incompatibility

Relative contraindications to SKP transplantation are center-specific. However, typical relative contraindications include the following (Freise et al., 1999):

- Cardiovascular disease requiring revascularization
- Obesity
- Current tobacco use
- Active substance abuse
- Poor compliance with medical care
- Age > 45

DONOR SELECTION

Donor selection is critically important to ensure optimal graft function and to lessen the risk of operative morbidity. SKP transplant procedures are almost exclusively performed with cadaveric grafts. Relative contraindications to donation of a cadaveric pancreas and kidney are listed below (Sollinger et al., 1998):

- Age > 45
- Preexisting renal disease
- Untreated hypertension with renal changes on biopsy
- Preexisting autoimmune diabetes mellitus (many donors become diabetic after brain death, and elevated glucose levels in the donor are not predictive of subsequent organ viability)
- Non–central nervous system malignancy
- Sepsis
- HIV, HBV, HCV infection
- Prolonged warm ischemic time

The single most important factor is the assessment of the organs by an experienced procuring surgeon. Further decisions regarding the suitability of the donor organs are made at laparotomy, at which time pancreatic fibrosis, trauma, or inflammation may preclude donation (Sollinger et al., 1998).

ORGAN PROCUREMENT

Pancreas procurement is generally accomplished in concert with the procurement of multiple other organs. The liver, duodenum, pancreas, and spleen can be removed separately or en bloc after cannulation of the portal vein (or inferior mesenteric vein) and aorta for organ perfusion. Division of the aorta, vena cava, inferior mesenteric vein (IMV), superior mesenteric vein (SMV), and superior mesenteric artery (SMA) are required for removal. The distal stomach and duodenum are stapled, divided, and delivered with the specimen (Sollinger et al., 1998).

The kidneys are generally removed en bloc via distal division of the ureters, and division of the aorta and vena cava on opposite sides of the renal vessels. Prior to removal, alpha blockade may be given to the patient to prevent vessel spasm, as well as heparin, mannitol, or furosemide (Lasix). All organs are flushed and stored in cold University of Wisconsin (UW) solution.

OPERATIVE PROCEDURE

ORGAN PREPARATION

Organs for transplantation undergo final preparation on the back table. Standard procedure includes the following:

- The duodenal segment is shortened, and stapled sides are oversewn with Lembert sutures.
- A splenectomy is performed and an iliac "Y" graft of donor artery is sewn end to end onto the splenic and SMA to provide for a singular anastomosis into the recipients iliac system (Sollinger et al., 1998).
- The kidney is trimmed of perinephric fat and vascular alterations are made as required for appropriate anastomosis.
- Exposure for transplantation is obtained through a midline laparotomy incision.
- Right medial visceral rotation is utilized for exposure to the right iliac system for pancreas transplant, followed by left medial rotation for exposure to the left iliacs for kidney transplantation.

VASCULAR AND URETERAL ANASTOMOSIS

Most pancreatic vascular anastomoses are performed with the iliac "Y" graft sewn to the recipient right common iliac artery and donor portal vein to the right iliac vein. An alternative venous anastomosis is to the recipient SMV or large tributary. This has the theoretical advantage of avoiding the unphysiologically elevated systemic insulin levels found with systemic (iliac) venous drainage (Stratta et al., 2000). Kidney grafts are anastomosed to the left iliac artery and vein. The donor ureter is sewn into the bladder mucosa on the anterolateral aspect of the filled bladder. A short extramucosal tunnel is approximated over the ureter to avoid future ureteral reflux.

EXOCRINE DRAINAGE

The manner of handling exocrine secretions has varied in the past. Initial attempts at enteric drainage were fraught with postoperative complications. This led to the widespread use of bladder drainage of exocrine secretions—a technique that has become predominant in the last decade. In this technique, the head of the pancreas is oriented caudally. The duodenum is opened longitudinally and anastomosed to the bladder in two layers.

Primary enteric drainage is regaining favor largely due to improved immunosuppression and preservation regimens and refined operative technique. Sollinger and colleagues (1998) found no significant differences in patient, pancreas graft, or kidney graft survival rates between bladder or enteric drainage at 1 and 3 years posttransplant. These investigators noted significantly fewer urologic complications in the enteric drainage group (Sollinger et al., 1998). Traditionally, the enteric drainage has been to the distal ileum, although diarrhea can be a significant problem. Some surgeons perform a more proximal anastomosis to the jejunum or to a Roux limb.

IMMEDIATE POST OPERATIVE CARE

Postoperative SKP transplant recipients are generally monitored in the intensive care unit during the immediate posttransplant period. Volume and electrolyte monitoring are early priorities. Other points to consider are the following:

- Central venous monitoring is preferred with a goal of avoiding over-hydration, as this exacerbates pancreatic edema.
- Urine output is replaced for approximately 24 hours. Foley catheter drainage is required, both for volume assessment and for bladder decompression to protect the anastomoses.

- Close attention is paid to serum glucose, potassium, calcium, and bicarbonate levels (Fabrega, Rivas, & Pollak, 1994).
- Exogenous insulin may be administered to "rest" the pancreatic allograft.
- Bowel function typically returns on postoperative day 4 or 5, after which the patient's diet can be advanced.
- Patients with known diabetic gastroparesis may benefit from a longer period of nasogastric tube decompression and possibly feeding through a nasoenteric tube.
- Perioperative antibiotics are customary for a variable amount of time; these are based on donor duodenal and preservation solution cultures (Fabrega et al., 1994).

IMMUNOSUPPRESSIVE REGIMENS

The pancreas is a relatively immunogenic organ, and rejection is a constant risk after transplantation. Interestingly, of all forms of pancreas transplantation, SKP allografts are immunologically well tolerated, as the kidney can be used to monitor the grafts for rejection. Early rejection episodes result in increased risk of recurrent rejection and eventual graft failure. Other points to consider are the following:

- Induction therapy with a depleting antilymphocyte antibody preparation has been standard, especially for solitary pancreatic transplantation; however, this induction therapy is more controversial in SKP transplantation (Gruessner, 1998).
- Anti-T-cell induction traditionally has been accomplished as part of quadruple immunosuppressive therapy with either monoclonal antibody (muromonab-CD3) or polyclonal antibody (antithymocyte globulin, Thymoglobulin) in concert with cyclosporine or tacrolimus, azathioprine or mycophenolic acid, and steroids.
- Rapamycin is a new immunosuppressive drug that is used in some centers, generally in combination with low-dose tacrolimus.
- Antibody induction has improved graft survival and has the added benefit of allowing delayed administration of nephrotoxic cyclosporine or tacrolimus in poorly functioning renal grafts. However, antibody induction is expensive, prolongs hospitalization, increases the risk of opportunistic infections, and has significant side effects of massive T-cell cytokine release (Gruessner, 1998). This cytokine release has, on occasion, been fatal.

REJECTION

In technically successful SKP transplantation, acute and chronic rejection is by far the greatest cause of graft loss, accounting for 60% of kidney and 44% of pancreatic losses, respectively. Animal studies suggest a rejection hierarchy: The kidney allograft is the most vulnerable, followed by the pancreas allograft and the duodenum (Gruessner & Sutherland, 1996). Biopsy-proven data to corroborate this rejection hierarchy in humans are lacking, largely because early rejection in the kidney serves as a surrogate marker of rejection for the pancreas.

DIAGNOSIS OF REJECTION

The diagnosis of rejection can be difficult. Clinical, laboratory, and radiologic data can be useful in making a diagnosis. Tissue biopsy is the gold standard by which a definitive diagnosis is made. Other points to consider are the following:

- Clinical manifestations of rejection of the kidney or pancreas include fever, oliguria, weight gain, edema, or graft tenderness (First, 1996), although most rejection episodes are asymptomatic in the early phase.
- A rise in serum creatinine is a useful serologic marker for kidney rejection and serves as a surrogate marker for pancreatic rejection.
- Beta 2 microglobulin is useful as a marker for immune activation with lymphocyte repopulation.
- Useful laboratory indicators of pancreatic rejection are lacking with the exception of the nonspecific 50% decrease in measured urinary amylase in bladder-drained grafts (Freise et al., 1999).
- Serum markers for pancreatic rejection in enteric-drained grafts are generally unreliable. Alteration in glucose metabolism occurs late in rejection, as the exocrine pancreas is rejected before the islets. Serum amylase is nonspecific. Other markers for exocrine pancreas rejection, such as serum anodal trypsinogen, pancreas secretory trypsin inhibitor, pancreas specific protein, and pancreatic elastase, have been studied, but they currently do not enjoy clinical confidence. Endocrine markers such as C peptide release to glucagon challenge and glucose disappearance rate are more specific than the exocrine markers, but they may appear too late to reverse the rejection episode (Gruessner & Sutherland, 1996).
- Radiologic studies can be used as adjuncts for the diagnosis of rejection.
- Ultrasound of the kidney may reveal graft enlargement, inhomogeneity of the renal cortex, or an increase in the arterial resistive index (First, 1996).

- Ultrasound has little role in identifying rejection of the pancreas.
- Nuclear scintigraphy may provide evidence of decreased organ perfusion, but it lacks sensitivity for pancreatic rejection. However, it may be useful in determining the likelihood of pancreatic graft survival after a rejection episode.
- Computerized tomography (CT) currently plays little role in diagnosing rejection.
- Magnetic resonance imaging (MRI) shows promise in aiding in the diagnosis of early rejection of the pancreas. Characteristic findings include a hypointense signal on T1 weighted images resembling muscular tissue and an increased signal on T2 images. MRI however, may lack sensitivity for more subtle rejection episodes (Pozniak, Propeck, Kelcz, & Sollinger, 1995).

The clinical assessment, serum markers, and radiologic studies, taken as a whole, may be sufficient to treat rejection in a given scenario. However, the definitive diagnosis of rejection is made by core needle or operative biopsy.

- Renal biopsy is fairly easy to perform and can be done surgically or under ultrasound or CT guidance.
- Nonoperative biopsy of the pancreas can also be performed under ultrasound or CT guidance or via cystoscopy for bladder-drained grafts. Both techniques share similar success in gaining adequate tissue, but ultrasound-guided percutaneous biopsy is preferred because of ease and decreased cost. (Laftavi et al., 1998).
- Further biopsy options include laparoscopic and open procedures, although these are rarely required.

TREATMENT OF REJECTION

The treatment of allograft rejection in SKP patients depends on severity, prior response to rejection therapy, and, to some extent, the organs involved. If rejection is irreversible, operative removal of the rejected organ(s) is required.

Kidney Allografts

Mild rejection of renal allografts can often be reversed with a short course of methylprednisolone for 3 to 4 days, followed by a steroid taper. This strategy has a 70% success rate in reversing graft rejection (First, 1996).

More severe rejection or steroid resistance can be treated with a 7- to 14-day course of anti-T-cell polyclonal or monoclonal antibody therapy. This strategy has a greater than 90% success rate.

Pancreas Allografts

Similar treatment strategies for pancreatic rejection can be attempted, although pancreatic rejection tends to be more steroid resistant. A combination of steroid and anti-T-cell therapy is usually successful in reversing rejection of the pancreas allograft. Failure to reverse a rejection episode leads to graft loss.

LONG-TERM CARE

The key to successful management of the SKP transplant recipient is constant surveillance. Weekly clinic visits are scheduled with the clinical coordinator, nephrologist, and transplant surgeon during the first month after transplantation. After the first month, patients typically are referred back to their primary care providers for routine follow-up care. The transplant surgeon and nephrologist provide a detailed discharge summary and an updated medication list. Visits to the transplant center decrease over time according to center specific protocols.

FOLLOW-UP TESTS

Follow-up laboratory work varies among transplant centers. Typical tests include the following:

- First two postoperative weeks: biweekly complete blood count (CBC), chemistry profile (including electrolytes), beta-2 microglobulin, immunosuppressant levels (tacrolimus, sirolimus, cyclosporine)
- Postoperative week 3 through weeks 12 to 24: weekly CBC, chemistry profile, beta-2 microglobulin, immunosuppressant levels
- Postoperative months 6 through 12: bimonthly CBC, chemistry profile, beta-2 microglobulin, immunosuppressant levels
- After month 12: monthly CBC, chemistry profile, beta-2 microglobulin, immunosuppressant levels (for remainder of patient's life)

COMPLICATIONS

Transplantation of the kidney and pancreas is a major surgical procedure and, as such, exposes patients to complications associated with abdominal surgery such as wound infection, dehiscence, ileus, pneumonia, and line sepsis. There is an increased risk for opportunistic infection and malignancy due to immunosuppression. Additionally, there are potential infectious, metabolic, and technical complications specific to the transplant procedure itself. Complications vary by exocrine drainage site.

INFECTION

Cytomegalovirus

The two forms of cytomegalovirus (CMV) infection are viremia and tissue invasive disease, the later of which is less common but more serious. The incidence of viremia and tissue invasive disease is highest in CMV seronegative patients who receive organs from a CMV sero-positive donor (Rubin, 1993).

Typically, SKP recipients receive ganciclovir postoperatively for CMV prophylaxis. The duration of the prophylactic regimen varies with the patient's risk. High-risk recipients (seronegative recipient/seropositive donor) are generally treated for at least 6 months to 1 year, whereas low-risk patients are treated for 3 to 6 months.

CMV disease typically presents as fever, low white count, and increased beta-2 microglobulin without a proportionate rise in creatinine. Gastrointestinal ulceration is common in tissue invasive disease. Diagnosis is made by serology (positive anti-CMV IgM), detection of the virus by culture or antigenemia, or identification of viral inclusions on biopsy of affected organs.

Treatment requires intravenous ganciclovir and/or CMV hyperimmune globulin and reduction in immunosuppression (see chapter 2).

METABOLIC COMPLICATIONS

Common metabolic complications include dehydration, metabolic acidosis, hyperkalemlia, and hypomagnesemia. The combination of high postoperative urine output and exocrine fluid losses for bladder-drained pancreatic allografts predisposes patients to profound dehydration. Additional loss of bicarbonate from the pancreas into the urine leads to metabolic acidosis. Both the loss of bicarbonate and metabolic acidosis can require readmission in the early postoperative period. Patients are encouraged to maintain adequate oral hydration, and oral bicarbonate supplements are often required (Fabrega et al., 1994). Hyperkalemia may be due to acidosis or diminished renal function. Hypomagnesemia is common with tacrolimus or cyclosporine administration.

PANCREAS–SPECIFIC COMPLICATIONS

Hyperglycemia or hypoglycemia can occur with postoperative pancreatic graft inflammation or rejection; however, these are generally very late signs of graft distress. Normal glucose metabolism should not be used as evidence of graft health.

Allograft pancreatitis and hyperamylasemia are seen in the postoperative period proportionate to the general viability of the donor organ. Reperfusion injury is associated with donor instability, older donor age, and increased ischemic time. Constipation and bowel obstruction are also causes of graft pancreatitis in enterically drained glands.

Reflux pancreatitis develops in 11% to 17% of recipients with bladder-drained allografts (Hickey et al., 1997). Treatment with Foley catheter drainage is usually effective.

Anastomotic leaks occur with enteric- and bladder-drained grafts in 5% and 16% of recipients, respectively (Sollinger et al., 1998). Resultant large fluid collections should be drained and operative repair seriously considered. Bladder leaks can initially be treated with Foley catheter decompression. If this intervention is unsuccessful, either operative repair or enteric conversion should be attempted. Enteric leaks, though less frequent, are associated with greater morbidity and are more likely to result in graft loss.

Graft thrombosis, a serious complication, occurs in 3–10 % of grafts (Fabrega et al., 1994). The pancreas is a relatively low flow organ. The incidence of graft thrombosis is lowest in SKP patients who are typically uremic and coagulopathic. Venous thrombosis usually precedes arterial thrombosis.

Splenic vein thrombosis treated with anticoagulation therapy is generally successful and results in good long-term graft function. However, anticoagulation therapy is not effective for recipients of a pancreas graft alone (Kuo et al., 1997). Propagation of the clot into the portal vein is likely to render the graft nonviable and leads to whole graft thrombosis and graft necrosis. In these cases, the pancreas should be removed.

UROLOGIC COMPLICATIONS

Bladder-drained pancreatic grafts are associated with urologic complications secondary to altered urinary pH and mucosal injury due to pancreatic digestive enzymes. Enteric conversion of these grafts is required in approximately 20% of recipients; hence the current impetus to perform primary enteric drainage of exocrine secretions (Sollinger et al., 1998).

Significant gross *hematuria* occurs in 9% to 28% of patients with bladder drainage. Hematuria often heralds other complications, such as anastomotic leak, graft pancreatitis, rejection, thrombosis, and an infectious process such as CMV duodenitis. Catheter placement is advisable to avoid clot-induced urinary retention and to facilitate irrigation while underlying causes are investigated. If drainage and irrigation fail, cystoscopy is useful diagnostically and therapeutically. In severe cases, enteric conversion can be performed for anastomotic bleeding. Graft pancreatectomy may be required in emergency situations.

Urinary tract infections are exceedingly common after bladder drainage and often require readmission to the hospital. In addition to the usual flora, *Staphylococcus epidermidis, Enterococcus, Pseudomonas,* and *Candida* are frequent etiologic agents. Appropriate antibiotic therapy based on culture and sensitivity data is usually successful (Hickey et al., 1997).

Urethral complications, such as urethritis, urethral disruption, and urethral stricture, are associated with bladder-drained exocrine secretions. Foley catheter drainage can be initially attempted, but if this fails, enteric conversion is indicated.

KIDNEY-SPECIFIC COMPLICATIONS

Renal graft complications in SKP transplant recipients are less common. Acute tubular necrosis requiring dialysis in the postoperative period occurs in only 4% of recipients. The low rate of renal graft dysfunction is attributed to the generally shorter ischemic times and younger donor age associated with simultaneous pancreas transplantation. Ureteral leaks and strictures are relatively rare; each occur in less than 1% of recipients. Because of the kidney's higher blood flow, graft thrombosis is uncommon. Lymphoceles are not uncommon and, if present despite percutaneous aspiration, require either laparoscopic or open reperitonealization.

WHEN TO CALL THE TRANSPLANT CENTER

The risks of transplantation and immunosuppression are typically explained in detail by the surgeon, nephrologist, and clinical coordinator. Educational booklets or slide presentations are frequently used to supplement patient and family education. Patients and their primary care providers typically have access to the transplant staff 24 hours a day. General communication with the transplant service is prudent if the recipient develops any of the following:

- Fever greater than 100.5°F
- Decrease in urine output
- Increase in weight greater than 2 to 3 pounds. over a 24-hour period
- Vomiting
- Diarrhea
- Requirement for any new prescription or over-the-counter medications that may interact with immunosuppression regimen

CONCLUSION

Success with simultaneous kidney pancreas transplantation has improved over the past decade with advances made in immunosuppressive regimens as well as in the surgical technique. This procedure is usually reserved for type 1 diabetics with end-stage renal disease, although select cases of type 2 diabetes have been reported. Challenges for physicians and nurses caring for this patient population include early identification of the subtle signs and symptoms of rejection and infection. Symptoms of pancreas graft rejection are difficult to evaluate because many tests are inconclusive. Close communication between community health care providers and transplant center personnel is very important to successful long-term outcomes of graft and patient survival.

REFERENCES

Diabetes Control and Complications Trial Research Group. (1993). The effect of intensive treatment of diabetes on the development and progression of long-term complications in insulin-dependent diabetes mellitus. *New England Journal of Medicine, 329,* 977–986.

Fabrega, A. J., Rivas, P. A., & Pollak, R. (1994). Pancreas–kidney transplantation for intensivists: Perioperative care and complications. *Journal of Intensive Care Medicine, 9,* 281–289.

First, M. R. (1996). Clinical diagnosis of renal allograft rejection. In K. Solez, L. C. Racusen, & M. E. Billingham (Eds.). *Solid organ transplant rejection: Mechanisms, pathology, and diagnosis* (pp. 431–443). New York: Marcel Dekker.

Freise, C. E., Narumi, S., Stock, P. G., & Melzer, J. S. (1999). Simultaneous pancreas–kidney transplantation: An overview of indications, complications, and outcomes. *Western Journal of Medicine, 170*(1), 11–18.

Gruessner, A. C., & Sutherland, D. E. (1999). Anaylses of pancreas transplant outcomes for United States cases reported to the United Network for Organ Sharing (UNOS) and non-US cases reported to the International Pancreas Transplant Registry (IPTR). *Clinical Transplantation,* 51–69.

Gruessner, R. W. (1998). Antibody induction therapy in pancreas transplantation. *Transplantation Proceedings, 30*(4), 1556–1559.

Gruessner, R. W. G., & Sutherland, D. E. R. (1996). Clinical diagnosis in pancreatic allograft rejection. In K. Solez, L. C. Racusen, & M. E. Billingham (Eds.). *Solid organ transplant rejection: Mechanisms, pathology, and diagnosis* (pp. 455–499). New York: Marcel Dekker.

Hickey, D. P., Bakthavatsalam, R., Bannon, C. A., O'Malley, K., Corr, J., & Little, D. M. (1997). Urologic complications of pancreatic transplantation. *Journal of Urology, 157*(6), 2042–2048.

Kuo, P. C., Wong, J., Schweitzer, E. J., Johnson, L. B., Lim, J. W., & Bartlett, S. T. (1997). Outcome after splenic vein thrombosis in the pancreas allograft. *Transplantation, 64*(6), 933–935.

Laftavi, M. R., Gruessner, A. C., Bland, B. J., Foshager, M., Walsh, J. W., Sutherland, D. E., & Gruessner, R. W. (1998). Diagnosis of pancreas rejection: Cystoscopic transduodenal versus percutaneous computed tomography scan-guided biopsy. *Transplantation, 65*(4): 528–532.

Libman, I., Songer, T., and LaPorte, R. (1993). How many people in the U.S. have IDDM? *Diabetes Care, 16*(5): 841–842.

Pozniak, M. A., Propeck, P. A., Kelcz, F., & Sollinger, H. (1995). Imaging of pancreas transplants. *Radiology Clinics of North America, 33*(3), 581–594.

Rubin, R. H. (1993). Infectious disease complications of renal transplantation. *Kidney International, 44*(1), 221–236

Sollinger, H. W., Odorico, J. S., Knechtle, S. J., D'Allesandro, A. M., Kalayoglu, M., & Pirsch, J. D., (1998). Experience with 500 simultaneous pancreas-kidney transplants. *Annals of Surgery, 228*(3), 284–296.

Stratta, R. J. (1999). Optimal immunosuppression in pancreas transplantation. *Transplantation Proceedings, 31*(1–2), 619–621.

Stratta, R. J., Gaber, A. O., Shokouh-Amiri, M. H., Reddy, K. S., Egidi, M. F., Grewal, H. P., & Graber, L. W. (2000). A prospective comparison of systemic-bladder versus portal-enteric drainage in vascularized pancreas transplantation. *Surgery, 127*(2), 217–226.

Sutherland, D. E. R. (1998). Pancreas and pancreas-kidney transplantation. *Current Opinions in Nephrology and Hypertension, 7,* 317–325.

Sutherland, D. E., & Gruessner, A. (1995). Long-term function (> 5 years) of pancreas grafts from the International Pancreas Transplant Registry database. *Transplantation Proceedings, 27*(6), 2977–2980.

United Network for Organ Sharing. (2001). *Transplant Patient DataSource: Adult graft and patient survival rates for kidney/pancreas transplants performed: National results.* Retrieved February 25, 2001, from http://www.unos.org

United Network for Organ Sharing. (2001). *Critical data: Waiting list.* Retrieved Janurary 23, 2002, from http://www.unos.org/Newsroom/cridtata_main.htm

U.S. Department of Health and Human Services. (2000). *Annual report of the U.S. Scientific Registry for Transplant Recipients and the Organ Procurement and Transplantation Network: Transplant data, 1990–1999.* Rockville, MD: Author.

9

Lung and Heart–Lung Transplantation

Steve Nathan and Linda Ohler

Although surgical procedures, immunosuppression, and follow-up care have helped increase the survival rates and quality of life of patients, lung and heart–lung transplantation continue to challenge clinicians. Internationally, the volume of heart–lung transplantation has dropped significantly from 241 cases in 1989 to 103 cases in 1998 (Hosenpud et al., 1999). The 1-year survival for single-lung and bilateral-lung transplantation are similar, at 75% (Hosenpud et al., 1999). Interestingly, 3 years after transplantation, bilateral-lung transplants have an approximately 50% survival, as compared to 40% for single-lung recipients. Eight-year survival rates are 40% and 30%, respectively, for bilateral- and single-lung transplants. Heart–lung survival statistics demonstrate a 5-year survival rate of 40% and a 10-year survival rate of 30% (Hosenpud et al., 1999). These differences in survival between single and bilateral transplants may be due to patient selection for the procedure rather than a function of the procedure itself, because younger patients are often recipients of the latter procedure.

INDICATIONS FOR LUNG OR HEART–LUNG TRANSPLANTATION

The most common diagnoses for which lung transplantation is performed include the following (Hosenpud et al., 1999; Maurer, Frost, Estenne, Higenbottam, & Glanville, 1998):

- Chronic obstructive pulmonary disease (COPD)
- Alpha-1 antitrypsin-induced emphysema
- Idiopathic pulmonary fibrosis (IPF)
- Cystic fibrosis (CF)
- Primary pulmonary hypertension (PPH)
- Eisenmenger's syndrome

Other disease entities potentially leading to lung transplantation include the following (Hosenpud et al., 1999):

- Bronchiectasis
- Sarcoidosis
- Lymphangioleiomyomatosis (LAM)
- Eosinophilic granunuloma of the lung

Single-lung transplantation is most often the treatment of choice for COPD and IPF. Cystic fibrosis and other bronchiectasis patients require bilateral-lung transplantation because of the high risk of transmission of infection. Bilateral-lung transplants are sometimes performed in younger COPD patients, such as those with alpha-1 antitrypsin deficiency, and patients with pulmonary hypertension. Heart–lung transplantation is reserved for Eisenmenger's syndrome. Determinations about the specific type of transplant to be performed depend on the outcomes of individualized testing.

EVALUATION FOR LUNG OR HEART–LUNG TRANSPLANTATION

Candidates for lung or heart–lung transplantation are carefully screened for their suitability as a candidate. Potential candidates should meet the following guidelines (Maurer et al., 1998; Trulock, 1997, 2000):

- End-stage pulmonary disease despite optimal medical therapy
- Life expectancy < 2–3 years
- Ambulatory with potential for rehabilitation
- > 70% or < 120% of ideal body weight

- Good psychosocial support system
- Satisfactory psychological profile
- Adequate insurance coverage

The recommended age criteria for recipients (Maurer et al., 1998):

- Heart–lung transplantation   < 55 years
- Bilateral-lung transplantation   < 60 years
- Single-lung transplantation   < 65 years

Contraindications to lung transplantation include the following:

- Active malignancy in past 2 years
- Cigarette smoking within past 6 months
- Creatinine clearance < 50 mg/mL/min
- Significant disease involving another organ system
- Nonadherence to medical regimens
- Drug or alcohol dependency
- Significant coronary disease
- Severe left ventricular dysfunction (may be considered for heart–lung transplantation)
- Untreatable infection
- Active hepatitis B infection
- Hepatitis C infection with abnormal liver tests
- Untreated tuberculosis
- Human immunodeficiency virus (HIV) infection

Relative contraindications (evaluated on an individual basis):

- Ventilator dependence
- Previous thoracic surgery
- Current use of steroids > 20 mg/day
- Symptomatic osteoporosis
- Severe musculoskeletal disease

The transplant evaluation is best done with tests performed in the order that is most likely to preclude candidacy. Evaluations done in systematic and individualized stages are most efficient and cost effective.

STAGE 1: REFERRAL

As part of the referral stage, the following items should be covered:

- Medical records obtained from referring physician
- Records reviewed with a transplant pulmonologist

- Telephone screening of patient
- Oxygen needs for travel
- Accommodations at transplant center
- Insurance coverage
- Educational needs

STAGE 2: SCREENING

Screening includes the following:

- History and physical by a transplant pulmonologist
- 6-minute walk
- Pulmonary function tests (PFTs)

The 6-minute walk may suggest that a patient is too well or too ill for transplantation. The results of this test are useful in determining the next steps in the evaluation process.

Patient Education

Education is important at this stage because it assists the patient and family in understanding the purpose of extensive testing prior to lung transplantation. Education also helps the patient and family make an informed decision about transplantation. Understanding the process and discussing risks and benefits early in the transplant evaluation can help the patient and family determine questions to ask of physicians and nurses. Table 9.1 suggests topics to be discussed with patients and their families as the evaluation process begins.

STAGE 3: PROCEDURES AND TESTS

Tests to determine candidacy for lung transplantation include the following (Maurer et al., 1998):

Pulmonary Assessment
- Ventilation-Perfusion (VQ) Scan
- Computed tomography scan (CT) of the chest
- PFTs
- Arterial blood gases (ABG)

TABLE 9.1 Suggested Educational Topics for Potential Lung Candidates

Evaluation process for lung, heart–lung transplantation
- Tests
- Consultations

Outcomes of lung transplantation

Risks and benefits of lung, heart–lung transplantation

Surgical procedure

Hospital care

Rejection/infection

Immunosuppressants

Follow-up care

Quality-of-life issues

Return to work

Cardiac Assessment
- Coronary angiography for patients > 45 years old
- Right heart catheterization to determine pulmonary vascular resistance
- Electrocardiogram (EKG)
- Multiple gated acquisition (MUGA)
- Echocardiogram

Renal Function
- 24-hour urine for creatinine clearance

Infectious Disease Assessment
- Tuberculosis skin test
- Cytomegalovirus (CMV) IgG, IgM
- Ebstein-Barr virus (EBV) IgG, IgM
- Hepatitis screen
- Varicella antibody titer
- Herpes simplex 1 and 2
- Immunization history
- Travel history

Tests of the Immune System
- Panel of reactive antibodies (PRA) to determine allosensitivities
- Human leukocyte antigens (HLA) with specificities if PRA is elevated
- ABO blood type

Miscellaneous Testing
- Mammogram for women
- Pelvic exam for women
- Prostate-specific antigen (PSA) for males
- Bone density scan
- Sigmoidoscopy/colonoscopy

Blood Tests
- CBC
- Chemistries
- Liver function tests

Consultations should be held in the following areas:

- Psychosocial Evaluation
  - History of substance abuse
  - Compliance/adherence issues
  - Emotional stability
- Financial/insurance assessment
- Dietitian, if necessary
- Surgeon
- Cardiologist (if necessary)
- Infectious disease specialist, if necessary

STAGE 4: MULTIDISCIPLINARY MEETING

A multidisciplinary meeting is held weekly at most transplant centers to discuss potential candidates for transplantation. The case is presented by a pulmonologist or lung transplant coordinator, and all consultants are invited to attend. A complete medical history is presented on each patient followed by tests results. Scans and X rays are reviewed by team members. Occasionally, additional testing is determined to be necessary. The type of transplant is determined based on the underlying disease, patient age, and test results. Thus, the patient is determined to be a candidate for single-lung, bilateral-lung, or heart–lung transplantation at this meeting.

STAGE 5: LISTING A PATIENT FOR LUNG OR HEART–LUNG TRANSPLANTATION

Candidates are listed with a national computer system at the United Network for Organ Sharing (UNOS). This system includes 11 regions with local organ procurement organizations (OPOs) working within UNOS.

Patients are listed according to their size and blood type. Organs are allocated on a local basis, with consideration given to length of time on the list, blood type, and size.

Other important points:

- Blood type and size are the major determining factors for organ suitability.
- There is no prioritization for the allocation of lungs.
- Patients with IPF are given 3 months of additional time on the waiting list due to the generally poor prognosis associated with this condition.
- Waiting times for lung or heart–lung transplantation can vary from region to region.
- Median wait times for lung transplantation range from 337 to 848 days (Pierson et al., 2000).
- From 20% to 25% of patients die awaiting a suitable lung or heart–lung donor (Pierson et al., 2000).

CARE OF THE CANDIDATE AWAITING LUNG OR HEART–LUNG TRANSPLANTATION

Most transplant programs require candidates for lung transplantation to participate in pulmonary rehabilitation programs 2 or 3 times a week while awaiting transplantation. Pulmonary rehabilitation programs include exercise, education, psychosocial support, and chest physiotherapy. These programs are designed to optimize functional capacity, decrease symptoms, and restore patients to their highest level of self-care (Resnikoff & Ries, 1998).

SURGICAL PROCEDURES

There are three anastamoses that are performed:

- Pulmonary artery
- Pulmonary veins
- Bronchus in the case of single- and bilateral-lung transplants and the trachea in the case of heart–lung transplants

Structures that are sacrificed as part of the surgical procedure include the following:

- *Pulmonary lymphatics.* This can have some ramifications with regards to the ability of patients to clear pleural effusions in the posttransplant period. Also, the lymphatics function to clear microbes from the pulmonary parenchyma. The lack of lymphatics posttransplant is one of many reasons why lung recipients are at high risk for infections.
- *Bronchial circulation.* This is a very inexact part of the human anatomy with multiple variants. As such, it is tedious and time consuming to reanastamose. Lack of bronchial circulation in the posttransplant period may predispose recipients to the development of ischemia of the airways. The integrity of the airways is initially dependent on retrograde pulmonary venous flow until revascularization can be reestablished.
- *Pulmonary nerves.* The consequences of this denervation are that the cough reflex distal to the anastamosis is abrogated.

SINGLE-LUNG TRANSPLANTATION

Single-lung transplantation is the most common transplant procedure. It is usually performed through a thoracotomy incision.

BILATERAL-LUNG TRANSPLANTATION

- Each lung is implanted with a bronchial anastamosis, as opposed to the earlier double-lung transplant procedure, in which both lungs were implanted as a block with a tracheal anastamosis.
- Bilateral-lung transplants are usually accomplished through a subcostal incision. This allows for better exposure of bronchial collaterals posteriorly, which can be extensive, especially in cystic fibrosis patients. If adequate hemostasis from these is not obtained, postoperative bleeding can be problematic.
- In the past, double-lung transplant procedures were accomplished through a median sternotomy incision.
- The advantage of the bilateral- versus the double-lung procedure is that the former can often be accomplished without the use of cardiopulmonary bypass (CPB). In patients with significant pulmonary hypertension, CPB is usually unavoidable, as patients are unable to be maintained with single-lung perfusion.

HEART–LUNG TRANSPLANTATION

The least common of all thoracic transplant procedures, heart–transplantation is performed through a median sternotomy and involves the standard vascular anastamosis and a tracheal anastamosis.

IMMEDIATE POSTOPERATIVE CARE

HEMODYNAMIC

The major principle of postoperative hemodynamic support is to maintain patients on the slightly "dry" side to reduce the incidence and/or severity of reperfusion edema. However, this should not however be at the expense of requiring pressor support, although a significant percentage of lung recipients will require such support in the early posttransplant period. This is especially true for patients who had significant pretransplant pulmonary hypertension and who required cardiopulmonary bypass for the procedure. Prolonged hypotension may predispose to bronchial complications and place the bronchial anastamosis at risk as blood flow to the bronchi is already somewhat compromised because of the lack of bronchial circulation.

Causes of hypotension in the early post lung transplant period include:

- Volume depletion
- Pleural bleeding
- Post by-pass effect
- Syndrome of low systemic vascular resistance (SVR)/high cardiac output. This is thought to be due to massive cytokine release effect
- Dynamic hyperinflation of the native lung. This is specific to single-lung COPD recipients with overinflation of the native lung, resulting in a shift of the mediastinum and hemodynamic compromise. The clue to this diagnosis is the demonstration of serial shift of the mediastinum on chest X ray.

Management focus on "deflating" the native side through ventilator manipulations involves:

- Reducing/eliminating positive end-expiratory pressure (PEEP)
- Increasing the Inspiration/Expiration (I/E) ratio by increasing the inspiratory flow rate and/or reducing the tidal volume or respiratory rate

In some cases, independent lung ventilation may be indicated. The best solution for this problem is to get the patient extubated and breathing spontaneously. Unfortunately, most of these patients are too early post-transplant or are not stable enough to warrant extubation.

Less common problems associated with post-operative hypotension include:

- Labile pulmonary artery pressures. This is seen in patients with pre-existing pulmonary hypertension.
- Right ventricular outflow obstruction. This rare entity has been described in patients with severe preexisting pulmonary hypertension, primarily secondary to Eisenmenger's syndrome.

VENTILATORY SUPPORT

Patients initally are maintained on volume-controlled ventilation after the surgery. Low levels of PEEP usually are used to prevent atelectasis. Some COPD patients may require the elimination of PEEP if they develop evidence of dynamic hyperinflation of the native lung.

Patients can be extubated as soon as they are deemed clinically stable; this can be within 24 hours of the procedure in uncomplicated cases. Prolonged weaning trials usually are not necessary.

Patients who had hypercapnea prior to transplantation cannot be expected to be extubated with normal pCO_2 levels. The pCO_2 may take a few weeks to normalize. It is acceptable to extubate such patients even with pCO_2 level in the 60s or 70s provided their acidosis is compensated. A useful strategy in such patients is to place them on pressure support ventilation prior to extubation to enable them to target their own pCO_2 level.

Most of these patients will have high serum bicarbonate levels reflective of a compensatory metabolic alkalosis. Acetazolamide to correct the metabolic alkalosis can be considered but should be used with caution and only in those patients who are felt to have a primary component to their metabolic alkalosis.

It is routine to maintain patients with severe pulmonary hypertension on mechanical ventilation for 3 to 5 days. The reason for this is that they are prone to marked swings in pulmonary artery pressures, which can be associated with hemodynamic instability and respiratory compromise. It is usual to heavily sedate patients to prevent any agitation that may precipitate increased pulmonary pressures.

Paralytic agents are best avoided because they may predispose patients to the development of critical illness myopathies, especially because transplant patients are already receiving high-dose steroids.

Differential diagnosis of allograft complications while on the ventilator includes the following:

Hypoxia Posttransplant
- Reperfusion pulmonary edema
- Mucous plugging and atelectasis
- Pneumonia
- Acute rejection
- Vascular anastamotic problem

Failure to Wean
- Retained secretions/mucous plugging
- Parenchymal process (such as reperfusion injury/pneumonia)
- Myopathy
- Phrenic nerve paresis
- Pain/anxiety
- Blunted hypercapneic response

ANCILLARY SUPPORTIVE MEASURES

Chest physiotherapy is important in helping to facilitate the clearance of secretions. This is especially vital in lung transplant recipients, who do not have a cough reflex distal to the anastamosis. Therefore, the cough reflex in response to secretions is diminished.

It may be worthwhile to avoid chest physiotherapy in the subgroup of patients with severe pulmonary hypertension since this may add to pain/anxiety and may precipitate elevations in pulmonary pressures. This in turn may result in or exacerbate reperfusion edema.

Once patients have been extubated, chest physiotherapy can be supplemented or replaced with the use of flutter valves and incentive spirometers. It is always a goal to ambulate patients as soon as possible after extubation to facilitate expectoration of secretions and reversal of any atelectasis.

PAIN CONTROL

Pain control is important for patient comfort and to facilitate deep breathing, compliance with physical therapy, breathing devices, and pulmonary rehabilitation. Standard narcotic medications, patient-controlled analgesia, and epidural anesthetics can all be used in lung transplant recipients.

Thoracotomy (single-lung transplants) incisions tend to result in more pain than sternotomy (heart–lung transplants) or subcostal incisions (bilateral–lung transplants). A thoracotomy involves dividing the chest muscles, dissecting nerve fibers, and spreading the ribs. Postoperatively, movement by the patient exacerbates the pain associated with this surgical approach. A sternotomy involves an incision through the sternum–a structure that has no nerve supply. After the sternotomy, the sternum is reapproximated with wires. Postoperatively, movement by the patient typically does not produce pain in the sternal area.

NUTRITION SUPPORT

Many lung transplant recipients are malnourished as a consequence of their underlying primary lung disease, especially cystic fibrosis and COPD patients. Early nutritional support is therefore very important to facilitate postoperative recovery.

REHABILITATION

Pulmonary rehabilitation should be started as soon as possible after extubation. Many lung transplant patients are severely deconditioned from their underlying disease even when they have participated actively in pulmonary rehabilitation prior to transplant.

Interestingly, deconditioning rather than breathing problems becomes a limiting factor in exercise. Thus, early aggressive rehabilitation is important.

BRONCHOSCOPY

Bronchoscopy is an important tool in the management of lung transplant recipients. Patients are usually first bronchoscoped in the operating room after the procedure is complete to determine the internal integrity of the bronchial anastamosis and to clear any secretions and blood that may have pooled during the procedure. Bronchoscopy is then performed as deemed clinically appropriate. Some transplant programs have a protocol of surveillance bronchoscopies. However, there is no data in the literature attesting to improved outcomes with surveillance bronchoscopies. It is often worthwhile to perform a bronchoscopy prior to extubation, and it may be necessary to perform serial bronchoscopies on patients who are intubated for periods of time, for optimal pulmonary toilet.

Indications for bronchoscopy include the following:

Intubated
- Excess secretions/mucous plugs
- Unexplained parenchymal infiltrates
- Failure to wean
- Prolonged airleak (to check integrity of bronchial anastamosis)

Extubated
- Failure to clear secretions despite appropriate chest physiotherapy
- Unexplained parenchymal infiltrates
- Low or decreasing pulmonary function tests
- Unexplained fever or leukocytosis

IMMUNOSUPPRESSION REGIMENS

Pretransplant/Intraoperative

Most programs will dose patients with a calcineurin inhibitor (tacrolimus or cyclosporine) and/or azathioprine prior to the transplant. However, as with much of the immunotherapy that is employed in lung transplantation, there is no data to support the efficacy of this approach.

It is standard for patients to receive a bolus of solumedrol (500 mg–1 g) when the pulmonary artery is unclamped. This is given more out of concern for reperfusion injury rather than out of concern for hyperacute rejection.

Immediate Posttransplant Period

Steroids.

In the early days of lung transplantation, every attempt was made to avoid steroids in the early posttransplant period because it was felt that this interfered with healing of the bronchial anastamosis. This has since been refuted, and it is now standard to administer steroids from the outset. Solumedrol 125 mg intravenously every 12 hours for 6 doses is usually employed before starting patients on oral prednisone at 1 mg/kg (but usually not more than 60 mg) per day.

Cytolytic therapy.

The use of cytolytics remains controversial. They gained favor in the early days of lung transplantation when it was considered necessary to avoid steroids in the early posttransplant period. There are no data in the literature to suggest that patients who receive cytolytics do any better than those who do not. Although the incidence of episodes of acute rejection may be reduced, the increased incidence of infections may counterbalance any beneficial effects. Similarly, there are no definitive data to suggest that cytolytics will reduce the incidence of chronic rejection.

Calcineurin inhibitors.

Both cyclosporine and tacrolimus are used in lung transplant recipients. There are some data to suggest that tacrolimus may be preferable, but some of these studies compared tacrolimus to earlier formulations of cyclosporine. Both are given immediately posttransplant either intravenously or via the nasogastric tube. Tacrolimus especially is well absorbed when given via the oral route.

Antimetabolites.

Either azathioprine or mycophenolate mofetil can be used.

Long-term Immunotherapy

Lung recipients are usually maintained on triple immunotherapy with a calcineurin inhibitor, an antimetabolite, and prednisone. Prednisone can usually be tapered to the 5 to 10 mg per day/alternate day range. Unlike other solid organs, discontinuation of steroids is less likely to meet with success because of the high incidence of chronic rejection (bronchiolitis obliterans).

INFECTION

The lung transplant is especially prone to the development of infection. There are several factors that place the allograft at higher risk compared to recipients of other solid organs:

- The lung is the only organ with a direct communication with the outside environment
- Blunted cough reflex
- Impaired mucociliary clearance
- Early alterations in surfactant
- Lack of pulmonary lymphatics

- Higher levels of immunosuppression
- Native lung infection/prior colonization

Bacterial

Antibacterial prophylaxis in lung transplant recipients is typically more aggressive than other solid organ recipients. Aside from the factors listed above, it is often prudent to assume that the donor may have aspirated at some stage of the terminal course or may have started to develop a nosocomial pneumonia. Antibacterial prophylaxis in the recipient should be implemented with these risks in mind and should include broad spectrum coverage.

Viral

Cytomegalovirus is a common infection in lung transplant recipients. CMV prophylaxis with ganciclovir is usually given to at risk recipients for anywhere from a few weeks to 6 months posttransplant.

Fungal

Candida, aspergillus and pneumocystis are the fungal pathogens of concern. Antifungal prophylaxis include

- Oral itraconazole or fluconazole
- Mycelex troches/nystatin swish and swallow (Candida)
- Inhaled amphotericin B (usually 15–25 mg daily or twice a day)
- Low-dose systemic amphotericin B
- Bactrim (trimethoprim sulfamethoxazole)

COMPLICATIONS

The temporal relationship to the transplant procedure has bearing on which complications the allograft may be at risk for.

Early Postoperative Period (first few days to first few weeks)
- Bleeding
- Reperfusion injury
- Infections
- Acute rejection

Intermediate Postoperative Period (weeks to months)
- Acute rejection
- Infections
- Bronchial strictures

Late Postoperative Period (months to years)
- Bronchiolitis obliterans
- Infections
- Acute rejection
- Malignancies (especially post-transplant lymphoproliferative disease)

REPERFUSION INJURY

Also referred to as reimplantation response or primary graft failure, reperfusion injury usually occurs immediately to a few days posttransplant. Of uncertain etiology, it may be related to ischemia or preservation injury and may be associated with high pretransplant pulmonary pressures.
Clinical manifestations include:

- Diffuse allograft infiltrates
- Poor gas exchange
- Frank edema fluid from the endotracheal tube

No specific therapy is required besides supportive care. Inhaled nitric oxide may be useful. Mortality may be significant (40%–60%) (Christie et al., 1998; King et al., 2000).

REJECTION

Acute allograft rejection is extremely common in lung transplant recipients. Most patients will have at least one episode of rejection within the first few months. Hyperacute rejection is extremely rare. Acute rejection may be asymptomatic. but clinical manifestations include:

- Shortness of breath/hypoxia
- Infiltrate on chest X ray (especially early acute rejection)
- Fever, leukocytosis
- Decrease in spirometric indices (especially later episodes)

DIAGNOSIS OF REJECTION

If the index of suspicion is high and other conditions (e.g., infection) have been excluded, then a clinical diagnosis may suffice. In this situation, pulsed steroids can act diagnostically as well as therapeutically. The diagnosis is usually confirmed with transbronchial biopsies. A minimum of 5 biopsies is recommended to optimize the sensitivity. The pathologic hallmark of acute rejection is perivascular lymphocytic cuffing. Thoracoscopic or open lung biopsies are usually not necessary. Table 9.2 provides the classification of rejection (Yousem et al., 1996).

Treatment is usually pulsed solumedrol (500–1,000 mg IV daily for 3 days), with subsequent prednisone taper. Recalcitrant acute rejection is unusual. Options for these situations include

1. Alterations in immunosuppressive therapy
   • Methotrexate
   • Substitute tacrolimus for cyclosporine
   • Substitute mycophenolate or sirolimus for azathioprine
   • Cytolytic therapy
2. Photopheresis
3. Total lymphoid irradiation

Prognosis is usually excellent. Recurrent episodes of acute rejection have been linked to the subsequent development of chronic rejection.

TABLE 9.2 Working Formulation for Classification and Grading of Pulmonary Allograft Rejection

A. Acute rejection
          Grade 0: None
          Grade 1: Minimal
          Grade 2: Mild
          Grade 3: Moderate
          Grade 4: Severe

B. Active airway damage without scarring
C. Chronic airway rejection—bronchiolitis obliterans
          Active
          inactive
D. Chronic vascular rejection—accelerated graft vascular sclerosis
E. Vasculitis

Source: Yousem et al., 1996

CHRONIC REJECTION (BRONCHIOLITIS OBLITERANS)

Chronic rejection, or bronchiolitis obliterans, is very common, with approximately 50% of recipients ultimately afflicted. Clinical manifestations include:

- Progressive serial decrement in lung function
- Apparent upper respiratory tract infection
- Progressive dyspnea on exertion

Chronic rejection usually occurs after the first year, but it can occur ealier. It can be associated with recurrent infections. Many patients will develop bronchiectasis and subsequent colonization/infection, with pseudomonas and other pathogens typical of bronchiectatic patients (Boehler, Kesten, Weder, & Speich, 1998).

The course is variable. Some patients can have stabilization in their lung function; others will have an intractable progressive deterioration and ultimately die from this condition. Bronchiolitis is the most common cause of death in lung transplant recipients after the first year.

Diagnosis

Pathologically chronic rejection is manifested by the obliteration of the small bronchioles (bronchiolitis obliterans). Unlike acute rejection, the yield of biopsies obtained via bronchoscopy is very low (about 20%) for bronchiolitis obliterans. Thoracoscopic or open lung biopsy is useful in diagnosis, but avoided unless there is a suspicion of their pathology.

BRONCHIOLITIS OBLITERANS SYNDROME

As defined by the International Society for Heart and Lung Transplantation, bronchiolitis obliterans syndrome (BOS) is an otherwise unexplained > 20% decrement in a patient's Forced Expiratory Volume (FEV1) from previously established maximal FEV1 (Cooper et al., 1993). BOS is further defined as:

Mild BOS: FEV1 66%–80% of baseline value
Moderate BOS: FEV1 51%–65% of baseline value
Severe BOS: FEV1 50% or less of baseline value

This has allowed clinicians to diagnose patients without subjecting them to the morbidity of a thoracoscopic or open lung biopsy. Such procedures were done frequently before BOS was defined, but in most cases they did not alter the patient's management.

Treatment

There is no cure for bronchiolitis obliterans. Attempts should be made to stabilize the progressive loss of lung function, and in a minority of cases some reversal may be achieved. The therapeutic options for this are the same as those for recalcitrant acute rejection (see above).

Prognosis

The prognosis has not been well delineated. One study showed a 66%, 44%, 37%, and 10% survival at 1, 3, 5, and 10 years, respectively (Reichenspurner et al., 1995).

LONG-TERM CARE

The key to success is constant vigilance. Patients should return to the clinic after discharge on a frequent basis, with a gradually tapering schedule of clinic visits over time. After the first year, patients should routinely return for follow-up visits at the transplant center every 3 months.

At each clinic visit, the following should be obtained:

- Blood work, including trough levels of tacrolimus or cyclosporine
- Chest X ray
- Spirometry

WHEN TO CALL THE TRANSPLANT CENTER

Patients are instructed to call the transplant center if they develop any of the following symptoms:

- Fever. Patients are instructed to record their temperature daily
- Symptoms of upper respiratory tract infection
- Increased shortness of breath
- Productive cough
- Decrease in spirometry. Patients are instructed to record their FVC and FEV1 on their own home spirometer on a daily basis. They are instructed to call if either of these two indices are decreased 10% below their baseline. Causes of reduction in spirometry:

- Acute rejection
- Bronchial stricture
- Chronic rejection
- Infections
- High glucose
- High blood pressure readings

CONCLUSION

Collaborative care between physicians and nurses in the community and the transplant center is important to successful outcomes after lung or heart–lung transplantation. Notifying the transplant center of any problems, hospital admissions, or questions is essential. Because of potential drug interactions, it is important to discuss treatment interventions with the transplant physician. Trough levels of immunosuppressive agents should be monitored at the transplant center or a laboratory using the same assay. Often clinical presentations and diagnostic test results make it difficult to differentiate between infection and rejection. Therefore, discussions with the transplant center will help to determine the interventions needed.

REFERENCES

Boehler, A., Kesten, S., Weder, W., & Speich, R. (1998). Bronchiolitis obliterans after lung transplantation: A review. *Chest, 114*(5), 1411–1426.

Christie, J. D., Bavaria, J. E., Palevsky, H. I., Litzky, L., Blumenthal, N. P., Kaiser, L. R., & Kotloff, R. M. (1998). Primary graft failure following lung transplantation. *Chest, 114*(1), 1–60.

Cooper, J. D., Billingham, M., Egan, T., Hertz, M. I., Higenbottam, T., Lynch, J., Mauer, J., Paradis, I., Patterson, G. A., & Smith, C. (1993). A working formulation for the standardization of nomenclature and the clinical staging of chronic dysfunction in lung allografts. *Journal of Heart and Lung Transplantation, 12*(5), 713–716.

Hosenpud, J. D., Bennett, L. E., Keck, B. M., Fiol, B., Boucek, M., & Novick, R. J. (1999). The registry of the International Society for Heart and Lung Transplantation: Sixteenth official report, 1999. *Journal of Heart and Lung Transplantation, 18*(7), 611–626.

King, R. C., Binns, O. A., Rodriguez, F., Kanithanon, R. C., Daniel, T. M., Spotnitz W. D., Tribble, C. G., & Kron, I. L. (2000). Reperfusion injury significantly impacts clinical outcome after pulmonary transplantation. *Annals of Thoracic Surgery, 69*(6), 1681–1685.

Maurer, J. R., Frost, A. E., Estenne, M., Higenbottam, T., & Glanville, A. (1998). International guidelines for the selection of lung transplant candidates. *Journal of Heart and Lung Transplantation, 17*(7), 703–709.

Paradis, I. L., Duncan, S. R., Dauber, J. H., Yousem, S., Hardesty, R., & Griffith, B. (1992). Distinguishing between infection, rejection, and the adult respiratory distress syndrome after human lung transplantation. *Journal of Heart and Lung Transplantation, 11*(4, Pt. 2), S232–S236.

Pierson, R. N., Milstone, A. P., Lloyd, J. E., Lewis, B. H., Pinson, C. W., & Ely, E. W. (2000). Lung allocation in the United States, 1995–1997: An analysis of equity and utility. *Journal of Heart and Lung Transplantation, 19*(9), 846–851.

Reichenspurner, H., Girgis, R. E., Robbins, R. C., Conte, J. V., Nair, R. V., Valentine, H., Berry, G. J., Morris, R. E., Theodore, J., & Reitz, B. A. (1995) Obliterative bronchiolitis after lung and heart–lung transplantation. *Annals of Thoracic Surgery, 60*(6), 1845–1853.

Resnikoff, P. M., & Ries, A. L. (1998). Pulmonary rehabilitation for chronic lung disease. *Journal of Heart and Lung Transplantation, 17*(7), 643–650.

Trulock, E. P. (1997). Lung transplantation. *American Journal of Respiratory Critical Care Medicine, 155*(3), 789–818.

Trulock, E. P. (2000). *Indications, selection of recipients, and choice of procedure for lung transplantation.* Retrieved January 10, 2001, from www.medscape.com/UpToDate

Yousem, S. A., Berry, G. J., Cagle, P. T., Chamberlain, D., Husain, A. N., Hruban, R. H., Marchevsky, A., Ohori, N. P., Ritter, J., Stewart, S., & Tazelaar, H. D. (1996). Revision of the 1990 working formulation for the classification of pulmonary allograft rejection: Lung Rejection Study Group. *Journal of Heart and Lung Transplantation, 15*(1, Pt. 1), 1–15.

10

Liver Transplantation

John D. Pirsch and Mary J. Douglas

For the patient with end-stage liver disease, liver transplantation is the only therapeutic option that will prolong life. The first liver transplantation procedure was performed by Thomas Starzl in 1963, but survival for greater than 1 year was not achieved until 1967 (Runyon, 1997). This procedure has now become routine, with excellent outcomes in terms of survival and quality of life (Neuberger, 2000). Current 1-, 3-, and 5-year patient survival rates are 88%, 79%, and 74%, respectively. Current 1-, 3-, and 5-year graft survival rates are 81%, 71%, and 66%, respectively (United Network for Organ Sharing [UNOS], 2000, *SR and OPTN Annual Report*). This chapter addresses the indications for liver transplantation, the evaluation process, and the perioperative and postoperative care of the liver transplant recipient.

INDICATIONS FOR LIVER TRANSPLANTATION

Liver transplantation is indicated for acute and chronic liver failure from multiple etiologies. Indications for liver transplantation are outlined in Table 10.1.

TABLE 10.1 Indications for Liver Transplantation

Chronic advanced cirrhosis

Primarily parenchymal disease
        Postnecrotic cirrhosis (viral, drug-related)
        Alcoholic cirrhosis
        Cystic fibrosis
        Autoimmune disease

Primarily cholestatic disease
        Biliary atresia
        Primary biliary cirrhosis (PBC)
        Primary sclerosing cholangitis (PSC)
        Cryptogenic cirrhosis

Primarily vascular disease
        Budd-Chiari syndrome
        Veno-occlusive disease

Acute fulminant hepatic failure
        Viral hepatitis
        Drug-induced
        Metabolic liver disease

Inborn errors of metabolism
        Glycogen storage disease
        Alpha-1-antitrypsin deficiency
        Wilson's disease
        Hemochromatosis

Primary hepatic malignancies

Retransplantation

Source: Powelson & Cosimi, 1999

ACUTE LIVER FAILURE

- Acute liver failure (ALF) is defined as an acute hepatic deterioration (not preceded by evidence of chronic liver disease) that has progressed from the onset of jaundice to the development of hepatic encephalopathy in less than 8 weeks (Benhamou, 1991). Before the availability of liver transplantation, the mortality rate of patients with ALF was greater than 80% (Shakil, Kramer, Mazariegos, Fung, & Rakela, 2000).

- Patients with ALF have the highest priority for donor organs. Currently, 6% of all adult liver transplantation procedures are performed for ALF (Shakil et al., 2000). More than 90% of these transplant recipients survive (Abecassis, Blei, Flamm, & Fryer, 2000).

Diagnosis of ALF

- Patients with impending ALF initially will present with vague symptoms such as anorexia or malaise.
- Liver function tests typically are not performed until the patient develops jaundice. Marked elevations of alanine aminotransferase (ALT), aspartate aminotransferase (AST), bilirubin, and prothrombin time indicate the severity of the liver dysfunction.

Fulminant Liver Failure

- Patients with fulminant liver failure require hospitalization in a facility with expertise in the management of ALF and access to liver transplantation services.
- Patients with progressive hepatic encephalopathy may require intubation and ventilatory support.
- Histamine antagonists or proton-pump inhibitors are commonly given to reduce the risk of gastrointestinal (GI) bleeding.
- Hepatic encephalopathy can cause brain swelling and herniation; therefore, intracranial pressure monitoring may also be required.

Transplant Criteria

Criteria for determining whether a patient may need a liver transplant include the following:

- Factor 5 level < 30%
- pH < 7.3
- International normalized ratio (INR) > 6.5
- Stage 3 or 4 encephalopathy
- Lack of response to medical therapy within 24 to 48 hours

Temporary Support

Temporary hepatic support may include the use of

- Fresh frozen plasma
- Recombinant factor 7

- N-acetylcysteine
- Plasmapheresis
- Dialysis
- Artificial and bioartificial liver support systems
- Hepatocyte transplantation
- Extracorporeal liver perfusion (Abecassis et al., 2000)

CHRONIC LIVER FAILURE

Chronic liver failure (CLF) is the most common diagnosis for which liver transplantation is performed. Chronic liver diseases include the following:

Chronic Hepatocellular Disease
- Hepatitis B, C, or D
- Alcoholic liver disease
- Autoimmune hepatitis

Chronic Cholestatic Disease
- Primary biliary cirrhosis
- Primary sclerosing cholangitis
- Biliary atresia

Metabolic Liver Disease
- Hemochromatosis
- Wilson's disease
- Alpha-1-antitrypsin deficiency

Inborn Errors of Metabolism
- Primary hereditary oxalosis
- Urea cycle defects (Penko & Tirbaso, 1999)

HEPATOCELLULAR CARCINOMA

Liver transplantation may be considered for treatment of hepatocellular carcinoma. The best outcomes are achieved in patients with

- Single lesions less than 5 cm in diameter or
- Multiple lesions, each of which is less than 3 cm in diameter (Carithers, 2000)

MOST COMMON INDICATIONS

Among adults, the most common indications for liver transplantation are alcoholic liver disease, hepatitis B and C, autoimmune disease, primary biliary cirrhosis, primary sclerosing cholangitis, and primary hepatocellular carcinoma. The most common indications for liver transplantation in infants and children are biliary atresia and metabolic disease (Penko & Tirbaso, 1999).

EVALUATION OF THE POTENTIAL LIVER TRANSPLANT CANDIDATE

PHYSIOLOGICAL ASSESSMENT

Patients referred for liver transplantation undergo a rigorous evaluation process that includes the following.

Assessment of the Hepatic System
- Tests to assess patency of the hepatic vessels (may also help detect hepatocellular carcinoma)
  - Ultrasonography
  - High-resolution computed tomography (CT) scan
  - Magnetic resonance imaging
- Liver biopsy: not always needed; can often provide a definitive diagnosis in certain patients with acute liver failure.

Other common diagnostic tests are listed in Table 10.2.

Assessment of the Gastrointestinal (GI) System
- May be indicated, depending on the etiology of the liver disease.
- Upper endoscopy is helpful in the assessment of portal hypertension.
- Colonoscopy may be useful as a baseline or as a potential marker for ulcerative colitis in patients with primary sclerosing cholangitis (PSC), and as a way to rule out colon carcinoma.
- Endoscopic retrograde cholangiopancreatography (ERCP) is particularly indicated for patients with cholestatic liver disease such as PSC. These patients may require frequent ERCP procedures for intrahepatic biliary strictures, stent placement to enhance biliary drainage, bile duct brushings, and biopsies. Patients with sclerosing cholangitis and accompanying ulcerative colitis have a cumulative risk of developing colorectal dysplasia/carcinoma of 9%, 31%, and 50% after 10, 20, and 25 years of disease duration, respectively (Broome, Lofberg, Veress, & Eriksson, 1995).

TABLE 10.2 Liver Transplantation: Diagnostic Tests

Hepatic
- Hepatitis panel (A, B, and C)
- Antismooth muscle antibody
- Antinuclear antibody
- Antimitochondrial antibody
- Alpha-1-antitrypsin
- Ceruloplasmin
- Copper
- Total iron binding capacity
- Iron saturation
- Ferritin
- Liver biopsy*

Gastrointestinal
- Upper endoscopy
- Colonoscopy
- Endoscopic retrograde cholangiopancreatography

Cardiopulmonary
- Electrocardiogram
- Chest radiograph
- Echocardiogram
- Stress thallium or dobutamine stress echocardiogram
- Right and left heart catheterization (for patients with cardiac risk factors and pulmonary hypertension)
- Pulmonary function tests (for patients with history of tobacco use or prior pulmonary disease)

Infectious disease
- Human immunodeficiency virus
- Cytomegalovirus
- Epstein-Barr virus

* as indicated

CONTRAINDICATIONS

Contraindications to liver transplantation are typically categorized as absolute or relative and may vary from center to center.

Absolute contraindications typically include the following (Carithers, 2000):

- Uncontrolled systemic infection
- Malignancy outside the hepatobiliary system
- Absence of viable splanchnic venous inflow system
- Active drug or alcohol abuse
- Advanced cardiopulmonary disease
- Severe psychiatric or neurological disorders
- Acquired immunodeficiency syndrome-related complex

Note: A few transplant centers offer transplantation to human immun-odeficiency virus (HIV)–seropositive patients. Given that this option is not available at all liver transplant centers, HIV-seropositive patients may have to travel greater distances to centers that accept HIV-seropositive individuals.

Relative contraindications include

- Inability to comprehend or comply with the intensive posttransplant regimen
- Age

As the age of the U.S. population increases, more patients over the age of 70 are referred for liver transplantation (Rudich & Busuttil, 1999). Recent studies have indicated that there are no significant differences in either mortality or morbidity between elderly and younger liver transplant recipients (Pirsch et al., 1991; Rudich & Busuttil, 1999). Therefore, many transplant centers evaluate patients on the basis of physiological, rather than chronological, age.

PSYCHOSOCIAL ASSESSMENT

- The psychosocial evaluation typically includes an assessment of the patient's lifestyle, social support system, and the ability to understand and comply with a complex medical regimen.
- Preexisting psychiatric disorders must be identified and treated.
- Any history of substance abuse must be explicitly addressed. Most transplant centers and many third-party payers require a 6- to 12-month period of abstinence from alcohol before a patient can be placed on the waiting list. Once listed, the consequences for the resumption of drinking vary. Candidates may be permanently removed from the waiting list or required to accrue another period of sobriety. The majority of centers remove the candidate from the waiting list, require further treatment for alcoholism, and reevaluate

the individual at a later time (typically in 6 months). A substance abuse counselor can facilitate the rehabilitation process (Everhart & Beresford, 1997; Weinrieb, Van Horn, McLellan, & Lucey, 2000).

- Social work, psychiatric, and neuropsychological consultations may be required to assess the patient's ability to understand the complex, long-term follow-up mandated by liver transplantation.
- The financial assessment typically includes an intake evaluation to assess the patient's ability to meet all financial obligations involved in transplantation. Although the liver transplant surgery may be covered by insurance or other methods of payment, many problems may arise regarding the patient's long-term ability to finance posttransplant care and medications. All of these issues must be carefully assessed and addressed with the patient before placement on the waiting list.

To summarize, the decision to place a patient on the liver transplant waiting list requires a comprehensive assessment of the etiology and staging of liver disease, any complications related to cirrhosis, potential contraindications, and the patient's psychosocial status. Once this information is obtained, each individual case is typically presented to a liver transplantation selection committee for a final decision regarding placing the patient on the waiting list.

ETHICAL ISSUES

One of the major ethical issues associated with liver transplantaton is whether patients with alcohol-induced liver disease should be eligible for this life-saving procedure (Nolan, 1995). Some early investigators found no difference in survival rates between alcoholic and nonalcoholic liver transplant recipients (Starzl et al., 1988). Others have argued that patients who have not assumed responsibility for maintaining their health should be ineligible for liver transplantation (Moss & Siegler, 1991). Superimposed on this debate is the issue of discrimination. Moss and Siegler (1991) maintain that alcoholism occurs across all socioeconomic strata, therefore, it is not discriminatory to keep alcoholic patients off the waiting list. Others, however, believe that such decisions discriminate against the poor, because individuals from lower socioeconomic strata have less ability to pay for alcoholic treatment programs (Killeen, 1993). Cohen and Benjamin (1991) point out that alcoholic patients could be excluded from liver transplantation only if a certain level of moral virtue were required of *all types* of transplant recipients. Given that this is not the case, they argue that the only fair approach is to evaluate all patients in need of a scarce resource by the same standard.

Another facet of this ethical dilemma is the issue of recidivism among patients who undergo transplantation for alcohol-induced liver disease. Overall, studies indicate a mean relapse rate of 15% (Bunzel & Laederach-Hofmann, 2000; Keeffe, 2001). A recent survey of U.S. liver transplant programs examined the rate of relapse to drinking at 2 years posttransplant. The mean rate of relapse of any type was 14%; however, the mean rate of relapse to addictive or uncontrolled drinking with medical or social consequences was 5% (Everhart & Beresford, 1997). Future recidivism studies must also take into consideration the fact that there are subgroups of individuals within the total population of alcohol-addicted patients referred for liver transplantation (Beresford & Everson, 2000). Individuals with polysubstance abuse typically have a poor response to treatment interventions. Patients with isolated alcohol addiction, on the other hand, are more likely to respond to therapy (Beresford, 1997).

UNOS LISTING CRITERIA

In order to receive a cadaveric allograft, the candidate must be placed on a local waiting list maintained by an organ procurement organization (OPO) and on the national UNOS waiting list. In November 2001, the Organ Procurement and Transplantation Network and UNOS approved a new policy for matching donated livers with patients on the waiting list (UNOS 2001, Policy Notice Memo). It is anticipated that this policy, implemented in February 2002, will save more lives of patients on the waiting list by ranking these patients by their short-term risk of death without a liver transplant.

MODEL FOR END-STAGE LIVER DISEASE

The Model for End-Stage Liver Disease (MELD) will be used for adult liver transplant candidates. Each candidate will be assigned a numerical score calculated by a formula that uses routine laboratory tests; this score will reflect how urgently each candidate is in need of a liver transplant within the next 3 months. Under the MELD policy, the former liver transplant statuses of 2A, 2B, and 3 will be replaced with a continuous scale. The MELD policy will not affect the former Status 1 category; this category will remain in place. (Status 1 patients are critically ill with either fulminant liver failure or a new, but nonfunctioning, liver allograft. Their life expectancy is less than 7 days without liver transplantation or re-transplantation).

The MELD scoring system will facilitate a more precise ranking of patients so that those in greatest need will be assigned the highest priority, rather than allocating livers to patients who have accumulated more waiting time but who are much more stable.

MELD scores will range from 6 (less ill) to 40 (gravely ill). These scores will fluctuate as a candidate's laboratory test results change over the waiting period. As the MELD score increases, laboratory tests will be performed more frequently to ensure that they reflect the candidate's current clinical condition. If two patients with the same MELD score are offered an organ, waiting time will be used as a tiebreaker. Candidates on the liver transplant waiting list at the time the MELD policy is implemented will be "grandfathered" into the new system and given credit for accrued waiting time.

PEDIATRIC END STAGE LIVER DISEASE MODEL

The Pediatric End Stage Liver Disease (PELD) model ranks liver transplant candidates under age of 18. Similar to the MELD system, the PELD model uses specific criteria to arrive at a numerical score. The PELD model also takes into consideration the growth and development needs of children. Children with rare medical conditions may be eligible for a modified score. The former pediatric status 1 will remain in place; however, the former pediatric 2B and 3 statues will be replaced by the new PELD policy. (There is no pediatric Status 2A.)

CARE OF THE LIVER TRANSPLANT CANDIDATE

The waiting time for a liver transplant can be lengthy. This period is often associated with anxiety for both the patient and family. Interventions such as support groups, patient and family counseling, and pharmacological therapy are useful in mitigating stressors and enhancing patient satisfaction (van Thiel, 1998).

The prevention and management of complications associated with chronic liver disease requires substantial commitment and attention on the part of the clinician (Abecassis et al., 2000). Table 10.3 lists complications that may develop during the waiting period and potential treatment options.

DONOR IDENTIFICATION

The major challenge facing the transplant community is the shortage of donor organs. Improvements in patient survival after liver transplantation have expanded the indications for this life-saving therapy and have led to a greater imbalance between donor organ supply and demand. Approaches to overcome this problem include the use of marginal donors, living-related donors, and split liver transplantation (Neuberger, 2000). Marginal donors may include older donors, hepatitis B core antibody carriers, hepatitis C carriers, and donors who succumb to cardiovascular complications. Most often, marginal donors are used for patients with great medical urgency and are accepted on a case-by-case basis by individual transplant centers.

Initial donor evaluation typically includes the following tests (UNOS, 2000, *Organ Distribution*):

- Liver enzymes
- Total and direct bilirubin
- Blood urea nitrogen (BUN)
- Creatinine
- Electrolytes
- Complete blood count (CBC)
- Prothrombin time
- Blood type
- Serologies for HIV, hepatitis, cytomegalovirus (CMV), rapid plasma reagin, and human T-lymphotropic virus

Donor height, weight, gender, age, cause of death, social history, and hospital course are also evaluated. A liver biopsy may also be obtained. If steatosis is > 30%, there is an increased likelihood of initial poor liver function or primary nonfunction.

RECIPIENT OPERATIVE PROCEDURE

The recipient operation consists of the hepatectomy of the native liver followed by implantation of the donor liver. The recipient liver is removed while the donor liver is prepared on the back table. The donor liver is then brought into the operative field. Typically, an anastomosis between the donor hepatic veins and the recipient inferior vena cava (IVC) is performed via the piggyback technique. The portal vein anastomosis is completed next. The liver is flushed with Ringer's lactate and albumin solution

TABLE 10.3 Management of Pretransplant Complications

Ascites
- Low-sodium diet
- Fluid restriction
- Daily weights
- Diuretics
  - Furosemide (Lasix), spironolactone (Aldactone)
- Large volume paracentesis
- Transjugular intrahepatic portosystemic shunt (TIPS)

Hepatic encephalopathy
- Correct precipitating event
- Protein intake 0.75–1 g/kg
- Medications
  - Lactulose, zinc, metronidazole, neomycin
- Stage 3/4
  - Elective endotracheal intubation

Spontaneous bacterial peritonitis
- Antibiotics
  - Cefotaxime (Claforan)
- Prevent renal failure
- Possible prophylaxis with norfloxacin, ciprofloxacin, TMP/SMZ (Bactrim)

Gastrointestinal hemorrhage
- Achieve hemostasis
  - Octreotide acetate (Sandostatin)
  - Endoscopic therapy
    - Banding, sclerotherapy
  - Mechanical tamponade
- Prevent rebleeding
- Maintenance therapy
  - Propranolol (Inderal)
  - Repeated endoscopic therapy
  - Transjugular intrahepatic portosystemic shunt procedure

via the hepatic artery to remove the University of Wisconsin (UW) solution. The infrahepatic IVC of the liver is ligated. The clamps are then released, and the liver is perfused. The use of venous–venous bypass is center- and case-specific. After the portal flow is secured and the graft reperfused, attention is then directed to the hepatic arterial anastomosis.

Once the liver is arterialized with satisfactory hepatic artery flow and hemostasis is achieved, bile duct reconstruction is performed. This may be through a choledochocholedochostomy and use of a T-tube stent or a Roux-en-Y anastomosis if the recipient bile duct is diseased (Kremer, Broelsch, & Henns Bruns, 1994).

IMMEDIATE POSTOPERATIVE CARE

Surgical and medical complications following liver transplantation are common. In the immediate postoperative period, the most feared complication is primary nonfunction (PNF). PNF occurs in up to 3% of grafts (Neuberger, 2000) and is associated with hemodynamic instability, acidosis, and fibrinolysis. PNF must be differentiated from early graft dysfunction that is reversible.

Ischemic injury, rejection, and vascular complications also predominate in the early posttransplant period. In the postoperative setting, good liver function is clinically manifested by an alert recipient who demonstrates normalizing INR, bilirubin, and ammonia. Conversely, poor initial hepatic dysfunction leads to prolonged intubation, coagulopathy, and multisystem organ failure. Although some livers may recover, retransplantation in this setting should be seriously considered.

Other early concerns are thrombosis of the hepatic artery or of the portal vein that can lead to biliary obstruction, liver infarction, or both. Hepatic artery thrombosis can also occur late in the recovery period. With hepatic artery occlusion, bile duct necrosis inevitably occurs. This is usually heralded by sepsis with multiple biliary abscesses caused by decreased arterial blood flow to the biliary tree. Ultrasonography and spiral CT scans are noninvasive modalities that have a reported sensitivity of more than 90% for detecting vascular complications. Angiography is helpful in equivocal cases (Savitsky, Uner, & Votey, 1998).

Postoperative bleeding may be a significant problem under normal circumstances with a functioning graft. Coagulopathy should be reversed by the time of abdominal closure (Abecassis et al., 2000). In the presence of oliguria, hypotension, or severe drop in hematocrit, postoperative bleeding must be considered.

Other medical complications in the early postoperative period may include acute rejection, preservation injury, infection, and drug toxicity. Laboratory values that are closely monitored include ammonia, prothrombin time, INR, AST, ALT, and bilirubin.

IMMUNOSUPPRESSIVE REGIMENS

The goal of immunosuppressive therapy after transplantation is to pre-vent allorecognition and subsequent destruction of transplanted tissue. There are four major types of immunosuppressive agents in use today: antilymphocyte therapy, antimetabolites, corticosteroids, and calcineurin inhibitors (Pirsch, 1998). Triple therapy is generally initiated with subse-quent reduction to double therapy in selected patients. The use of these agents is transplant center-specific depending on experience, underlying disease process, and general clinical condition of the transplant recipient (see chapter 4).

REJECTION

TYPES OF REJECTION

Three main types of rejection may occur: hyperacute, acute, and chronic rejection.

Hyperacute Rejection
- Occurs within minutes to days posttransplant.
- Is due to preformed IgG antibodies in the recipient that react against class 1 human leukocyte antigens (HLA) in the transplanted organ.
- Causes loss of organ function as a result of antibody deposit, com-plement activation, and vascular destruction. Preformed antibodies to the donor can be detected by cross-matching the donor and recip-ient prior to the transplant. However, because of the limited time for organ preservation, cross-matching is not performed in clinical liver transplantation.
- Is extremely rare in liver transplantation.

Acute Rejection
- Is the most common form of rejection.
- Occurs most frequently within 6 months of transplantation; Approximately 60% to 80% of liver transplant recipients will have at least one rejection episode.
- Is mediated by T cells that infiltrate the allograft and cause tissue destruction.
- Treatment of acute rejection with increased doses of immunosup-pressants is usually successful.

Chronic Rejection
- Histologically, the main characteristic of chronic rejection is intimal hyperplasia of the small- and medium-sized arteries that results in slowly progressive ischemia in the transplanted organ.
- In liver transplantation, this process leads to the progressive loss of bile ducts in the portal triads known as ductopenic rejection. Loss of bile ducts can lead to cholestasis and the possible need for retransplantation.
- Many cases of ductopenia may be treated successfully with administration of tacrolimus and mycophenolate mofetil early in the course (Gavlik et al., 1997; Sher et al., 1997).

SIGNS AND SYMPTOMS

The clinical signs and symptoms of rejection include:

- Fever
- Right upper quadrant pain
- Anorexia
- Ascites
- Decreased bile output
- Elevated (typically) bilirubin, transaminase, alkaline phosphatase (ALP), white blood cell (WBC), and eosinophil levels.

Any variance from the patient's baseline values deserves further workup. A history and physical with a review of systems, along with a review of medications and compliance should be initiated. Also:

- Ultrasound of the liver is typically performed as the initial diagnostic procedure. This test assesses blood flow and is useful in determining the presence of dilated biliary ducts.
- If no explanation for increase in laboratory values is found, a liver biopsy may be indicated to rule out infection or recurrent disease.
- A cholangiogram and abdominal CT scan may be necessary to rule out leaks, obstruction, fluid collection, or abscess formation.

POSTTRANSPLANTATION CARE

ROUTINE MONITORING

During the first 6 postoperative months, as the risk of rejection diminishes, immunosuppressive medications are usually reduced. Frequent patient assessment is imperative.

Laboratory Tests

Typically, tests are obtained 2 to 3 times per week immediately posttransplant; the interval between tests is gradually extended to every 1 to 2 months thereafter. Routine monitoring helps to detect early deterioration of graft function as well as possible problems with compliance. Lapses in follow-up may allow graft dysfunction to develop and go undetected for several months. Transplant recipients are encouraged to assume responsibility for obtaining and recording results of their routine laboratory tests and reporting these to their transplant center.

Routine laboratory assessment should include

- CBC with platelets
- BUN
- Creatinine
- Potassium
- Chloride
- Carbon dioxide
- Glucose
- Sodium
- Liver function tests: ALT, AST, total bilirubin, gamma-glutamyl-transferase (GGT), ALP, albumin

MEDICATIONS

At each outpatient visit, it is important to review all of the patient's medications, including any over-the-counter (OTC) medications or herbal supplements.

TRANSPLANT-RELATED COMPLICATIONS

In addition to monitoring allograft function, the patient's primary health care provider may have to assess and treat the patient for the following transplant-related complications:

- Hypertension (may be secondary to immunosuppressant drugs)
- Renal dysfunction
- Posttransplant vasculopathy
- Steroid-induced diabetes
- Hyperlipidemia; hypercholesteremia
- Obesity
- Osteoporosis

Recipients may also experience neurocognitive and/or psychosocial problems after transplantation (see chapter 13).

MANAGEMENT OF COMPLICATIONS

The underlying principle for the management of posttransplant complications is close follow-up. Complications that can result in graft dysfunction include biliary stricture, biloma formation, hepatic artery thrombosis, rejection, or infection (especially recurrent hepatitis C). Multiple differential diagnoses may be possible, and more than one cause for transplant dysfunction may exist. Treatment of graft dysfunction requires extensive care that is best provided by the transplant center of record. Any intervention requires close daily monitoring to ensure an appropriate therapeutic response.

Infection

Types of infection.

Transplant recipients are susceptible to a variety of infections.

- In the immediate postoperative period, most infections are related to the surgical procedure and usually involve wound infections, bacteremia, urinary tract infections, or pneumonia
- Between 30 and 90 days, fever is most often a sign of graft rejection or CMV infection. Infection with CMV is common after transplant, particularly in CMV seronegative recipients who received a CMV seropositive graft. Reinfection with a new CMV strain can also occur, especially during times of peak immunosuppression
- Epstein-Barr virus (EBV) infection may occur early after transplantation and is usually related to heightened immunosuppression in the previously seronegative host.
- Opportunistic infections are relatively uncommon 6 months posttransplantation; however, herpes simplex virus, herpes zoster virus,

and occasionally CMV infections may occur at any time in the late posttransplant course. Less common opportunistic infections, such as toxoplasmosis and cryptococcosis, may occur, but their incidence has been greatly reduced with the prophylactic use of trimethoprim/sulfamethoxazole (TMP/SMZ).

Prophylactic protocols.

- Most transplant centers use prophylactic protocols to prevent opportunistic CMV infections including intravenous ganciclovir in the immediate postoperative period, followed by high-dose oral acyclovir or oral ganciclovir for at least 3 months. Valganciclovir is also used by many centers.
- In the past, *Pneumocystis carinii* pneumonia was a frequent complication of transplantation. Routine prophylaxis with trimethoprim/sulfamethoxazole (TMP/SMZ) has nearly eliminated the occurrence of pneumocystis infection in transplant patients. Dapsone or pentamidine may be given to patients with allergies to sulfa products. Prophylaxis against pneumocystis infection should be continued throughout the first posttransplant year.

Diagnosis and treatment of infection.

- Fever in the later posttransplant period is often a sign of infection, generally either urinary or respiratory.
- Initial evaluation should include a careful history, physical examination, and appropriate laboratory tests based on the presenting signs and symptoms.
- The primary care provider in consultation with the transplant center can treat most minor infections.
- Careful attention should be directed to possible drug interactions with the patient's immunosuppressive regimen (see chapter 4).
- Patients with fevers of unknown etiology should be referred to the transplant center for evaluation before any antibiotic therapy is administered.

Management of immunosuppressants.

- During episodes of infection, adjustment of immunosuppressive medication can be difficult and is best managed by the transplant team.
- For most long-term transplant recipients, the dose of immunosuppressive medications can be reduced during acute infection without substantially increasing the risk of rejection.

- Mild infection may require discontinuation of antimetabolite (aza-thioprine or mycophenolate) therapy.
- For moderately severe infections, both antimetabolite and calcineurin inhibitors may have to be withdrawn. Corticosteroid therapy is gen-erally continued.
- For the most severe of infections, hydrocortisone is administered intravenously every 8 hours until the infection is under control.
- Close monitoring of the allograft function during infectious com-plications is essential (see chapter 2).

CARDIOVASCULAR DISEASE

Cardiac Vasculopathy

One of the leading causes of death in liver transplant recipients greater than 5 years posttransplantation is cardiac vasculopathy (Neuberger, 2000). Therefore, routine follow-up of the transplant patient should focus on risk factors that are amenable to treatment, such as diet, physical inactiv-ity, smoking, diabetes, and hypertension.

Hypertension

- Hypertension develops in 50% to 80% of patients following trans-plantation. In most patients, hypertension is associated with cyclosporine, tacrolimus, and corticosteroid use. Cyclosporine and tacrolimus cause afferent arterial vasoconstriction or renal artery constriction, which in turn may stimulate the release of endothelin (Pirsch, 1998). The corresponding decrease in renal blood flow may result in activation of the renin angiotensin system.
- Loop diuretics are commonly used to treat hypertension, particu-larly in patients with hypertension related to sodium retention.
- Beta-blockers, preferably those that do not affect lipid levels, are use-ful for posttransplant hypertension; however, they may be relatively contraindicated in patients with diabetes or severe peripheral vas-cular disease.
- Calcium channel blockers may also be used to treat postoperative hypertension. Verapamil and diltiazem may increase the cyclosporine level; therefore, the patient's cyclosporine levels need to be closely monitored.

RENAL INSUFFICIENCY

Calcineurin inhibitors are associated with renal impairment. In a recent study of 139 liver transplant recipients who had survived five years or more, 108 patients (78%) had mild to moderate chronic renal failure, defined as serum creatinine level > 125 µM/L (Fisher, Nightingale, Gunson, Lipkin, & Neuberger, 1998). The risk of nephrotoxicity may be lessened by close monitoring of renal function, reducing calcineurin inhibitors to minimal effective doses, controlling hypertension, and using calcium channel antagonists (Bennett, DeMattos, Meyer, Andoh, & Barry, 1996).

HYPERLIPIDEMIA

Hyperlipidemia is extremely common following transplantation and likely contributes to the mortality from coronary artery disease. Risk factors for hyperlipidemia include age, renal dysfunction, diuretic and beta-blocker use, diabetes, male gender, and obesity. In addition, posttransplant hyperlipidemia is exacerbated by the use of corticosteroids, cyclosporine, and sirolimus.

MALIGNANCY

The increasing number of successful long-term transplant patients has heightened concern about the development of malignancies posttransplantation. The effects of immunosuppressive drug therapy on the immune system increase the risk of cancer following transplantation. This is particularly true in the liver transplant population with the increased incidence of lymphomas noted (Penn, 1996). Routine surveillance for malignancies is important in the long-term follow-up process.

Skin Carcinoma

The incidence of skin cancer among the general population is increasing rapidly, with over 1 million nonmelanoma skin cancers occurring each year. The incidence of squamous and basal cell carcinomas has doubled in the last 20 and 25 years, respectively.

Skin cancers are the most common malignancy following transplantation. Cutaneous malignancies may result from activation and/or proliferation of oncogenic viruses secondary to decreased immune surveillance or from the direct mutagenic effects of immunosuppressive medications

(Sheiner et al., 2000). The incidence of skin cancer reported in recent single-center studies ranges from 2% to 5% (Haagsma et al., 2001; Jain et al., 1998). In terms of clinical presentation and behavior, skin cancer can range from small, isolated, and easily curable tumors to numerous, aggressive, uncommon and life-threatening neoplasms. Metastatic skin cancer occurs in 5% to 7% of cases and is often fatal. Among Cincinnati Transplant Tumor Registry patients, 5.4% died as a direct result of skin cancer (Otley & Pittelkow, 2000).

Factors that are associated with increased risk of skin cancer following transplantation include

- Longer duration of immunosuppression
- More intense immunosuppression
- More extensive ultraviolet radiation exposure
- Increased age
- Presence of human papillomavirus infection
- Easily burned skin
- CD4 lymphocytopenia
- Increased age (Otley & Pittelkow, 2000; Penn, 1996).

Recipients at high risk for the development of skin cancer include patients with

- A history of skin cancer or actinic keratosis before transplantation
- Fitzpatrick skin types I (inability to tan), II (tendency to burn often), or III (tendency to burn sometimes)
- A freckled complexion, blue eyes, red or blonde hair
- A history of extensive sun exposure (Otley & Pittelkow, 2000).

Liver transplant recipients are encouraged to perform skin self-examination on a monthly basis. Those with a history of squamous cell carcinoma or melanoma should also perform lymph node self-examination. Recommendations for dermatologic follow-up intervals for liver transplant recipients are as follows (Otley & Pittelkow, 2000):

No history of skin cancer or actinic keratosis	Yearly
History of actinic keratosis	Every 6 months
History of 1 nonmelanoma skin cancer	Every 6 months
History of multiple nonmelanoma skin cancers	Every 4 months
History of high-risk squamous cell carcinoma or melanoma	Every 3 months
History of metastatic squamous cell carcinoma	Every 2 months

Liver transplant recipients are also encouraged to adopt the following sun-protective practices:

- Wear protective clothing and wide-brimmed hats.
- Limit outdoor activities between 10:00 A.M. and 4:00 P.M.
- Apply sun screen lotion with a sun protection factor (SPF) of 15 or higher.
- Apply lip balm that contains SPF.
- Avoid suntanning (natural or artificial) (Otley & Pittelkow, 2000).

Hepatocellular Carcinoma

Should hepatocellular carcinoma be present in the native liver on explantation, a CT scan and alpha fetoprotein levels should be obtained every 3 to 6 months.

METABOLIC BONE DISEASE

Metabolic bone disease (osteoporosis) is common after transplantation and is a significant cause of long-term morbidity and mortality. Osteoporosis may develop secondary to the underlying hepatic disease that led to transplantation and may be accelerated by corticosteroid use after transplantation. Bone loss is rapid after transplantation; the rate of bone loss is the greatest in the first 6 posttransplant months.

Liver transplant recipients have an increased risk of metabolic bone disease because of altered metabolism of vitamin D in the liver (Pirsch, 1998). Bone disease is especially prevalent in patients who required liver transplantation for primary biliary cirrhosis.

Two new antiresorptive agents have been approved for the treatment of osteoporosis. These include alendronate (Fosamax) and nasal calcitonin (Miacalcin). Both of these agents can be used in the transplant population.

Evaluation for metabolic bone disease should include measurement of bone density and parathyroid, vitamin D, gonadal, and thyroid hormone levels. All patients should have a calcium intake of approximately 1,000 to 1,500 mg a day, along with vitamin D supplementation. Postmenopausal women should be considered for hormone replacement therapy.

BLOOD DYSCRASIAS

Leukopenia is common in the early posttransplantation period. It is most likely due to drug-related bone marrow suppression. Patients with systemic illness including fever and leukopenia that develops within the first 6 months following transplant should be tested for CMV infection.

RECURRENT DISEASE

Recurrent disease rates vary after liver transplantation depending on the disease process involved. Even if recurrence is diagnosed, the effect on long-term graft survival can be minimal.

Metabolic Abnormalities

- When the metabolic abnormality is primarily within the liver, transplantation will be curative for the metabolic disease (Neuberger, 2000).
- Primary biliary cirrhosis recurs in 20% and 45% of allografts at 5 and 15 years, respectively (Wiesner & Neuberger, 2000).
- Autoimmune hepatitis can recur if steroids are withdrawn; however, this usually responds to resumption of steroid therapy.
- Recurrence of primary sclerosing cholangitis (PSC) occurs in up to 20% of patients, but it appears to have little effect on patient survival (Gow & Chapman, 2000).

Hepatitis A

Hepatitis A may recur, but long-term graft survival is unaffected.

Hepatitis B

- Predictors for hepatitis B virus recurrence include a high level of viral replication prior to transplantation (i.e., HBeAg and hepatitis B virus DNA detectable by molecular hybridization), absence of coinfection with hepatitis C or D virus, and orthotopic liver transplantation for cirrhosis (Rosen & Martin, 2000).
- Hepatitis B virus is known to recur posttransplantation if hepatitis B immune globulin or lamivudine (Epivir) are not used prophylactically. At this time, there is a lack of consensus about the dose of hepatitis B immune globulin that is necessary to prevent recurrence

of this disease. Development of resistant mutant forms of the virus is an increasing problem with the use of lamivudine. Treatment of recurrent hepatitis B infection is center-specific.

Hepatitis C

Hepatitis C is the leading cause of end-stage liver disease and the most common indication for orthotopic liver transplantation worldwide. The recurrence of infection with hepatitis C after transplantation is almost invariable, but the extent of graft damage is variable. Cirrhosis at 5 years occurs in 8% to 25% of liver transplant recipients (Wiesner & Neuberger, 2000).

- Risk factors for severe recurrent hepatitis C include genotype 1b, high pretransplant levels of hepatitis C virus-RNA, and higher levels of immunosuppression (Neuberger, 2000).
- The signs and symptoms of acute graft rejection and recurrent hepatitis C infection are similar. Rejection, however, tends to occur in the first 3 months posttransplant whereas recurrent hepatitis C infection is more likely to occur later in the posttransplant period (Keeffe, 2001).
- Treatment approaches include preemptive antiviral therapy in hepatitis C-positive candidates, early posttransplant antiviral therapy prior to histological documentation of recurrence, and treatment of established recurrence (Rosen & Martin, 2000). Treatment of recurrent hepatitis C with a combination of interferon and ribavirin has shown promise (Gopal et al., 2001; Keeffe, 2001). Biochemical, histological, and viral responses to combination therapy have been reported (Szabo, Katz, & Bonkovsky, 2000). Many patients, however, cannot tolerate combination therapy due to severe side effects; dose reductions or discontinuation of therapy (temporary or permanent) may be required (Ben-Ari et al., 2000; DeVera et al., 2001).

It is likely that as liver transplantation survival rates improve even further, disease recurrence will increase accordingly. New strategies will be required to mitigate this problem.

NEWER APPROACHES TO LIVER REPLACEMENT

Despite concerted efforts to increase organ donation, organ procurement rates have remained relatively constant. As a result, the demand for donor livers far exceeds the supply. Between 1988 and 1997, the number of liver donors and liver transplantation procedures increased 2.4-fold. During this same period, however, the number of patients on the liver transplant waiting list increased 15.6-fold, and the number of patients who died on the waiting list increased 5.8-fold. This disparity between the number of available cadaver organs and the ever-increasing number of liver transplant candidates has spurred the expanded use of marginal donors and the development of alternative surgical approaches such as cadaver split-liver and adult living donor liver transplantation (Keeffe, 2000).

EXPANDED USE OF MARGINAL DONORS

The expanded use of marginal donors includes the following:

- Use of older donors
- Use of donor livers from patients with mild, chronic hepatitis C for hepatitis C virus (HCV)-positive recipients
- Use of donor livers from patients with positive hepatitis B virus (HBV) core antibody for HBV-positive recipients (Keefe, 2001)

Older Donors

In recent years, there has been a considerable increase in the overall percent of donors over age 50. As with all organs, increasing donor age is associated with poorer graft function (Keefe, 2001). One-, 3-, and 5-year graft survival rates for recipients of livers from donors age 50 to 64 are 78%, 64%, and 56%, respectively. For the same posttransplant intervals, the 1-, 3- and 5-year graft survival rates for recipients of livers from donors age 18 to 34 are 85%, 75%, and 69%, respectively. One-, 3-, and 5-year patient survival rates for recipients of livers from donors age 50 to 64 are 86%, 73%, and 67%, respectively. For the same posttransplant intervals, patient survival rates for donors age 18 to 34 are 89%, 81%, and 75%, respectively (UNOS, 2000, *Annual Report*).

Hepatitis C–Positive Donors

HCV-positive recipients who receive HCV-positive grafts appear to have good short- and medium-term outcomes (Keefe, 2001; Vargas et al., 1999). A preliminary analysis of the UNOS database indicates that the use of HCV-positive donor livers in HCV-positive candidates was associated with comparable graft and patient survival to the use of HCV-negative allografts (Rosen & Martin, 2000).

Hepatitis B–Positive Donors

There is limited experience regarding long-term outcomes of HBV-positive candidates who receive allografts from HBV core antibody-positive donors. However, it is well known that such allografts frequently transmit HBV to HBV-negative recipients (Keeffe, 2000).

ALTERNATIVE SURGICAL APPROACHES

Cadaver Split-Liver Transplantation

This technique involves transplanting two recipients from a single adult cadaver liver. Typically, the right lobe is implanted into an adult recipient, and the left lobe or left lateral segment is implanted into a pediatric recipient (Keeffe, 2001). Both ex vivo (splitting the liver after removal from the cadaver) and in vivo (splitting the liver in the cadaver prior to procurement) techniques have been used. Initial outcomes of split-liver transplantation were poor. More recently, however, Rela and colleagues (1998) reported graft and patient survival of 88% and 90%, respectively, at a median follow-up of 12 months (range: 6–70 months).

Living Donor Transplantation

The number of living liver donors has increased from 14 in 1990 to 347 in 2000 (UNOS, 2001, *Number of U.S. Organ Donors*). Approximately 52% of living liver donors are in the 18 to 34-year age range; 42% are in the 35 to 49 year age range (UNOS, 2000, *SR and OPTN Annual Report*). The longest surviving liver transplant recipient of a living related donor graft was transplanted in November 1989 (UNOS, 2001, *Living Donation*). Two factors that have been associated with the success of living donor liver transplantation are the liver's distinct segmental anatomy and its capacity to regenerate (Seaman, 2001).

Donor selection.

The work-up for a potential living donor is extensive and typically consists of a phased evaluation that begins with a number of psychosocial interviews. The medical evaluation is initiated with a thorough history and physical examination and blood type compatibility. The selection protocol continues with progressively more invasive laboratory, radiologic, and graft evaluations. Donor informed consent is an essential element of the evaluation process and involves multiple educational sessions with potential donors, recipients, and family members (Renz & Busuttil, 2000; Seaman, 2001).

Donor outcomes.

Potential donor complications include hemorrhage, bile duct injury, infection, pulmonary embolus, and risks associated with general anesthesia and reoperation. Compared to left lateral segment resections, right lobe resections entail greater parenchymal dissection and increased risk of bleeding and bile duct leak (Seaman, 2001). Overall donor morbidity and mortality rates are approximately 10% and 0.5%, respectively (Keeffe, 2001; Renz & Busuttil, 2000).

Recipient outcomes.

A recent survey of 30 North American liver transplant programs performing a total of 208 adult-to-adult living donor procedures indicated an overall complication rate of 30% and an mortality rate of 13% (Renz & Busuttil, 2000).

WHEN TO CALL THE TRANSPLANT CENTER

Community health care providers can treat many minor problems that may occur in liver transplant recipients. However, a call to the transplant center of record is warranted if any of the following issues develop:

- Clinical signs and symptoms of rejection:
  - Fever
  - Right upper quadrant pain
  - Anorexia
  - Nausea, vomiting, diarrhea
  - Ascites
  - Fluctuating bile output (if bile drainage in place)
  Note: Routine laboratory work-up should include bilirubin, transaminase, ALP, albumin, WBC, BUN, creatinine, potassium, chloride, carbon dioxide, glucose, sodium, hematocrit, and platelets.)
- Fever of unknown origin
- Patient is uncertain of correct doses of immunosuppressants
- Addition or deletion of any prescription medications, OTC medications, or herbal supplements to assess for possible drug interactions

CONCLUSION

Liver transplantation offers the greatest hope of survival currently available for patients with acute and chronic liver disease for whom other available forms of therapy have failed. With the limited supply of donor organs, careful selection of patients for transplantation is required. The most difficult challenges remain with the timing of the transplant procedure and the long-term care of this select population.

REFERENCES

Abecassis, M., Blei, A. T., Flamm, S., & Fryer, J. P. (2000). Liver transplantation. In F. P. Stuart, M. M. Abecassis, & D. B. Kaufman (Eds.), *Organ transplantation* (pp. 169–207). Georgetown, TX: Landes Bioscience.

Ben-Ari, Z., Mor, E., Shaharabani, E., Bar-Nathan, N., Shapira, Z., & Tur-Kaspa, R. (2000). Combination of interferon-alpha and ribavirin therapy for recurrent hepatitis C virus infection after liver transplantation. *Transplantation Proceedings, 32*(4), 714–716.

Benhamou, J. P. (1991). Fulminant and sub-fulminant hepatic failure: Definition and causes. In R. Williams, & R. D. Hughes (Eds.), *Acute liver failure: Improved understanding and better therapy* (pp. 6–10). London: Mitre Press.

Bennett, W. M., DeMattos, A., Meyer, M. M., Andoh, T., & Barry, J. M. (1996). Chronic cyclosporine nephropathy: The Achilles' heel of immunosuppressive therapy. *Kidney International, 50*, 1089–1100.

Beresford, T. P. (1997). Predictive factors for alcoholic relapse in the selection of alcohol-dependent persons for hepatic transplant. *Liver Transplantation and Surgery, 3*, 280–291.

Beresford, T. P., & Everson, G. T. (2000). Liver transplantation for alcoholic liver disease: Bias, beliefs, 6-month rule, and relapse—But where are the data? [Editorial]. *Liver Transplantation, 6*(6), 777–778.

Broome, U., Lofberg, R., Veress, B., & Eriksson, L. S. (1995). Primary sclerosing cholangitis and ulcerative colitis: Evidence for increased neoplastic potential. *Hepatology, 22*, 1404–1408.

Bunzel, B., & Laederach-Hofmann, K. (2000). Solid organ transplantation: Are there predictors for posttransplant noncompliance? A literature review. *Transplantation, 70*(5), 711–716.

Carithers, R. L., Jr. (2000). Liver transplantation. *Liver Transplantation, 6*, 122–135.

Cohen, C., & Benjamin, M. (1991). Alcoholics and liver transplantation. *Journal of the American Medical Association, 265*(10), 1299–1301.

DeVera, M. E., Smallwood, G. A., Rosado, K., Davis, L., Martinez, E., Sharma, S., Stieber, A. C., & Heffron, T. G. (2001). Interferon-alpha and ribavirin for the treatment of recurrent hepatitis C after liver transplantation. *Transplantation, 71*(5), 678–686.

Everhart, J. E., & Beresford, T. P. (1997). Liver transplantation for alcoholic liver disease: A survey of transplantation programs in the United States. *Liver Transplantation and Surgery, 3*(3), 220–226.

Fisher, N. C., Nightingale, P. G., Gunson, B. K., Lipkin, G. W., & Neuberger, J. M. (1998). Chronic renal failure following liver transplantation: A retrospective analysis. *Transplantation, 66,* 59–66.

Gavlik, A., Goldberg, M. G., Tsaroucha, A., Webb, M. G., Khan, R. T., Weppler, D., Nery, J. R., Khan, M. F., Zucker, K., Viciana, A. L., Miller, J. A., & Tzakis, A. G. (1997). Mycophenolate mofetil rescue therapy in liver transplant recipients. *Transplantation Proceedings, 29,* 549–552.

Gopal, D. V., Rabkin, J. M., Berk, B. S., Corless, C. L., Chou, S., Olyaei, A., Orloff, S. L., & Rosen, H. R., (2001). Treatment of progressive hepatitis C recurrence after liver transplantation with combination interferon plus ribavirin. *Liver Transplantation, 7*(3), 181–190.

Gow, P. J., & Chapman, R. W. (2000). Liver transplantation for primary sclerosing cholangitis. *Liver, 20,* 97–103.

Haagsma, E. B., Hagens, V. E., Schaapveld, M., van den Berg, A. P., de Vries, D. G. E., Klompmaker, I. J., Slooff, M. J. H., & Jansen, P. L. M. (2001). Increased cancer risk after liver transplantation: A population-based study. *Hepatology, 34*(1), 84–91.

Jain, A. B., Yee, L. D., Nalesnik, M. A., Youk, A., Marsh, G., Reyes, J., Zak, M., Rakela, J., Irish, W., & Fung, J. J. (1998). Comparative incidence of de novo nonlymphoid malignancies after liver transplantation under tacrolimus using surveillance epidemiologic end result data. *Transplantation, 66*(9), 1193–2000.

Keeffe, E. B. (2000). Liver transplantation at the millennium: Past, present, and future. *Clinics in Liver Disease, 4*(1), 241–255.

Keeffe, E. B. (2001). Liver transplantation: Current status and novel approaches to liver replacement. *Gastroenterology, 120*(3), 749–762.

Killeen, T. (1993). Alcoholism and liver transplantation: Ethical and nursing implications. *Perspectives in Psychiatric Care, 29*(1), 7–12.

Kremer, B., Broelsch, C. E., & Henne-Bruns, D. (1994). *Atlas of liver, pancreas, and kidney transplantation.* New York: Georg Thieme Verlag.

Moss, A. H., & Siegler, M. (1991). Should alcoholics compete equally for liver transplantation? *Journal of the American Medical Association, 265*(10), 1295–1298.

Neuberger, J. (2000). Liver transplantation. *Journal of Hepatology, 32*(1, Suppl.), 198–207.

Nolan, M. T. (1995). Ethical issues in transplantation. In M. T. Nolan & S. M. Augustine (Eds.), *Transplantation nursing: Acute and long-term care* (pp. 361–373). Norwalk, CT: Appelton & Lange.

Otley, C. C., & Pittelkow, M. R. (2000). Skin cancer in liver transplant recipients. *Liver Transplantation, 6*(3), 253–262.

Penko, M. E., & Tirbaso, D. (1999). An overview of liver transplantation. *AACN Clinical Issues, 10*(2), 176–184.

Penn, I. (1996). Posttransplantation de novo tumors in liver allograft recipients. *Liver Transplantation and Surgery, 2,* 52–59.

Pirsch, J. D. (1998). Care of the transplant patient. *Clinical Symposia, 50*(1), 2–35.

Pirsch, J. D., Kalayoglu, M., D'Alessandro, A. M., Voss, B. J., Armbrust, M. J., Reed,

A., Knechtle, S. J., Sollinger, H. W., & Belzer, F. O. (1991). Orthotopic liver transplantation in patients 60 years of age and older. *Transplantation, 51*, 431–433.

Powelson, J. A., & Cosimi, A. B. (1999). Liver transplantation. In L. C. Ginns, A. B. Cosimi, & P. J. Morris (Eds.), *Transplantation* (pp. 324–368). Malden, MA: Commerce Place.

Rela, M., Vougas, V., Muiesan, P., Vilca-Melendez, H., Smyrniotis, V., Gibbs, P., Karani, J., Williams, R., & Heaton, N. (1998). Split liver transplantation: Kings' College Hospital experience. *Annals of Surgery, 227*(2), 282–288.

Renz, J. F., & Busuttil, R. W. (2000). Adult-to-adult living-donor liver transplantation: A critical analysis. *Seminars in Liver Disease, 20*(4), 411–424.

Rosen, H. R., & Martin, P. (2000). Viral hepatitis in the liver transplant recipient. *Infectious Disease Clinics of North America, 14*(3), 761–784.

Rudich, S., & Busuttil, R. (1999). Similar outcomes, morbidity, and mortality for orthotopic liver transplantation between the very elderly and the young. *Transplantation Proceedings, 31*, 523–525.

Runyon, B. A. (1997). Historical aspects of treatment of patients with cirrhosis and ascites. *Seminars in Liver Disease, 17*, 163–173.

Savitsky, E. A., Uner, A. B., & Votey, S. R. (1998). Evaluation of orthotopic liver transplant recipients presenting to the emergency department. *Annals of Emergency Medicine, 31*, 507–517.

Seaman, D. S. (2001). Adult living donor liver transplantation: Current status. *Journal of Clinical Gastroenterology, 33*(2), 97–106.

Shakil, A. O., Kramer, D., Mazariegos, G. V., Fung, J. J., & Rakela, J. (2000). Acute liver failure: Clinical features, outcome analysis, and applicability of prognostic criteria. *Liver Transplantation, 6*, 163–169.

Sheiner, P. A., Magliocca, J. F., Bodian, C. A., Kim-Schluger, L., Altaca, G., Guarrera, J. V., Emre, S., Fishbein, T. M., Guy, S. R., Schwartz, M. E., & Miller, C. M. (2000). Long-term medical complications in patients surviving > or = 5 years after liver transplant. *Transplantation, 69*(5), 781–789.

Sher, L. S., Cosenza, C. A., Michel, J., Makowka, L., Miller, C. M., Schwartz, M. E., Busuttil, R., McDiarmid, S., Burdick, J. F., Klein A. S., Esquivel, C., Klintmalm, G., Levy, M., Roberts, J. P., Lake, J. R., Kalayoglu, M., D'Alessandro, A. M., Gordon, R. D., Stieber, A. C., Shaw, B. W., Jr., Thistlethwaite, J. R., Whittington, P., Wiesner, R. H., Porayko, M., Bynon, J. S., Eckhoff, D. E., Freeman, R. B., Rohrer, R. J., Lewis, W. D., Marsh, J. W., Peters, M., Powelson, J., & Cosimi, A. B. (1997). Efficacy of tacrolimus as rescue therapy for chronic rejection in orthotopic liver transplantation: A report of the U.S. Multicenter Liver Study Group. *Transplantation, 64*, 258–263.

Starzl, T. E., Van Thiel, D., Tzakis, A. G., Iwatsuki, S., Todo, S., Marsh, J. W., Koneru, B., Staschak, S., Stieber, A., & Gordon, R. D. (1988). Orthotopic liver transplantation for alcoholic cirrhosis. *Journal of the American Medical Association, 260*(17), 2542–2544.

Szabo, G., Katz, E., & Bonkovsky, H. L. (2000). Management of recurrent hepatitis C after liver transplantation: A concise review. *American Journal of Gastroenterology, 95*(9), 2164–2170.

United Network for Organ Sharing. (2000). *SR and OPTN annual report: Graft and* patient survival rates at one, three, and five years. Retrieved October 26, 2001, from http://www.unos.org/frame_Default.asp?Catetory=Data

United Network for Organ Sharing. (2000). *SR and OPTN annual report: Living donor characteristics—1990 to 1999. Table 21: Liver Donors.* Retrieved November 4, 2001, from http://www.unos.org/Data/anrpt00/ar00_table21_01_lild.htm

United Network for Organ Sharing. (2001). *Living donation: An overview.* Retrieved October 28, 2001, from http://www.unos.org/Newsroom/critdata_living-donor.htm

United Network for Organ Sharing. (2001). *Number of U.S. organ donors by organ and donor type 1990–December 2000.* Retrieved October 28, 2001, from http://www.unos.org/Newsroom/critdata_livingdonor.htm

United Network for Organ Sharing. (2001). *Policy notice memo: OPTN/UNOS board endorses further development of liver urgency scale.* Retrieved January 19, 2002, from http://www.unos.org/newsroom/archive%5Fpolicy%F20010716%5Fmeld.htm

U.S. Department of Health and Human Services. (2000). *Annual Report of the U.S. Scientific Registry for Transplant Recipients and the Organ Procurement and Transplantation Network: Transplant Data, 1990–1999.* Rockville, MD: Author.

van Thiel, D. (1998). How to assess a patient's support system and personal abilities prior to liver transplantation. *Hepatogastroenterology, 45,* 1395–1397.

Vargas, H. E., Laskus, T., Wang, L. F., Lee, R., Radkowski, M., Dodson, F., Fung, J. J., & Rakela, J. (1999). Outcome of liver transplantation in hepatitis C virus-infected patients who received hepatitis C virus-infected grafts. *Gastroenterology, 117,* 149–153.

Weinrieb, R. M., Van Horn, D. H., McLellan, A. T., & Lucey, M. R. (2000). Interpreting the significance of drinking by alcohol-dependent liver transplant patients: Fostering candor is the key to recovery. *Liver Transplantation, 6*(6), 769–776.

Wiesner, R., & Neuberger, J. (2000, May). Recurrence of disease after liver transplantation. *Transplant 2000,* Symposium conducted at the meeting of the American Society of Transplantation, Chicago.

11

Intestinal Transplantation

Laurel Williams, Simon P. Horslen,
and Alan N. Langnas

Prior to intestinal transplantation, the only option for patients with intestinal failure was total parenteral nutrition (TPN). Although TPN can sustain life for months to years, it may result in several life-threatening complications such as liver disease, sepsis, and problems with the maintenance of intravenous access sites. Initial intestinal transplantation procedures in animals by Lillehei and colleagues in 1959 and multivisceral transplantation by Starzl and Kaupp in 1960 established the technical basis for these surgeries (Anderson, DeVoll-Zabrocki, Brown, Iverson, & Larson, 2000; Reyes et al., 1998). However, over the following three decades, the formidable barriers of the massive lymphocyte content and bacterial load within the intestine challenged the long-term success of these procedures (Okada & Wilmore, 1999).

The first recipients of intestinal transplantation in the 1960s did poorly because of infection, rejection and technical complications (Grant, 1997). The introduction of cyclosporine in the early 1980s improved survival rates somewhat. However, cyclosporine was not as successful in preventing rejection in intestinal transplantation as it was in heart and liver transplantation (Jan et al., 1999).

In 1988, Grant performed the first successful liver and intestinal transplant in a 41-year-old female (Grant, 1990). The patient was able to resume a normal diet and lifestyle 1 year posttransplantation. She survived for 6 years and died from recurrent pulmonary emboli secondary to a hyper-coagulable state. This patient's longer survival time and return to a more normal lifestyle encouraged other centers to overcome the challenges associated with transplantation of the intestine. The clinical application of intestinal transplantation, however, was radically changed with the intro-duction of tacrolimus in 1989 (Jan et al., 1999). Medical advancements made over the past 10 years, including new immunosuppressive regimens and refined surgical techniques, have made intestinal transplantation more successful and offer new options and hope for people with previ-ously fatal intestinal disease.

SURVIVAL RATES

The 1999 International Intestinal Transplant Registry Report provides data on 474 intestinal transplant procedures performed in 446 patients who have undergone intestinal (45%), intestine/liver (40%), and multi-visceral (15%) transplantation. These transplant procedures have been performed in 46 centers throughout the world, although most of them have been done in the United States (Goulet, 1999). The 1- and 5-year patient survival rates for each of these types of procedures is as follows:

- intestinal: 70% (1-year), 45% (5-year)
- intestine/liver: 65% (1-year), 45% (5-year);
- multivisceral: 50% (1-year), 30% (5-year) (Intestinal Transplant Registry, Patient Survival by Organs Transplanted)

United Network for Organ Sharing (UNOS) graft survival rates for intestinal transplantation procedures performed between 1990 and 1998 are as follows:

- 1-year: 64%
- 3-year: 49%
- 5-year: 37% (UNOS, *Graft Survival Rates*)

Patient survival rates for intestinal transplantation procedures per-formed during this same period are

- 1-year: 80%
- 3-year: 62%
- 5-year: 50% (UNOS, *Patient Survival Rates*)

Individual intestinal transplant programs in the United States have reported one-year patient and graft survival rates as high as 93% and 71%, respectively (Sudan, Kaufman et al., 2000).

QUALITY OF LIFE

Few studies have examined quality of life (QOL) in intestinal transplantation patients. In one single-center study of 27 pediatric and 4 adult patients who underwent isolated small intestine or combined liver/small intestine transplantation, 84% of the children returned to day care, preschool, or school at their appropriate age level. Many of these children also participated in extracurricular activities such as sports, dance, and scouting. Seventy-five percent of the adult recipients returned to work or school (Sudan, Iverson, et al., 2000). Rovera and colleagues reported that QOL in adult intestinal transplant recipients was similar to that of patients who were dependent on home parenteral nutrition and that QOL following transplantation improves with time (Rovera et al., 1998).

The transplant community continues to work diligently to improve the survival rates and quality of life for all patients with intestinal failure.

INDICATIONS FOR INTESTINAL TRANSPLANTATION

The indication for intestinal transplantation is irreversible intestinal failure with associated complications. Intestinal failure is defined as "gastrointestinal disease that leads to an inability to maintain sufficient fluid, electrolyte, and nutritional status for more than one month without TPN" (Mazariegos & Reyes, 1999, p. 371).

Intestinal failure may be divided into two categories, structural and functional. Structural intestinal failure is characterized by a reduction in the functioning intestinal mass (short bowel syndrome [SBS]). Functional intestinal failure is characterized by extensive mucosal lesions or severe dysmotility of the gut (Okada & Wilmore, 1999). Both structural and functional problems may cause disturbances of intestinal motility and absorption of water, electrolytes, calories, and other nutrients. The majority of patients referred for intestinal transplantation have structural problems such as SBS secondary to extensive bowel resection due to neonatal disorders, abdominal trauma, or disruption of the blood supply and ischemic changes to the intestine. Intestinal failure may occur at any age and requires prompt and early referral to an intestinal failure/transplant center.

Common structural disease processes include the following:

- Necrotizing enterocolitis (NEC)
- Midgut volvulus secondary to malrotation
- Gastroschisis
- Atresias/stenosis of the small bowel
- Crohn's disease
- Vascular accidents/mesenteric thrombosis/trauma
- Familial adenomatous polyposis (FAP) (see Table 11.1)

Functional problems include the following:

- Chronic intestinal pseudo-obstruction syndrome (CIPS) (see Münchausen by Proxy, below)
- Congenital enteritis (i.e., microvillus inclusion disease [MID])
- Total intestinal aganglionosis (Hirshsprung's disease)
- Radiation enteritis (see Table 11.2)

MÜNCHAUSEN BY PROXY

Münchausen by proxy (MBP) must be considered whenever pediatric patients present with a diagnosis of CIPS that cannot be supported by history or definitive diagnostic testing (Kosmach-Park, in press). MBP is a form of child abuse in which a parent falsifies a child's medical history, induces signs and symptoms of illness, and makes the child undergo extensive diagnostic or therapeutic procedures (Zitelli, Seltman, & Shannon, 1987).

CIPS is a relatively rare disorder with nonspecific diagnostic tests. Both MBP and CIP present as a group of symptoms that cannot be readily diagnosed. Therefore, a child who in actuality is a victim of MBP may mistakenly be diagnosed with CIP.

TYPES OF INTESTINAL TRANSPLANT PROCEDURES

There are several types of intestinal transplantation procedures, each with its respective indications:

Isolated Intestinal Transplantation
- Intestinal failure with dependence on TPN
- Recurrent and life-threatening septic episodes secondary to vascular access line infections

TABLE 11.1 Structural Intestinal Failure: Syndromes, Signs and Symptoms, Diagnostic Tests, Findings, and Treatment

Syndrome	Clinical manifestations	Diagnosis	Findings	Treatment
Necrotizing enterocolitis Ulceration and necrosis of GI tract (focal or diffuse) Often associated with prematurity Primarily affects distal small bowel and colon	Lethargy Temperature instability Apnea Shock Ileus Feeding intolerance Gastric retention of feedings Absence of bowel sounds Abdominal distention Bilious vomiting Gross or occult blood in stools Disseminated intravascular coagulation (Israel, 1996; Vanderhoof & Langnas, 1997)	Clinical presentation Plain abdominal radiography Metrizamide GI series Portal vein ultra-sonography	Nonspecific air fluid levels resembling intestinal obstruction Intestinal pneumatitis (linear streaks or bubbles of gas in bowel wall) Gas in portal venous system Localized or generalized pneumoperitoneum (if perforated) Intestinal dilatation Intraabdominal fluid Colonic stenosis (late complication)	Conservative medical management Broad-spectrum antibiotics Surgical resection if severe Transplantation

continued

Malrotation of the small intestine with midgut volvulus Etiology: failure of midgut to achieve normal anatomic position during embryonic development Leads to volvulus (twisting) of midgut, high intestinal obstruction, ischemia, gangrene Most common during infancy but can occur at any age; 90% of infants present by 2 months of age May mimic other forms of bowel obstruction	Anorexia Bilious vomiting and minimal abdominal distention (early stages) Vague fullness, right upper quadrant (with/without distention) Increased abdominal distention with tenderness and voluntary guarding associated with midgut ischemia Passage of blood-tinged mucus per rectum Lethargy Fever Tachycardia Erythema and edema of the abdominal wall Gangrene (Keljo & Squires, 1998; Wesson & Haddock, 1996)	Plain abdominal radiography Upper GI series Barium enema Oral contrast studies (if there is no indication of ischemia)	Indicative of high small intestinal obstruction; obstructed midgut may be filled with fluid and appear gaseous Partial duodenal obstruction and absence of duodenal loop; jejunum situated in right side of abdomen Cecum in abdominal position in upper or left abdomen	Emergency resection of ischemic bowel Transplantation

continued

TABLE 11.1 (continued)

Syndrome	Clinical manifestations	Diagnosis	Findings	Treatment
Gastroschisis Herniation of abdominal contents lateral to umbilical ring secondary to abdominal wall defect Incidence: 1:10,000 births	Defects situated to the right of the umbilicus Eviscerated mass of bowel loops Edematous or dusky bowel Bowel may be encased by thick fibrinous membranes Absence of peristalsis Absence of sac or remnant Small peritoneal cavity Extrusion of other organs (e.g., stomach, urinary bladder, kidneys, ovaries, uterus) within eviscerated mass 21% of patients may have additional defects (e.g., structural defects: vascular disruptions, renal and gallbladder agenesis) (Keljo & Squires, 1998; Taylor & Ross, 1996)	Prenatal ultrasonography Clinical presentation at birth		Parenteral nutrition Enteral nutrition if tolerated by mouth, nasogastric tube or gastrostomy Staged operative repair Transplantation

continued

TABLE 11.1 (continued)

Syndrome	Clinical manifestations	Diagnosis	Findings	Treatment
Omphalocele Herniation of abdominal viscera into base of umbilical cord Incidence: 2.5:10,000 births	Abdominal contents enclosed within membranous sac (intact or ruptured) Extrusion of liver in some cases Bowel may be normal in appearance 75% of patients have extraintestinal birth defects (e.g., trisomy 13 or 18; Beckwith-Wiedemann syndrome) (Keljo & Squires, 1998; Taylor & Ross, 1996)	Prenatal ultrasonography Clinical presentation at birth		Parenteral nutrition Enteral nutrition if tolerated by mouth, nasogastric tube or gastrostomy Primary closure most common Transplantation
Duodenal atresia Complete, congenital obstruction of lumen of duodenum 50% of intestinal atresias occur in duodenum Incidence: 1:20,000 to 1:40,000 births	Bile-stained emesis shortly after birth (secondary to complete obstruction) Nondistended abdomen Intermittent vomiting (with incomplete obstruction) Often associated with other abnormalities and genetic defects (Babyn & Stringer, 1996; Keljo & Squires, 1998; Milla, 1996; Wesson & Haddock, 1996)	Plain abdominal radiography	"Double bubbles" representing gas and fluid in stomach and proximal duodenum	Aggressive supportive care to maintain hydration, nutritional status, cardiovascular stability Nasogastric suctioning Surgical resection of atretic intestine Prolonged intravenous or enteral nutritional support required in some cases Transplantation

continued

TABLE 11.1 (continued)

Syndrome	Clinical manifestations	Diagnosis	Findings	Treatment
Jejunal and ileal atresia 36% of intestinal atresias occur in jejunum; 14% occur in ileum Incidence: 1:332 to 1:5000 births Prevalence: 2.8:10,000 live births	Jaundice Polyhydramnios Bile-stained or feculent vomiting Generalized abdominal distention Failure to pass meconium stool (70% of infants) Passage of meconium (30% of infants) Nonhemolytic, indirect hyperbilirubinemia, especially in patients with proximal obstruction (Keljo & Squires, 1998; Wesson & Haddock, 1996)	Plain prone and upright radiography Water soluble contrast studies if there is a potential for perforations	Multiple loops of distended bowel containing air-fluid levels Peritoneal calcifications indicative of prenatal perforation and meconium peritonitis Impacted meconium	Aggressive supportive care to maintain temperature and fluid balance Orogastric suction to decrease abdominal distention Resection of atretic portion of intestine with end-to-end anastomosis Prolonged intravenous or enteral nutritional support required in some cases Transplantation

continued

TABLE 11.1 *(continued)*

Syndrome	Clinical manifestations	Diagnosis	Findings	Treatment
Crohn's disease Chronic transmural inflammation that may involve any part of the GI tract, typically in a discontinuous manner; may be associated with extraintestinal features Typically affects ileum, colon, perianal region 25%–33% of patients present before age 20; 15% of patients have onset after age 50	Mild, crampy, colicky postprandial pain in right lower quadrant or suprapubic region Diarrhea Early satiety Low-grade fever Mucus and blood in stools Poor growth or weight loss prior to major GI symptoms Gross bleeding (patients with colonic involvement) Perianal fistulas, abscesses, fissures with skin tags Fibrostenotic narrowing, obstruction, constipation, and obstipation Extraintestinal manifestations: Skin lesions Aphthous stomatitis Digital clubbing Pelvic osteomyelitis Osteomalacia Gallstone formation Oxalate kidney stones Amyloidosis (rare) Thromboembolic complications Hepatobiliary disease	Barium contrast studies	Submucosal edema, pseudodiverticula Mucosal edema (blunting, flattening, thickening, distortion or straightening of the valvulae conniventes of small bowel) Separation of barium-filled bowel loops Deep transverse and longitudinal ulcerations with intervening edematous mucosa (characteristic "cobblestone" appearance) Multiple tight fibrotic strictures with intervening dilated segments of bowel ("string of sausages" appearance) "String sign" of narrowed terminal ileum due to edema and spasm	Drug therapy Antibiotics Corticosteroids Immunosuppressants Nonsteroidal anti-inflammatory drugs Restricted oral intake Nutritional therapy Aggressive nutritional support Elemental enteral feedings Total parenteral nutrition Surgical resection Transplantation

continued

TABLE 11.1 (continued)

Syndrome	Clinical manifestations	Diagnosis	Findings	Treatment
		Endoscopic biopsy	Multiple stellate fistulas with fine or broad radiating fistulous tracts	
			Deep transmural inflammation with formation of granulomas Endoscopic features of malignant stricture: rigidity of stricture edge, eccentric lumen, abrupt, shelflike margin, nodularity	
	(Kornbluth, Sachar, & Saloman, 1998; Leichtner, Jackson, & Grand, 1996)	Computed tomography	Marked transmural thickening; fistulas	
Ischemic lesions Mesenteric ischemia may result from functional or mechanical decreases in blood flow to all or part of the	Clinical manifestations depend on cause and extent of injury Superior mesenteric artery thrombosis (SMAT) • History of postprandial abdominal pain weeks to months preceding onset of severe abdominal pain	Angiography	SMAT: complete occlusion of SMA 1–2 cm from its origin; absence of collateral circulation or inadequate filling of collateral vessels (acute occlusion)	Broad-spectrum antibiotics Surgical resection Maintenance of fluid and electrolyte balance

continued

TABLE 11.1 (*continued*)

Syndrome	Clinical manifestations	Diagnosis	Findings	Treatment
small intestine and right half of colon Etiology may be due to traumatic injury, complications of abdominal surgery, or hematological disorders such as antithrombin 3 deficiency	Superior mesenteric artery embolism (SMAE) • Sudden severe abdominal pain with rapid, forceful bowel evacuation • Absent or minimal abdominal signs Nonocclusive mesenteric ischemia (NOMI) • Right-sided abdominal pain associated with passage of maroon or bright red blood in stool • Unexplained abdominal distention or GI bleeding • Occult blood in stool Mesenteric venous thrombosis (acute) (MVT) • Abdominal pain out of proportion to physical findings • Nausea, vomiting • Fecal occult blood • Abdominal tenderness, distention • Decreased bowel sounds		SMAE: rounded filling defect with nearly complete obstruction to flow NOMI: narrowing of origins of superior mesenteric artery (SMA) branches; irregularities in intestinal branches; spasm of the arcades; impaired filling of intramural vessels Acute MVT: thrombus in superior mesenteric vein (SMV); failure to visualize SMV or portal vein; slow/absent filling of mesenteric veins; arterial spasm; failure of arterial arcades to empty;	Nutritional support Maximization of absorptive capacity of remaining bowel Transplantation

continued

TABLE 11.1 (continued)

Syndrome	Clinical manifestations	Diagnosis	Findings	Treatment
	Mesenteric venous thrombosis (subacute) • Nonspecific abdominal pain (Brandt & Smithline, 1998; Thompson & Langnas, 2002)	Small bowel series	reflux of contrast into artery; prolonged blush of involved segment Acute MVT: thickening of bowel wall; separation of loops and characteristic "thumbprint" pattern	
		Computed tomography	Acute MVT: thickened bowel wall; enlarged CMV; central lucency in lumen of vein; sharply defined vein wall; diluted collateral vessels in a thickened mesentery	
		Plain abdominal films (to aid with differential diagnosis)		
		Tests for hypercoagulation disorders		

continued

TABLE 11.1 (continued)

Syndrome	Clinical manifestations	Diagnosis	Findings	Treatment
Familial adenomatous polyposis Autosomal, dominantly inherited disorder characterized by progressive development of hundreds to thousands of adenomatous polyps in large intestine Prevalence: 1:5,000 to 1:7,500 births Polyps usually not apparent until after puberty Symptoms typically begin 10 years after development of polyps	Nausea Diarrhea Abdominal pain Hematochezia Gardner's syndrome: triad of GI polyposis and extra-intestinal manifestations of bone and soft tissue tumors; may be associated with congenital hypertrophy of the retinal pigment epithelium (CHRPE) (Burt & Jacoby, 1999; Itzkowitz & Young, 1998; Winter, 1996)	Sigmoidoscopy Colonoscopy Air contrast barium enema Fiberoptic or video endoscopy Genetic testing to confirm diagnosis	Colonic adenomas Duodenal, especially periampullary, adenomas Gastric fundic gland hyperplasia Jejunal and ileal adenomas Ileal lymphoid polyps	Subtotal colectomy with ileorectal anastomosis Total proctocolectomy with ileostomy Colectomy with mucosal proctectomy and ileoanal pouch pull-through Medical management for small polyps Radiation Transplantation

continued

TABLE 11.2 Common Functional Disorders: Signs and Symptoms, Diagnostic Tests, Findings, and Treatment

Syndrome	Clinical manifestations	Diagnosis	Findings	Treatment
Chronic Intestinal Pseudo Obstruction Syndrome Enteric neuromuscular disease that requires tube feedings or parenteral support in order to maintain nutrition. Etiology: ineffective intestinal propulsion associated with myopathic or neuropathic disorders, developmental abnormalities, or systemic illness such as amyloidosis, myotonic dystrophy, or progressive systemic sclerosis	Signs and symptoms of intestinal obstruction without evidence of occluding lesion in intestinal lumen Abdominal pain and distention Vomiting (may be feculent) Steatorrhea Diarrhea Constipation Weight loss Succussion splash Hypertympany Visible bowel loops Loud borborygmi Palpable bladder Flattened growth curve Failure to thrive May be associated with megacystis, microcolon, megaloureters Esophageal involvement • Dysphagia • Chest pain	Specific diagnostic studies depend on suspected underlying disorder Imaging studies • Plain abdominal films • Barium studies of esophagus, stomach, small intestine and colon • Enteroclysis • Intravenous pyelography • Voiding cystogram • Esophagogastroduodenoscopy • Chest radiograph • Chest computed tomography Functional studies • Radionuclide gastric emptying and small bowel transit studies • Esophageal manometry	Findings vary with underlying disorder	Broad-spectrum antibiotics for treatment of stagnant loop syndrome Enteral feedings, purgatives, antidiarrheal agents Nasogastric suction for acute episodes Total parenteral nutrition for severe, intractable episodes Palliative surgery in selected cases Transplantation

continued

TABLE 11.2 (continued)

Syndrome	Clinical manifestations	Diagnosis	Findings	Treatment
Developmental abnormalities present in infancy or childhood; degenerative disorders present later	• Regurgitation • Reflux • Heartburn (Hyman, 1994; Schuffler, 1996)	• Gastroduodenal manometry • Cystometrogram Laboratory studies • Thyroid function studies • Antinuclear antibody and SCL-90 • Urinary porphobilinogen and porphyrins • Serum prophobilinogen deaminase • Serum CPK and adolase • Serologic tests for Chegas' disease Other tests • Autonomic function tests • Electromyogram • Nerve conduction velocity • Striated muscle biopsy • Magnetic resonance imaging of brain • Diagnostic laparotomy with biopsy		

continued

TABLE 11.2 (continued)

Syndrome	Clinical manifestations	Diagnosis	Findings	Treatment
Microvillus inclusion disease Autosomal recessive disorder Involves brush border membrane Patients present in infancy, typically within first 3 weeks	Intractable, high-output, secretory, nonbloody diarrhea that is unresponsive to withdrawal of oral diet Steatorrhea Vomiting Dehydration Metabolic acidosis (Davidson, 1996; Keljo & Squires, 1998; Oliva, Perman, Saavedra, Young-Ramasaran, & Schwarz, 1994; Petty, 1999)	Biopsy with electron microscopy Laboratory tests of small intestinal function	Localization of cytoplasmic inclusions to the microvillus membrane in villus cells; severe villous atrophy without crypt injury Abnormal fecal fat excretion, vitamin B_{12} absorption, and mucosal disaccharidase levels	Parenteral feeding only Somatostatin analogue octreotide may control diarrhea Transplantation
Total intestinal aganglionosis (congenital megacolon; Hirschsprung's disease) Congenital absence of ganglion cells in submucosal and myenteric plexuses of distal intestine	Little or no passage of meconium Constipation Vomiting Perforation of appendix or colon Abdominal distention Empty rectum on digital examination Rectal impaction Gastric dysmotility	Plain abdominal radiograph	Diameter of retrosigmoid region or descending colon is more than 6.5 cm in length, the ascending colon is wider than 8 cm or the cecal diameter is greater than 12 cm Absence of gas in pelvis with infant in prone position	Restore fluid and electrolyte balance Enteral feedings as tolerated Total parenteral nutrition Perform adequate evacuation of colon with warm saline enemas

continued

TABLE 11.2 *(continued)*

Syndrome	Clinical manifestations	Diagnosis	Findings	Treatment
Incidence: 1:5,000 live births; higher incidence in males; most cases occur in full-term infants	Enterocolitis (abdominal distention; explosive, watery stools; fever; hypovolemic shock); may be associated with other anomalies (hydrocephalus, ventricular septal defect, imperforate anus, Meckel diverticulum, polyposis, central hypoventilation syndrome, Down's syndrome, renal/urologic problems) Later onset symptoms: Severe constipation Recurrent fecal impactions Anemia Malnutrition (Kirschner, 1996; Phillips & Pemberton, 1998; Wesson & Haddock, 1996)	Proctosigmoidoscopy	Normal but empty rectum; no evidence of obstruction	Broad-spectrum antibiotics for enterocolitis
		Barium enema	Rectal diameter narrower than the sigmoid colon	Surgical resection of aganglionic section(s)
		Anal manometry	Contraction of internal sphincter in response to balloon distention of rectum	Transplantation (especially in children with long segments of colon affected by this disease)
		Intestinal biopsy and acetylcholinesterase	Increased acetylcholinesterase staining	

continued

TABLE 11.2 (*continued*)

Syndrome	Clinical manifestations	Diagnosis	Findings	Treatment
Radiation enteritis Incidence in children: unknown; associated with treatment for pelvic rhabdomyosarcomas, retroperitoneal soft tissue sarcomas, and Wilm's tumor with extension into abdomen Incidence in adults: 2.4% to 25% of patients treated for pelvic or abdominal malignancy Increased risk of enteritis associated with previous abdominal surgery and concomitant radiation and chemotherapy	Children: Early (during radiation therapy) • Colicky abdominal pain • Vomiting • Diarrhea Delayed (months after completion of radiation) • Vomiting • Diarrhea • Abdominal distention with radiologic evidence of obstruction Very late (years after completion of radiation) • Strictures • Fistula • Obliterative arteritis • Fibrosis • Protein-losing enteropathy • Malabsorptive syndromes • Electrolyte disturbances Adults Early (1st or 2nd week of radiation therapy) • Nausea, vomiting • Diarrhea	Clinical presentation Evidence of malabsorption Small bowel barium radiograph	Early phase: mucosal edema; dilated loops of hypotonic small intestine; separation of intestinal loops; thickening and straightening of mucosal folds; spiked appearance of mucosa; severe spasm Late/chronic phase: mucosal edema; separation of intestinal loops; excessive secretions; narrowed, fixed, tubular, poorly distensible segments with no mucosal markings; Rectosigmoid colon: straightened and ahaustral segments; ulcerations	Restoration/maintenance of fluid and electrolyte balance Nutritional support Elemental diet Parenteral nutrition Low-fat, lactose-free diet Antispasmodic agents Cholestyramine Sulfasalazine Corticosteroids Broad-spectrum antibiotics for malabsorption due to small

continued

TABLE 11.2 *(continued)*

Syndrome	Clinical manifestations	Diagnosis	Findings	Treatment
	• Proctocolitis (tenesmus, diarrhea, mucoid rectal discharge) • Rectal bleeding • Abdominal cramping Late Small intestine: • Colicky abdominal pain due to obstruction • Nausea, vomiting • Malabsorption • Weight loss • Fistulas between intestine and pelvic or abdominal organs • Pelvic abscesses • Diarrhea, steatorrhea Rectum: • Proctitis (tenesmus, constipation, bloody, mucoid rectal drainage) (Dubois & Earnest, 1998; Hirsch & Kleinman, 1996)	Small bowel biopsy Angiography Colonoscopy: useful in evaluation of mucosal lesions beyond reach of sigmoidoscope Computed tomography: useful in differential diagnosis of nonspecific barium findings	Villus blunting with dilation of lymphatics and moderately dense, round cell infiltrates in lamina propria Abnormalities in smaller branches of mesenteric vasculature Edema, granularity and friability; pale, opaque mucosa; prominent submucosal telangiectatic vessels	intestinal stasis with bacterial overgrowth Presacral sympathectomy for intractable pelvic pain Surgical intervention for • Obstruction • Perforations • Fistulas Transplantation

- Inability to place or difficulty in locating central venous access
- Progressive yet still reversible liver disease
- Poor quality of life or failure to thrive

Intestinal and Liver Transplantation
- Intestinal failure with dependence on TPN
- TPN-induced hepatic dysfunction progressing to end-stage liver disease

Multivisceral Transplantation
- Inability to remove bowel and liver without removing pancreas
- Stomach dysmotility

CONTRAINDICATIONS TO INTESTINAL TRANSPLANTATION

Contraindications to intestinal transplantation may be characterized as absolute or relative. Absolute contraindications include the following:

- Multiorgan system failure
- Uncontrolled sepsis
- Human immunodeficiency virus (HIV) infection
- Malignancy outside of intestines with metastasis
- Severe, unresolvable cardiac, respiratory, or cerebral complications

Relative contraindications include

- Severe physical debilitation
- Psychosocial issues such as current, active drug abuse or noncompliance

TRANSPLANT EVALUATION PROCESS

Evaluation of the patient with intestinal failure requires a thorough, multidisciplinary team assessment. Specific testing varies among transplant centers and typically takes 3 to 5 days to complete. With children, blood tests may be spread over several days in order to limit the amount of blood that is drawn on any given day (Anderson et al., 2000). The goals of the evaluation process are to

- Confirm the diagnosis (etiology and extent of disease)
- Review all body systems to ascertain risks to the patient and therapeutic medical or surgical interventions required to maintain or stabilize the patient (see Table 11.3)

- Determine the appropriate long-term therapy (i.e., surgical or medical management)
- Educate the patient and family about the procedure, risks, benefits, alternatives, and associated costs
- Ascertain support systems and resources for the patient and family (see Table 11.3)

THE WAITING LIST

In May 2001, there were 167 patients on the UNOS intestinal transplantation waiting list (UNOS, *Patients on the UNOS National Patient Waiting List*). Approximately 74% of these candidates were pediatric patients. Of these, 75% were in the 0 to 5 years age group (UNOS, *Number of Patient Registrations*). Median 1999 waiting times ranged from 85 days for candidates in the 35 to 49-year age group to 396 days for candidates between 1 and 5 years of age (UNOS, *Number of Registrations*). The length of the waiting period is influenced by medical status, blood type and body size.

PREOPERATIVE CARE OF THE TRANSPLANT CANDIDATE

During the waiting period, management of the intestinal transplant candidate includes the following:

1. Maintenance of adequate nutrition
   - Optimize TPN
   - Optimize enteral feedings (when possible)
   - Administer supplemental fat-soluble vitamins, trace elements, carnitine, and so on
2. Prevention and treatment of infection
   - Provide meticulous line care
   - Treatment and prophylaxis of bacterial overgrowth
3. Prevention of vascular complications
   - Provide meticulous line care
   - Minimize number of line sites
4. Prevention of hepatic complications
   - Provide enteral feeding as tolerated
   - Cycle TPN
   - Decrease lipid content of TPN
   - Administer ursodeoxycholic acid for cholestasis
   - Manage hepatic complications such as coagulopathy, bleeding, and so on

TABLE 11.3 Common Tests Performed During Evaluation Process

Medical/surgical consultations
- Gastrointestinal (thorough history and physical examination)
- Surgical
- Dental
- Nutritional
- Others as indicated (e.g., pulmonary, cardiology, neurology, etc.)

Laboratory tests
- Blood typing
- Liver function tests
- Prothrombin time; partial thromboplastin time; clotting factors
- Alpha-fetoprotein
- Alpha-1 antitrypsin phenotype
- Iron studies (serum B_{12}, folate, red blood cell folate, mean corpuscular volume, mean corpuscular hemoglobin concentration, iron, ferritin)
- Electrolytes, blood urea nitrogen (BUN), creatinine, calcium, magnesium, phosphorous, zinc
- Complete lipid profile
- Complete blood count with differential and platelet count
- Tissue typing

Infectious disease screening tests
- Hepatitis C virus
- Hepatitis B virus
- Human immunodeficiency virus
- Cytomegalovirus
- Epstein-Barr virus
- Blood cultures*
- Fungal cultures of stoma or rectum

Radiologic and other studies
- Chest radiograph
- Echocardiogram
- Electrocardiogram (age dependent)
- Gastrointestinal contrast studies (upper and lower)
- Abdominal ultrasonography with doppler flow study
- Doppler ultrasound of central vein patency

continued

TABLE 11.3 *(continued)*

Histological studies
• Bowel histology*
• Liver histology*

Metabolic Assessment
• D-xylose tolerance test
• Fecal fat analysis
• Nitrogen excretion studies

Nutritional assessment
• Dietary and weight history
• Growth–velocity determination
• Caloric requirements
• Evaluation of TPN (tolerance; vitamins, carnitine, minerals, trace elements, etc.)
• Weight, height, triceps skin-fold measurement; mid-arm circumference
• Bone age
• Intestinal motility studies

Psychosocial consultations
• Social worker
• Child developmental specialist
• Child life specialist
• Psychologist
• Psychiatrist
• Financial counselor

*As indicated
Anderson et al., 2000; Funovits, Altieri, Kovalak, & Staschak-Chicko, 1993;
Strom, Koehler, Mazariegos, & Reyes, 1999

   5. Use of oral stimulation for prevention of oral aversion
     • Consult with occupational therapy, speech therapy, feeding team
   6. Promote normal growth and development
     • Consult with physical therapy, speech therapy

During the waiting period, frequent communication between the candidate's local gastroenterologist and transplant center is essential, particularly with respect to ongoing monitoring of progressive liver disease. The height and weight of pediatric candidates are obtained every 2 to 4 weeks so that donor size requirements can be updated (Anderson et al., 2000).

DONOR AND RECIPIENT CONSIDERATIONS

SELECTION OF DONOR

A number of factors are considered in the donor selection process. These include
- Blood type
- Age (typically less than 50–55 years)
- Body size (height and weight typically 25% to 50% smaller than the recipient's height and weight, particularly for patients with short-bowel syndrome who have a loss of peritoneal domain [Vanderhoof & Langnas, 1997])
- Infectious disease status (free of active infection)
    - With respect to cytomegalovirus (CMV) status, some transplant centers will accept CMV-positive donors for CMV-positive recipients.
- Liver function status (for liver/small intestine or multivisceral transplantation)

PREPARATION OF THE DONOR

Most donors are cadaveric. Preoperatively, a bowel cleanser (e.g., polyethylene glycol 3350 and electrolytes for oral solution [GoLYTELY]) may be administered via a nasogastric tube (Funovits, Alteri, Kovalak, & Staschak-Chicko, 1993). Muromonab-CD3 or antithymocyte globulin may also be given.

PREPARATION OF THE RECIPIENT

Cleansing and selective decontamination of the recipient's intestine may be initiated with the administration of a bowel cleanser and prophylactic antibiotics.

SURGICAL PROCEDURE

Surgical procedures for the various types of intestinal transplantation procedures are outlined below (See Figures 11.1 and 11.2).

ISOLATED INTESTINAL TRANSPLANTATION

- Midline incision
- Removal of native intestine as indicated

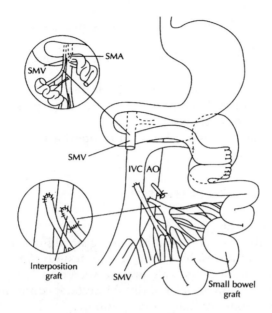

Figure 11.1 Isolated Small Bowel Transplantation.

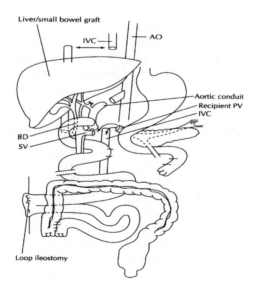

Figure 11.1 Transplantation of the Combined Liver-Small Bowel Graft.

Figures 11.1 and 11.2 from: DeRoover, A., & Langnas, A. N. (1999). Surgical methods of small bowel transplantation and liver-small bowel transplantation. *Current Opinion in Organ Transplantation*, 4(4), 335–342. Copyright Lippincott, Williams & Wilkins. Used with permission.

- Anastomosis of the donor superior mesenteric artery to the recipient aorta
- Anastomosis of the donor jejunum to the recipient jejunum or duodenum
- Placement of a jejunostomy tube if indicated
- Anastomosis of the ileum to the native colon (if present) with creation of a loop or end ileostomy
- Venous drainage of donor bowel into superior mesenteric vein or inferior vena cava

LIVER AND INTESTINAL TRANSPLANTATION

- Midline or subcostal incision
- Removal of the liver and nonfunctioning small intestine
- Implantation of the en bloc liver/small intestine composite
- Native portal drainage into allograft or vena cava
- Establishment of proximal and distal intestinal continuity
- Creation of ostomy (usually loop ileostomy)

MULTIVISCERAL TRANSPLANTATION

- Midline or subcostal incision
- Removal of all native GI organs
- Implantation of en bloc organs (including stomach and colon)
- Establishment of proximal and distal intestinal continuity
- Creation of ostomy (usually loop ileostomy)

IMMEDIATE POSTOPERATIVE CARE

GRAFT FUNCTION

Monitoring of graft function involves

- Careful assessment of stomal output
- Observation of tolerance of enteral feedings
- Surveillance ileoscopy with biopsies

FLUID AND ELECTROLYTE BALANCE

Intestinal transplantation recipients are at risk for fluid volume deficit related to enteric losses and inadequate volume replacement. Intensive hemodynamic monitoring is required during the immediate postoperative period. Fluid and electrolyte management includes the following:

1. Strict measurement of intake and output
   - Enteric output includes losses from the ileostomy, nasogastric tube, jejunostomy tube and rectum; other losses occur via drains and wounds
   - There is minimal output on postoperative days 1–5 until the postoperative ileus resolves. After resolution of the ileus, ostomy outputs should range from 35–50 cc/kg.
   - Resolution of ileus typically occurs between postoperative day 4 and 5
   - Sudden increase in enteric or nasogastric losses (> 50 to 80 cc/kg/day) may indicate rejection or infection
     - Rejection may be associated with a loss of absorptive capacity and an increase in the secretory activity of the lumen
2. Daily weights
3. Frequent biochemical monitoring and subsequent adjustment of intravenous (IV) fluids and replacement of electrolytes
   - Hypovolemia may precipitate hyponatremia, hypokalemia, and metabolic acidosis
   - Immunosuppressive therapy may precipitate metabolic imbalances and hypomagnesemia (Funovits et al., 1993)

RENAL STATUS

There is potential for renal dysfunction secondary to hypovolemia and nephrotoxicity from immunosuppressive and antimicrobial therapies. Management of renal status includes

- Adequate hydration
- Close monitoring of immunosuppression and antibiotic levels
- Biochemical monitoring
- Strict measurement of intake and output with daily weights
- Short-term dialysis or continuous venous–venous hemodialysis if needed

NUTRITIONAL STATUS

Parenteral Nutrition

1. TPN is continued postoperatively (for approximately 4 to 6 weeks)
   - Caloric requirements are based on factors such as intubation status, postoperative complications, fever, rejection, and wound healing (Strohm, Koehler, Mazariegos, & Reyes, 1999)
   - Guidelines for caloric requirements for pediatric recipients:

0 to 1 year	90–120 kilocalories/kg/day
1 to 7 years	75–90 kilocalories/kg/day
7 to 12 years	60–75 kilocalories/kg/day
12 to 18 years	30–60 kilocalories/kg/day
	(Kerner, 1983)

   - Conditions that increase caloric requirements for pediatric patients receiving TPN include

Fever (12% increase for each degree over 37°C)	
Cardiac failure	(15%–25% increase)
Major surgery	(20%–30% increase)
Sepsis	(40%–50% increase)
Long-term growth failure	(50%–100% increase) (Kerner, 1983)

   - Potential complications that can interfere with the ability to provide optimal caloric requirements for pediatric transplant recipients include
     - Hyperglycemia secondary to corticosteroid boluses
     - Pancreatitis or renal insufficiency induced by drugs
     - Decreased motility and absorption secondary to allograft rejection (Strohm et al., 1999)

Enteral Nutrition

1. Enteral feedings (starting with elemental formulas) are started once graft motility is reestablished; indicators of graft motility include the
   - Presence of bowel sounds
   - Absence of abdominal distention
   - Quantity and quality of ileal output (Funovits et al., 1993)
2. Low-fat, low osmolar feedings are provided, occasionally directly into the jejunum.
   - Fat malabsorption may result from lymphatic disruption associated with surgery or from pancreatitis (Strohm et al., 1999).
3. Fat content and concentration are increased as tolerated.
4. Fiber, fluid replacement, or loperamide hydrochloride (Imodium) are added as required.

5. Stomal output and weight gain are closely monitored.
6. Calorie counts and nutritional consultations are obtained daily.
7. Oral stimulation is provided as indicated.
8. TPN is gradually decreased as enteral feedings are tolerated and increased; feeding tolerance is assessed by monitoring the patient's clinical state of hydration and routine biochemical markers.

SKIN INTEGRITY

Skin integrity is a potential problem due to high ostomy output, diarrhea, and lengthy intensive care unit (ICU) stays. Management of skin integrity includes

- Close inspection of skin/wound(s) sites, IV lines, and other tube sites
- Meticulous wound and skin care
- Dressing and ostomy appliance changes as indicated
- Enterostomal therapy consultation

PAIN MANAGEMENT

Short-acting, reversible narcotics are provided as needed. Pain medication requirements typically decrease rapidly within the first 24 hours. For some patients, however, larger doses of pain medication may be required over a longer period of time due to poor drug absorption associated with GI tract dysmotility (Funovits et al., 1993).

Pain management may be particularly challenging if the recipient has a long history of chronic illness and multiple prior surgical procedures. Pain management consultations are obtained as indicated, particularly for patients with chronic pain problems (such as patients with Crohn's disease).

INFECTION

Infection is a primary concern in the early postoperative period and is the leading cause of death in intestinal transplant recipients. Bacterial translocation (the migration of bacteria from the intestinal lumen to other tissues and organs) occurs during periods of stress (ischemia, reperfusion, rejection) and predisposes the recipient to infection (Abu-Elmagd et al., 1994; Todo et al., 1995).

Infections are common because of the

- Involved transplant procedure
- Lengthy operative time
- Potential for allograft rejection and posttransplant lymphoproliferative disease to precipitate breakdown of the mucosal barrier that results in bacteremia or fungemia (Mazariegos & Reyes, 1999)

Bacterial infections predominate during the first 4 to 6 weeks. Fungal infections can occur in the early postoperative period if additional surgery is required (e.g., reexploration for complications such as perforation, dehiscence, etc.), if the incision remains open, or if the patient is very debilitated or has experienced rejection episodes. Viral infections typically occur later in the postoperative course.

Types of Infection

The most common organisms seen in intestinal transplant recipients are

1. Bacterial
   - Gram-positive: streptococcus (e.g., enterococcus), staphylococcus (e.g., epidermitis)
   - Gram-negative: klebsiella, pseudomonas, enterobacter
2. Fungal
   - Candida
   - Aspergillus
3. Viral
   - Cytomegalovirus
   - Epstein-Barr virus
   - Adenovirus

Infection Prophylaxis

Prophylactic regimens vary among transplant centers; however, prophylaxis is typically provided for the following infections:

1. Pneumocystis carinii pneumonia
   - Sulfamethoxazole-trimethoprim (Bactrim, Cotrim, Septra)
   - Atovaquone (Mepron) or inhaled pentamidine (NebuPent) for patients with sulfa allergy or decreased white blood cell (WBC) count

2. Cytomegalovirus infections
   - IV ganciclovir, depending on donor and recipient serologic tests
   - Oral ganciclovir (Cytovene)
3. Fungal infections
   - Nystatin (Mycostatin) or gentian violet for oral candidiasis
   - Fluconazole (Diflucan)
   - Amphotericin B

Routine Vaccinations

1. Routine vaccinations are center- and patient-specific.
2. Depending on the recipient's level of immunosuppression and infection status, routine vaccines are typically resumed 3 to 12 months posttransplant.
3. Protocols regarding the administration of live vaccines, such as the oral polio, varicella, and measles, mumps, and rubella vaccines, are center-specific. Some centers avoid all live vaccines. The injectable polio vaccine is generally administered rather than the oral polio vaccine.
4. Annual influenza vaccines may be recommended for the recipient. Family members should receive an annual influenza vaccine (unless otherwise contraindicated).

Non-pharmacological Measures

In addition to the above prophylaxis, nonpharmacological measures that are used to prevent infection include

- Meticulous line care
- Frequent and thorough handwashing
- Maintenance of adequate nutrition
- Avoidance of people with obvious signs of infection
- Avoidance of potential sources of foodborne microbes (raw eggs, meat, and shellfish) (see chapter 2)

IMMUNOSUPPRESSION REGIMENS

Basic immunosuppression therapy for intestinal transplant recipients varies among transplant centers but generally includes some combination of the medications listed below (see chapter 4).

MAINTENANCE THERAPY

1. Calcineurin inhibitor: tacrolimus (Prograf)
   * Tacrolimus is more potent than cyclosporine and is readily absorbed by the intestinal graft, even if it is not functioning well (Funovits et al., 1993).
   * Common side effects: nephrotoxicity, hyperkalemia, hypertension, hyperlipidemia, diabetes, increased risk of infection
2. Corticosteroids: methylprednisolone (Solu-Medrol), prednisone (Deltasone), prednisolone
   * Common side effects: cataracts, osteopenia, hypertension, cushingoid appearance, irritability/mood swings; hyperglycemia, increase in appetite, acne

ADJUNCTIVE THERAPY

1. Mammalian target of rapamycin (mTOR) inhibitor
   * Sirolimus (Rapamune)
   * Common side effects: hypercholesterolemia, hyperlipidemia, low platelet count, neutropenia
2. Antiproliferative agent
   * Mycophenolate mofetil (CellCept)
   * Common side effects: GI upset; decreased white blood cell count

INDUCTION THERAPY

1. Interleukin-2 antagonists: basiliximab (Simulect); daclizumab (Zenapax)

SHORT-DURATION THERAPY FOR PERSISTENT OR ACUTE REJECTION

1. Monoclonal T-cell antibodies: muromonab-CD3 (Orthoclone OKT3)
   * Common side effects: cytokine release syndrome, viral infections
2. Polyclonal antilymphocyte antibodies: antithymocyte globulin (ATGAM); Antithymocyte globulin (Rabbit) (Thymoglobulin)
   * Common side effects: leukopenia, thrombocytopenia

REJECTION

Despite technical and pharmacological advances over the last decade, rejection continues to be a formidable problem. In the largest reported series, the overall incidence of treated rejection episodes in both children and adults was 93% (Abu-Elmagd et al., 1998; Reyes et al., 1998).

SURVEILLANCE

Rejection surveillance includes routine ileoscopy/endoscopy with biopsies. The frequency of these biopsies varies among transplant centers. A typical regimen might include twice weekly biopsies for 4 to 6 weeks, then weekly biopsies for 4 to 6 weeks, then biweekly biopsies for 4 to 6 weeks, then as indicated.

CLINICAL SIGNS AND SYMPTOMS

Common manifestations of rejection include

- High stomal output (more than 3 L/24 hours) or a significant decrease in stomal output
- Fever
- Sluggish or absent intestinal motility
- Decreased or absent bowel sounds
- Abdominal pain and/or distention
- Change in stomal color
- Irritability/mood changes

DIAGNOSIS

- Endoscopy or ileoscopy with biopsy
- Radiologic monitoring of gastric emptying and intestinal transit time
  - Normal gastric emptying time: 30 to 60 minutes
  - Normal intestinal transit time: 2 to 4 hours
  - Prolonged emptying time or rapid transit time is associated with poor intestinal function (Funovits et al., 1993)

TREATMENT

- Steroid bolus and taper
- Increased immunosuppression
- Initiation of monoclonal or polyclonal antibody therapy

LONG-TERM CARE AND FOLLOW-UP

The long-term care of the intestinal transplant recipient involves frequent monitoring to determine nutritional status, assess immunosuppression levels, and screen for and treat infections.

BIOCHEMICAL MONITORING

In the posttransplant patient, the following biochemical tests are frequently done in order to monitor

- Absorption of fluids and electrolytes and nutritional status (sodium, potassium, chloride, blood urea nitrogen, creatinine, magnesium, phosphorus, calcium, glucose, carbon dioxide and vitamin levels)
- Infection, blood loss, bone marrow suppression, and hemolysis (complete blood cell count, platelet count)
- Immunosuppression levels to determine if levels are therapeutic (e.g., tacrolimus levels)
- Liver function (bilirubin, alkaline phosphatase, aspartate aminotransferase, alanine aminotransferase, lactate dehydrogenase, total protein, and albumin)

NUTRITIONAL MANAGEMENT

1. Convert to age-appropriate whole protein feeding by 2 to 3 months; normal diet for age as tolerated.
   - Infant recipients may require gastrostomy tube feedings for up to 1 year posttransplant.
2. Initiate oral aversion techniques if patient has not been previously accustomed to oral feeding.
3. Reverse ileostomy between 3 to 12 months (per center-specific protocols).
4. Monitor vitamin and mineral status (particularly vitamins A and B_{12}, zinc, selenium, and red blood cell folate).

5. Readjust fluids, electrolytes, and oral supplements as needed.
6. Observe pediatric recipients for lactose intolerance and wheat allergies (Strohm et al., 1999).
7. Revert to enteral or total parenteral nutrition as required during episodes of rejection or infection or during periods of poor absorption or excessive stomal output (Strohm et al., 1999).
8. Monitor posttransplant growth of pediatric recipients:
   - Weight
   - Height
   - Weight/height ratio
   - Tricep skinfold measurement
   - Midarm muscle circumference (Strohm et al., 1999)

DIAGNOSIS AND TREATMENT OF INFECTION

Intestinal transplant recipients may be at increased risk of developing community acquired infections. In addition to a thorough history and physical examination and routine laboratory tests, evaluation of the febrile patient may also require

- Blood cultures
- Chest radiography
- Urine culture
- Serum titers for CMV, EBV DNA, CMV early antigen, CMV buffy coat (pp65)
- Arterial blood gases, if indicated.

Treatment of infections may include

- Acetominophen for fever
- Antibiotics if an infectious source is identified or if the patient appears septic
- Close monitoring or return of patient to transplant center, depending on level of illness

Non-steroidal anti-inflammatory agents are avoided due to their adverse effect on renal function. Certain antimicrobial agents either increase (e.g., erythromycin, clarithromycin) or decrease (e.g., isoniazid) serum cyclosporine and tacrolimus levels. The transplant center must be notified if any of these agents are prescribed (see chapter 2).

POSTTRANSPLANT LYMPHOPROLIFERATIVE DISEASE (PTLD)

The incidence of EBV-associated PTLD in pediatric and adult intestinal transplant recipients is 29% and 11%, respectively. PTLD is more common after multivisceral than isolated intestinal transplantation. Clinical manifestations frequently include

- Fever
- Gastrointestinal pain
- Gastrointestinal symptoms
- Lymphadenopathy or localized masses on abdominal imaging

Genomic EBV surveillance in peripheral blood has enhanced the diagnosis of PTLD. Treatment includes a reduction in immunosuppression and antiviral therapy (Mazariegos & Reyes, 1999; Nalesnik et al., 2000).

GRAFT VS. HOST DISEASE (GVHD)

GVHD occurs in patients receiving abundant lymphoid tissue such as bone marrow, intestine and other solid organs. In solid organ transplant recipients, GVHD is often associated with bone marrow aplasia or immunodeficiency (Crawford, 1993). The reported incidence of GVHD among intestinal transplant recipients ranges between 5% and 14% (Abu-Elmagd et al., 1998; Pinna et al., 2000; Reyes et al., 1998). It is caused by the T cells of the donor organ that are carried within the graft and are cytotoxic to the recipient's cells.

Clinical Manifestations

GVHD may be asymptomatic or may be associated with rejection. Signs and symptoms typically occur within 7 to 50 days posttransplant and include

- Fever
- Skin rash
- Diarrhea
- Weight loss

Diagnosis

The diagnosis of GVHD is difficult to make. Typically, skin and bowel biopsies are required; skin biopsy, however, may not be definitive. Other causes of these symptoms, such as drug toxicity, infection, PTLD, and TPN administration, must be ruled out.

Treatment

Treatment of GVHD includes high-dose steroids and increased immunosuppression. Surveillance endoscopies with biopsies may be performed. Spontaneous resolution may occur.

WHEN TO CALL THE TRANSPLANT CENTER

Health care providers should call the transplant center whenever the patient experiences any of the following:

- Persistent fever > 3 days
- Sepsis
- Sudden increase in or cessation of ostomy output
- Bloody ostomy output
- Change in color of stoma
- Stomal prolapse
- Inability to tolerate enteral feedings (nausea, vomiting, dehydration)
- Difficulty in maintaining nutritional status
- New onset snoring
- Lymphadenopathy
- Persistent headaches
- Patient unwell with no obvious cause

In addition, healthcare providers should check with the transplant center regarding the administration of any vaccines. Transplant personnel are most willing to answer any and all questions.

CONCLUSION

The increasing experience and improved outcomes of intestinal transplantation support the clinical use of this treatment modality. Currently, the potential morbidity and mortality of intestinal transplantation is greater than that of other transplant procedures. However, the benefit of long-term survival, enteral versus parenteral nutrition and improved quality of life outweighs those risks (Thompson & Langnas, 2002). Survival rates will continue to improve as the science of intestinal transplantation advances.

Early referral to transplant centers of excellence remains key to optimal patient outcomes.

ACKNOWLEDGMENTS

The authors gratefully acknowledge the support and editorial assistance of Deb Andersen, RN, and Joyce Rogue, RN, and secretarial assistance from Tamara Bernard, Sue Jones, and Tracy Krasser.

REFERENCES

Abu-Elmagd, K., Reyes, J., Todo, S., Rao, A., Lee, R., Irish, W., Furukawa, H., Bueno, J., McMichael, J., Fawzy, A. T., Murase, N., Demetris, J., Rakela, J., Fung, J. J., & Starzl, T. E. (1998).. Clinical intestinal transplantation: New perspectives and immunologic considerations. *Journal of the American College of Surgeons, 186*(5), 512–525.

Andersen, D., DeVoll-Zabrocki, A., Brown, C. Iverson, A., & Larsen, J. (2000). Intestinal transplantation in pediatric patients: A nursing challenge: Part 1. Evaluation for intestinal transplantation. *Gastroenterology Nursing, 23*(1), 3–9.

Babyn, P., & Stringer, D. A. (1996). Imaging: Part 2: Radiography—Plain film. In W. A. Walker, P. R. Durie, J. R. Hamilton, J. A. Walker-Smith, & J. B. Watkins. (Eds.), *Pediatric gastrointestinal disease: Pathophysiology, diagnosis, management* (2nd ed., vol. 2, pp. 1654–1673). St. Louis: Mosby.

Brandt, L. H., & Smithline, A. E. (1998). Ischemic lesions of the bowel. In M. Feldman, B. R. Scharschmidt, & M. H. Sleisenger (Eds.), *Gastrointestinal and liver disease: Pathophysiology, diagnosis, management* (6th ed., vol. 2, pp. 2009–2024). Philadelphia: W. B. Saunders.

Burt, R. W., & Jacoby, R. F. (1999). Polyposis syndromes. In T. Yamada (Ed.), *Textbook of gastroenterology* (3rd ed., vol. 2, pp. 1995–2022), Philadelphia: Lippincott, Williams & Wilkins.

Crawford, J. M. (1993). Graft-versus host disease of the liver. In V. K. Rustigi, & D. H. Van Thiel, D. H. (Eds.), *The liver in systemic diseases* (pp. 315–332). New York: Raven Press.

Davidson, G. P. (1996). Enteropathies of unknown origin. In W. A. Walker, P. Durie, J. R. Hamilton, J. A. Walker-Smith, & J. B. Watkins. (Eds.), *Pediatric gastrointestinal disease: Pathophysiology, diagnosis, management* (2nd ed., vol. 1, pp. 862–867). St. Louis: Mosby.

DeRoover, A., & Langnas, A. N. (1999). Surgical methods of small bowel transplantation and liver-small bowel transplantation. *Current Opinion in Organ Transplantation, 4*(4), 335–342.

Dubois, A., & Earnest, D. L. (1998). Radiation enteritis and colitis. In M. Feldman, B. F. Scharschmidt, & M. H. Sleisenger (Eds.), *Gastrointestinal and liver disease: Pathophysiology, diagnosis, management,* (6th ed., vol. 2, pp. 1696–1707). Philadelphia: W. B. Saunders.

Funovits, M., Alteri, K., Kovalak, J., & Staschak-Chicko, S. I. (1993). Small intestine transplantation: A nursing perspective. *Critical Care Nursing Clinics of North America, 5*(1), 203–213.

Goulet, O. (1999). Clinical results of intestinal transplantation. *Current Opinion in Organ Transplantation, 4*(4), 350–353.

Grant, D. (1990). Successful small-bowel/liver transplantation. *Lancet, 335,* 181–184.

Grant, D. (1997). Intestinal transplantation: Report of the International Registry. *Transplantation, 67*(7), 1061–1064.

Hirsch, B. Z., & Kleinman, R. E. (1996). Radiation enteritis. In W. A. Walker, P. Durie, J. R. Hamilton, J. A. Walker-Smith, & J. B. Watkins. (Eds.), *Pediatric gastrointestinal disease: Pathophysiology, diagnosis, management.* (2nd ed., vol. 1, pp. 915–919). St. Louis: Mosby.

Hyman, P. E. (1994). Chronic intestinal pseudo-obstruction. In P. E. Hyman & G. DiLorenzo (Eds.). *Pediatric gastromotility disorders,* (pp. 115–128). New York: Academy of Professional Information Services.

Intestinal Transplant Registry. (2001). Patient survival by organs transplanted. Retrieved May 5, 2001, http://www.lhsc.on.ca/itr/results

Israel, E. J. (1996). Necrotizing enterocolitis. In W. A. Walker, P. R. Durie, J. R. Hamilton, J. A. Walker-Smith, & J. B. Watkins. (Eds.), *Pediatric gastrointestinal disease: Pathophysiology, diagnosis, management,* (2nd ed., vol. 1, pp. 750–761). St. Louis: Mosby.

Itkowitz, S. H., & Young, S. K. (1998). Colonic polyps and polyposis syndromes. In M. Feldman, B. F. Scharschmidt, & M. H. Sleisenger. (Eds.), *Gastrointestinal and liver disease: Pathophysiology, diagnosis, management,* (6th ed., vol. 2, pp. 1865–1905). Philadelphia: W. B. Saunders.

Jan, D., Michel, J. L., Goulet, O., Sarnacki, S., Lacaille, F., Damotte, D., Cozard, J. P., Aigrain, Y., Brousse, N., Peuchmaur, M., Rengeval, A., Colomb, V., Jouvet, P., Ricour, C., & Revillon, Y. (1999). Up-to-date evolution of small bowel transplantation in children with intestinal failure. *Journal of Pediatric Surgery, 34*(5), 841–844.

Kelijo, D. J., & Squires, R. H., Jr. (1998). Anatomy and anomalies of the small and large intestine. In M. Feldman, B. F. Scharschmidt, & M. H. Sleisenger. (Eds.), *Gastrointestinal and liver disease: Pathophysiology, diagnosis, management* (6th ed., vol. 2, pp. 1419–1436). Philadelphia: W. B. Saunders.

Kerner, J. (1983). Caloric requirements. In J. Kerner (Ed.), *Manual of Pediatric Parenteral Nutrition* (pp. 63–67). New York: Wiley.

Kirschner, B. S. (1996). Hirschsprung's disease. In W. A. Walker, P. R. Durie, J. R. Hamilton, J. A. Walker-Smith, & J. B. Watkins (Eds.), *Pediatric gastrointestinal disease: Pathophysiology, diagnosis, management* (2nd ed., vol. 1, pp. 980–983). Philadelphia: W. B. Saunders.

Kornbluth, A., Sachar, D. B., & Salomon, P. (1998). Crohn's disease. In M. Feldman, B. F. Scharschmidt, & M. H. Sleisenger (Eds), *Gastrointestinal and liver disease: Pathophysiology, diagnosis, management* (6th ed., vol 2, pp. 1708–1734). Philadelphia: W. B. Saunders.

Kosmach-Park, B. (in press). Transplantation for loss of intestinal function. In. S. Smith & L. Ohler (Eds.), *Organ transplantation: Concepts, issues, practice and outcomes.* Medscape web site.

Leichtner, A. M, Jackson, W. D., & Grand, R. J. (1996). Crohn's disease. In W. A. Walker, P. R. Durie, J. R. Hamilton, J. A. Walker-Smith, & J. B. Watkins (Eds.), *Pediatric gastrointestinal disease: Pathophysiology, diagnosis, management* (2nd ed., pp. 692–711). Philadelphia: W. B. Saunders.

Mazariegos, G. V., & Reyes, J. (1999). An update of current clinical practices in pediatric organ transplantation. *Pediatrics in Review, 20*(11), 363–375.

Milla, P. J. (1996). The stomach and duodenum: Part 5: Motor disorders including pyloric stenosis. In W. A. Walker, P. R. Durie, J. R. Hamilton, J. A. Walker-Smith, & J. B. Watkins (Eds.), *Pediatric gastrointestinal disease: Pathophysiology, diagnosis, management* (2nd ed., vol. 1, pp. 543–553). St. Louis: Mosby.

Nalesnik, M., Jaffe, R., Reyes, G., Mazariegos, J. J., Fung, T. E., Starzl, T. E., & Abu-Elmagd, K. (2000). Posttransplant lymphoproliferative disorders in small bowel allograft recipients. *Transplantation Proceedings, 32,* 1213.

Okada, A., & Wilmore, D. (1999). Closing remarks. *Journal of Parenteral and Enteral Nutrition, 23*(5), S126–S127.

Oliva. N. M., Perman. J. A., Saavedra, J. M., Young-Ramasaran, J., & Schwarz, K. B. (1994). Successful intestinal transplantation for microvillus inclusion disease. *Gastroenterology, 106,* 771–777.

Petty, E. M. (1999). Gastrointestinal manifestations of specific genetic disorders. In T. Yamada (Ed.), *Textbook of gastroenterology* (3rd ed., vol. 2, pp. 2460–2503). Philadelphia: Lippincott, Williams & Wilkins.

Phillips, S. F., & Pemberton, J. H. (1998). Megacolon: Congenital and acquired. In M. Feldman, B. F. Scharschmidt, & M. H. Sleisenger (Eds.), *Gastrointestinal and liver disease: Pathophysiology, diagnosis, management* (6th ed., vol. 2, pp. 1810–1819). Philadelphia: W. B. Saunders.

Pinna, A. D., Weppler, D., Nery, J., Ruiz, P., Kato, T., Kahn, F., Levi, D., Nishida, S., DeFaria, W., Berho, M., & Tzakis, A. G. (2000). Intestinal transplantation at the University of Miami: Five years of experience. *Transplantation Proceedings, 32*(6), 1226–1227.

Reyes, J., Bueno, J., Kocoshis, S., Green, M., Abu-Elmagd, K., Furukawa, H., Barksdale, E. M., Strom, S., Todo, S., Fung, J. J., Irish, W., & Starzl, T. E. (1998). Current status of intestinal transplantation in children. *Journal of Pediatric Surgery, 33,* 243–254.

Rovera, G. M., DiMartini, A., Schoen, R. E., Rakela, J., Abu-Elmagd, K., & Graham, T. O. (1998). Quality of life of patients after intestinal transplantation. *Transplantation, 66*(9), 1141–1145.

Schuffler, M. D. (1998). Chronic intestinal pseudo-obstruction. In M. Feldman, B. F. Scharschmidt, & M. H. Sleisenger. (Eds.), *Gastrointestinal and liver disease: Pathophysiology, diagnosis, management* (6th ed., pp. 1820–1830). Philadelphia: W. B. Saunders.

Strohm, S. L., Koehler, A. N., Mazariegos, G. V., & Reyes, J. (1999). Nutrition management in pediatric small bowel transplant. *Nutrition in Clinical Practice, 14,* 58–63.

Sudan, D. L., Iverson, A., Weseman, R., Kaufman, S., Horslen, S., Fox, I. J., Shaw, B. W. Jr., & Langnas, A. N. (2000). Assessment of function and quality of life long-term after small bowel transplantation. *Transplantation Proceedings, 32,* 1211–1212.

Sudan, D. L., Kaufman, S. J., Shaw, B. Jr., Fox, I. J., McCashlsand, T. M., Schafer, D. F., Radio, S. J., Hinrichs, S. H., Vanderhoof, J. A., & Langnas, A. N. (2000). Isolated intestinal transplantation for intestinal failure. *American Journal of Gastroenterology, 95*(6), 1506–1515.

Taylor, L. A., & Ross, A. J. (1996). Abdominal masses. In W. A. Walker, P. R. Durie, J. R. Hamilton, J. A. Walker-Smith, & J. B. Watkins (Eds.), *Pediatric gastrointestinal disease: Pathophysiology, diagnosis, management* (2nd ed., vol. 1, pp. 227–240). Philadelphia: W. B. Saunders.

Thompson, J. S., & Langnas, A. N. (2002). Small intestinal insufficiency and the short bowel syndrome. In G. Zindema (Ed), *Shackelford's surgery of the alimentary tract* (5th ed. vol. 5, 295–315). Philadelphia: W. B. Saunders.

Todo, S., Reyes, J., Furukawa, J., Abu-Elmagd, K., Lee, R. G., Tzakis, A., Rao, A. S., & Starzl, T. E. (1995). Outcome analysis of 71 clinical intestinal transplantations. *Annals of Surgery, 222*(3), 270–280.

United Network for Organ Sharing. (2000). *Graft survival rates at three months and at one, three, and five years,* Table 97: Intestinal Transplants. Retrieved May 28, 2001, from http://www.unos.org/Data/anrpt00/ar00_table97_01_in.htm

United Network for Organ Sharing. (2001). *Number of patient registrations on the national transplant waiting list by age.* Retrieved May 28, 2001, from http://www.unos.org/Newsroom/critdata_wait.htm

United Network for Organ Sharing. (2000). *Number of registrations and median waiting times (in days) to transplant: Registrations added during 1990 to 1999.* Retrieved May 28, 2001, from http://www.unos.org/Data/anrpt00/ar00_table100_01_in.htm

United Network for Organ Sharing. (2000). *Patient survival rates at three months and at one, three and five years. Table 98: Intestine Transplants.* Retrieved May 28, 2001, from http://www.unos.org/Data/anrpt00/ar00_table98_01_in.htm

United Network for Organ Sharing. (2001). *Patients on the UNOS National Patient Waiting List.* Retrieved May 28, 2001, from http://www.unos.org/Frame_default.asp?Category=Newsdata

Vanderhoof, J., & Langnas, A. (1997). Short-bowel syndrome in children and adults. *Gastroenterology, 113*(50), 1768–1778.

Wesson, D. E., & Haddock, G. (1996). The intestine Part 1: Congenital abnormalities. In W. A. Walker, P. R. Durie, J. R. Hamilton, J. A. Walker-Smith, & J. B. Watkins (Eds.), *Pediatric gastrointestinal disease: Pathophysiology, diagnosis, management* (2nd ed., vol. 1, pp. 555–563). Philadelphia: W. B. Saunders.

Winter, H. S. (1996). Intestinal polyps. In W. A. Walker, P. R. Durie, J. R. Hamilton, J. A. Walker-Smith, & J. B. Watkins (Eds.), *Pediatric gastrointestinal disease: Pathophysiology, diagnosis, management* (2nd ed., vol. 1, pp. 891–906). Philadelphia: W. B. Saunders.

Zitelli, B. J., Seltman, M. F., & Shannon, M. R. (1987). Münchausen's syndrome by proxy and its professional participants. *American Journal of Diseases in Children, 141*(10), 1099–1102.

12

Islet Cell Transplantation

Linda Ohler and David Harlan

HISTORICAL PERSPECTIVES

Pancreas transplantation has been a treatment option for patients with type 1 diabetes mellitus (T1DM) for approximately 20 years. The procedure currently carries an 80% probability of prolonged insulin independence for at least one year. Pancreas transplantation is a major surgical procedure that carries many potential complications. Approximately 2% of pancreatic cells are needed to control blood sugar, whereas 98% of pancreatic cells function to manufacture and/or deliver digestive enzymes to the gut and play no role in glucose control (Pick & Jameson, 2000). The idea of transplanting only the insulin producing cells has been an attractive one. Thus, transplanting the entire pancreas using highly invasive surgery may not be necessary if islet cell transplantation is effective. Islet cell transplantation could be developed to achieve success commensurate with that of the whole organ transplant without the risks associated with surgery.

Islet cell transplantation has the potential of normalizing blood glucose levels and halting the progression of diabetic complications (Kenyon, Ranucoli, Massetti, Chatzipetrou, & Ricordi, 1998). Islet cell transplantation has been used as an alternative to pancreas transplantation for select patients for over a decade. Although only 8% to 12% of the 405 patients receiving islet cell transplants between 1990 and 2000 achieved insulin independence for more than 1 year, Shapiro and colleagues in Edmonton, Canada, have recently reported improved results (Pick & Jameson, 2000; Shapiro et al., 2000). The Edmonton group adapted the islet cell procedure in at least four ways. First, they modified the islet isolation technique developed by Ricordi Lacy and Scharp (1989) (Hering & Ricordi, 1999). Second, they infused more islets than previous groups have used. Third, they infused the islets immediately following their isolation rather than keeping them in a culture for a period of time. Fourth, they employed a steroid free immunosuppression protocol. Triple therapy immunosuppression regimens utilized in solid organ transplantation often include calcineurin inhibitors and glucocorticoids. These drugs are known to have diabetogenic effects. The Edmonton group therefore surmised the drugs could damage or kill sensitive islet cells. By using a steroid free protocol with low-dose calcineurin inhibitors and sirolimus, researchers are finding improved outcomes for this type of transplant. Although standard therapy for islet cell transplantation is available in transplant centers, the new Edmonton protocol, as it has become to be called, will be tested in select centers in the United States. This research is currently available for type 1 diabetics only. Criteria for islet cell transplant candidates at the National Institutes of Health closely follows that from the Edmonton group.

POTENTIAL CANDIDATES

- Type 1 diabetes mellitus > 5 years
- Brittle diabetes as defined by (any one of the following):
  - Episodes of hypoglycemia unawareness, defined as the inability to sense a low blood sugar until it falls to less than 54 mg/dL
  - Failure of an intensive insulin regimen to adequately control blood sugar levels as judged by an endocrinologist unassociated with the protocol
  - More than two hospitalizations in the past year due to poor glycemia control
  - Progressive secondary complications despite an intensive insulin regimen

CONTRAINDICATIONS TO ISLET
TRANSPLANTATION PROTOCOL

- Obesity, as defined as a body mass index (BMI) greater than 28 kg/m^2
- Cardiac disease

- Evidence of advanced diabetic nephropathy (creatinine clearance less than 60 cc/kg/min or 24 hour urine albumin > 300 mcg/day)
- History of nonadherence
- Liver disease or structural abnormality
- History of malignancy
- Active infection
- Evidence of residual islet cell function
- Anemia or other hematologic abnormality (low platelet or white cell count)
- Pregnant, breastfeeding, or intent for future pregnancy
- Age > 65
- Alcohol, tobacco, or other substance abuse
- Psychological unsuitability for what remains a very experimental procedure
- Insulin requirements of > 0.7iU/kg/day

SCREENING CANDIDATES FOR ISLET CELL TRANSPLANTATION

1. Complete history and physical by transplant physician/primary investigator
2. Routine blood tests
   - Viral studies
3. Routine urine tests
4. Diagnostic tests
   - Abdominal ultrasound
   - Chest X ray
   - Electrocardiogram
   - Arginine-stimulated C-peptide
   - Cortisol test

Once a patient is determined to be good candidate for islet cell transplantation, the patient is listed with the United Network for Organ Sharing (UNOS) according to weight and blood type. When a potential cadaveric donor is identified, the patient is brought to the transplant center and placed on an insulin drip while investigators perform the islet isolation. If an insufficient number of islets is obtained, the insulin drip is discontinued and the patient is sent home on the previous insulin regimen. Patients must be prepared emotionally for this disappointment. A patient may be called to the transplant center several times before there is a sufficient yield of islets for the procedure.

THE ISLET CELL PROCEDURE

The procedure described in this chapter is experimental. The following is an outline of recommended steps.

1. Patient is brought to the hospital and started on an insulin drip.
2. Blood glucose levels are monitored hourly while awaiting islet procurement for the procedure.
3. Ideal pancreata for islet isolations have a cold ischemia time less of than 6 hours. However, cold ischemic times of up to 12 hours are acceptable.
4. Islets are infused as soon as possible following their isolation, but no later than 24 hours after the aortic cross-clamp time.
5. A minimum of 10,000 islet equivalents (IEQ) per kg body weight should be infused. Most likely this will require two separate procedures.
6. For the first islet infusion, at least 4,000 IEQ/kg body weight should be infused. If a second dose is required, then sufficient islets in that second dose are infused to achieve a total transplanted islet mass of 10,000 IEQ/kg body weight.
7. Once islet yield is determined to be sufficient and of good quality, the patient is given low dose tacrolimus and sirolimus orally. Intravenous daclizumab is also given at this time.
8. Prophylactic antibiotics are administered prior to the islet transplant.
9. Patient is transported to special procedures in the radiology department.
10. Patient is given a sedative and local anesthesia.
11. Radiologist cannulates the portal vein using ultrasound guidance.
12. Endocrinologist infuses islet cells into the cannulated vein.
13. Procedure takes about 60 minutes.

Most patients will require islet cells from two donors before insulin independence is achieved. Following the first infusion of islets, the patient usually remains on an insulin drip for 24 hours with hourly blood glucose checks. Once stabilized, the insulin drip can be discontinued. Following the initial islet infusion, the recipient's requirement for insulin is reduced by 33% to 50% in most cases.

Potential Complications of the Procedure
- Bleeding
- Infection
- Spasm or clots in the portal vein
- Moderate discomfort at infusion site
- Damage to liver, gall bladder or intra-abdominal vessels
- Elevation in antibody titres potentially limiting the patient's suitability for future organ transplants

MEDICATIONS

Medications used to suppress the immune system have known side effects (see chapter 4). Conventional immunosuppression has been associated with nephrotoxicity, hypertension, infection, malignancies, and adverse effects on the islet cells. This research is being done without steroids, using low-dose tacrolimus and therapeutic doses of sirolimus.

1. Low-dose tacrolimus. Initially, 1.0 mg bid, then titrate the dose to desired trough levels.
   - Follow trough levels.
   - Maintain levels within 3.0–6.0 ng/mL range.
2. Sirolimus initially at 0.1 mg/kg body weight.
   - Follow trough levels.
   - Maintain levels within 8.0–12.0 ng/mL range.
3. Dacluzimab 1.0 mg/kg body weight IV every other week for a total of 5 doses. Therapy begins immediately prior to the first islet infusion and continues for 4 doses after the infusion. Daclizumab is also given prior to the second infusion of islet cells and continues for 4 doses after the final infusion of cells.
4. CMV prophylaxis: ganciclovir 500 mg tid
5. Mycelex troches or nystatin to prevent thrush
6. PCP prophylaxis: trimethoprim/sulfamethoxazole double strength (DS) 1 tablet 3 times a week for 6 months or inhaled pentamadine monthly.

The second islet infusion follows the same procedure.

MONITORING REJECTION

Determining rejection remains a challenge to clinicians. There are several tests to watch, but none has been determined useful for detecting rejection.

- Elevated blood glucose levels certainly indicate a potential problem
- C-peptide levels
- Hemoglobin A1C

Other experimental assays are being studied.

FOLLOW-UP AFTER THE FIRST INFUSION OF ISLETS

Patients are usually discharged from the hospital within 48 hours after the first islet infusion. This, of course, depends on each individual. Indeed, several patients in Edmonton have had this procedure performed on an outpatient basis (personal communication, James Shapiro, MD, January 2001). Monitoring the patient while awaiting the second infusion includes the following:

- Blood sugars before and 2 hours after every meal as well as before retiring at night
- VS, Weight daily
- Infusions of dacluzimab every other week for a total of 5 doses
- Monitoring tacrolimus and sirolimus levels 2 to 3 times weekly
- Review of medications with each visit
- Observation for signs and symptoms of rejection or infection
- Enoxaparin 30 mg subcutaneously bid for 7 days following the islet infusion to decrease the risk of thrombosis
- Abdominal ultrasound at 12 hours and 1 week after the infusion to insure portal vein patency and rule out subcapsular bleed

SECOND INFUSION OF ISLETS

The same procedure is followed with the second infusion of islet cells as with the first. Timing between infusions is dependent on islet cell availability and may occur within a week or months after the first transplant. Most patients will require insulin while awaiting the second transplant and must be monitored for side effects of immunosuppressive drugs, for infection, and rejection. Patients are admitted to the hospital, started on an insulin drip, and prepared for the second infusion of islets cells. The same procedure is followed as with the first infection. Once the second infusion has occurred, the insulin drip is slowly weaned and the patient may be prepared for discharge.

Long-term follow-up of these patients will include the following:

- Monitoring of immunosuppressive therapy
- Islet cell function
- Monitoring fasting and postprandial blood sugars
- Monitoring for signs of rejection and infection
- Annual routine physicals that include
  - Pap smear and mammogram for women
  - Prostate-specific antigen for men

- Regular dental follow-up
- Annual ophthalmologic evaluation
- Close observation for skin cancers

PATIENT EDUCATION ABOUT SELF-CARE AFTER TRANSPLANTATION

Patients and their families require a strong self-care education program after transplantation. This education begins at the time of evaluation for transplantation and continues throughout the long-term follow-up phases. Every opportunity to interact with the patient should include teaching. Most islet cell recipients and their families are well versed in diabetes, but transplantation brings additional learning needs that include medications, rejection, infection, complications, travel, and return to work. Table 12.1

TABLE 12.1 Education Topics for Patients Being Evaluated for Islet Cell Transplantation

1. Participation in research
2. Informed consent process
3. Goals of islet cell transplantation
4. Current outcomes of islet cell transplantation
5. Candidacy for islet cell transplantation
6. Testing required
7. Being listed for transplantation
   - Role of United Network for Organ Sharing
   - Role of local organ procurement organization
8. Waiting
   - Taking care of yourself
   - Staying in touch with your transplant physician and coordinator
9. The call
   - Being notified that islet cells may be available for you
   - Recognizing that there may be several calls to the hospital before the transplant is done.
10. The transplant
    - Procedure
    - Hospital stay
11. Medications after transplantation
12. Care between transplants
13. The second transplant
14. Long-term follow-up care

includes topics for pretransplant education for patients being evaluated for transplantation. Discharge teaching topics are included on Table 12.2, and long-term follow-up points are covered in Table 12.3.

TABLE 12.2 Topics for Discharge Teaching After the First Islet Cell Transplant

1. Care of the infusion site
2. Medications and side effects
3. Insulin requirements
4. Signs of rejection
5. Signs of infection
6. Preventing infection
    - Foods to avoid (raw fish, raw meat, and raw eggs)
    - Indoor construction
    - Pet sources for infection
    - Family sources of infection
7. When to call the coordinator or transplant physician on call
8. Follow-up schedule after discharge
    - Importance of blood work
    - What is a trough level
    - Timing of blood work
9. Staying prepared for the second transplant
10. Sexual activities after transplantation

TABLE 12.3 Long-term Follow-up Care

1. Continued blood work
2. Monitoring immunosuppression
3. Monitoring daily self care
4. Signs and symptoms of infection and rejection
5. Routine follow-up tests
6. Annual physical exams
7. Sexual activities
8. Traveling after a transplant

CONCLUSIONS

As we continue to examine outcomes related to new methods for islet isolation and transplantation in a steroid free environment, we will also be evaluating the quality of life of patients participating in this protocol. Although initial results are promising, it is much too soon to determine how successful this procedure will be in limiting the requirements for insulin in type 1 diabetics. Primary care physicians, nurses, and endocrinologists in the community are encouraged to work closely with the transplant center in identifying and treating potential complications of this procedure. Contacting the patient's transplant coordinator or physician to report problems or concerns will increase the collaborative process needed in long term follow up of these patients. Transplant centers welcome questions and observations from colleagues in the community.

REFERENCES

Hering, B., & Ricordi, C. (1999). Islet transplantation for patients with type 1 diabetes mellitus. *Graft, 2,* 12.

Kenyon, N. S., Ranuncoli, A., Masetti, M., Chatzipetrou, M., & Ricordi, C. (1998) Islet cell transplantation: Present and future perspectives. *Diabetes Metabolic Reviews, 14*(4), 303–313.

Pick, A., & Jameson, J. L. (2000). Advances in islet cell transplantation: Use of glucocorticoid-free immunosuppressive regimen. Harrison's online www.medscape.com/HOL/articles/2000/10/hol42/ho/42.html/ accessed 10/22/00.

Ricordi, C., Lacy, P. E., & Scharp, D. W. (1989). Automated islet isolation from human pancreas. *Diabetes, 38,* (Suppl. 1), 140–142.

Shapiro, A. M. J., Lakey, J. R. T., Ryan, E. A., Korbutt, G. S., Toth, E., Warnock, G. L., Kneteman, N. M., & Rajotte, R. V. (2000). Islet transplantation in seven patients with type 1 diabetes mellitus using a glucocorticoid-free immunosuppressive regimen. *New England Journal of Medicine, 343*(4), 230–238.

13

Psychosocial Issues

Wayne Paris, Isao Fukunishi, Linda Wright,
Martha Markovitz, and Gayla Calhoun-Wilson

With the introduction of cyclosporine, a new era in transplantation began. Improved immunosuppression was partly responsible for the exponential growth in the number of transplant programs. More importantly, the increased frequency of organ transplantation has been accompanied by improved long-term survival. Despite this improvement, however, many transplant recipients, family members, and living donors are confronted with a number of psychosocial challenges. The purpose of this chapter is to identify salient psychosocial issues associated with the various phases of solid organ transplantation. Pretransplant issues will be discussed in terms of the stressors and coping strategies associated with the evaluation and waiting periods. Recipient issues will be discussed in terms of the early posttransplant phase through long-term adaptation. Psychosocial issues pertaining to living donation will be discussed from the perspectives of both the living donor and the recipient.

PRETRANSPLANT PHASE

STRESSORS

The stressors that patients face during the pretransplant period can be divided into two categories: those associated with the transplant evaluation phase and those pertaining to the waiting period itself.

Transplant Evaluation Phase

Although the evaluation process for each type of organ transplantation is unique, the stressors that confront patients during this time period are often similar. One of the major stressors that patients experience is fear that they will not be accepted for transplantation. As patients undergo the rigorous physiological and psychosocial evaluation process, they may fear that a previously undiagnosed comorbidity will eliminate them from further consideration for transplantation. Patients may be reluctant to report emotional problems out of the mistaken belief that these problems will make them less desirable transplant candidates.

The evaluation process is particularly stressful for patients who have been substance abusers (alcohol, tobacco, or drugs). Many transplant centers require that these patients undergo periodic substance abuse screening; patients are placed on the transplant list only after a documented period of abstinence (e.g., 6 months) (Cupples, 1995).

Transplant Waiting Period

Once they are actually placed on the organ waiting list, many candidates initially experience a period of relief and euphoria. This elation often wanes, however, and anxiety typically increases as the waiting period lengthens and the candidate's physical condition deteriorates. Major stressors associated with this period include:

- Fears regarding physiological well-being (e.g., progressive physical deterioration; fear of developing complications that would result in removal from the waiting list, fear of rehospitalizations, fear of death)
- Inability to work, dependence on others, and spousal role reversal. Patients often try to maintain a positive self-image in face of their decreasing ability to perform their former roles. However, progressive disability often leads to low self-esteem and social isolation.
- Deaths of fellow candidates on the waiting list. Many transplant centers have monthly support group meetings for candidates and, over the course of the waiting period, patients and family members often develop strong bonds with one another.
- Relocation to a distant transplant center. Some patients must make temporary living arrangements to be closer to the transplant center. This relocation may result in prolonged absence from family members, especially school-age children. Candidates often experience guilt about not being able to help their family members at home.

- Guilt about wishing for a donor organ. Some candidates may reinterpret this wish as "wishing for another person's death" and develop feelings of guilt and self-recrimination. Other candidates may fantasize about "drunk drivers" or "donor weather" that increases the risk of automobile accidents and the availability of donor organs. Such thoughts may also precipitate guilt feelings.
- "False alarms." Many candidates are given electronic pagers so that they can be easily contacted by the transplant center when a donor organ becomes available. However, the pager number may be misdialed by other individuals; each time the pager goes off, the candidate immediately thinks "my donor organ has arrived." On other occasions, the candidate may actually be called in to the transplant center, only to be sent home when it is determined that the donor organ is not suitable.
- Sexual dysfunction. Many end-stage diseases and the medications used to treat them cause sexual dysfunction. This dysfunction further impacts the candidate's self-esteem and relationships (Cupples, 1995).

Parents of pediatric transplant candidates face many of the same stressors as adult transplant candidates. Perhaps the most severe stressor, however, is watching the child's condition worsen progressively. Parents are aware of the fact that the sickest children typically receive transplants first; therefore, their child must deteriorate in order to obtain priority status on the waiting list (Gold, Kirkpatrick, Fricker, & Zitelli, 1986).

PRETRANSPLANT PHASE

COPING STRATEGIES

Transplant candidates use a variety of coping mechanisms during the pretransplant period. In general, the larger and more diversified the candidate's repertoire of coping mechanisms, the more successfully the individual can manage the stressors associated with transplantation. A number of studies have examined how transplant candidates cope with the stressors of the pretransplant period. Bright, Craven, and Kelly (1990) noted that formal support groups were useful in helping lung transplant candidates cope with their lack of control. These candidates and family members also used their informal support networks to share information and resources. However, candidates who relied primarily on denial found that this coping mechanism was challenged by frequent contact with other transplant candidates.

In one of the earliest studies of its kind, Cardin and Clark (1985) found that heart transplant candidates used denial to cope with survival statistics by focusing solely on survival rates. Muirhead and colleagues reported that heart transplant candidates used positive coping mechanisms such as maintaining a positive attitude and seeking social support rather than negative coping mechanisms (e.g., confrontation, passive acceptance, or escapism) (Muirhead et al., 1992). In their longitudinal study of coping mechanisms used by heart transplant candidates during the first year on the waiting list, Cupples, Nolan, Augustine, and Kynoch (1998) found that the five most frequently used coping strategies were thinking positively, trying to keep life normal, keeping a sense of humor, praying or trusting in God, and trying to distract oneself.

Stressors during the pretransplant period can challenge even the most well-adapted candidate. Symptoms that the candidate's coping abilities are deteriorating include the following:

- Inability to identify or share feelings
- Inability to use support systems
- Self-deprecating statements
- Feelings of powerlessness, hopelessness, withdrawal, or resignation (Cardin & Clark, 1985)

Prompt referral to a mental health professional may be required to help the candidate whose coping skills are overwhelmed by the magnitude of pretransplant stressors.

RECIPIENT ISSUES

THE EARLY POSTTRANSPLANT PHASE

Particularly in the early posttransplant phase, life may not be as the recipient expected, with some degree of continuing physical disability, vulnerability to infection as a result of immunosuppressant therapy, and periodic physical crises. The early posttransplant phase may be accompanied by delirium, anxiety, depression, or adjustment disorders. Psychotherapeutic approaches to these problems include cognitive, traditional and behavioral therapy as well as psychopharmacologic interventions.

Disorders

Delirium.

Posttransplant delirium and other organic brain syndromes have been reported following heart (Mai, McKenzie, & Kostuk,1986), lung (Craven, 1990), liver (de Groen, Aksamit, Rakela, Forbes, & Drom, 1987), and kidney (Fricchione, 1989) transplantation. Liver transplant recipients appear to be at greatest risk for posttransplant delirium. Initially, episodes of hepatic encephalopathy may place these recipients at increased risk, but neurological functioning usually improves with a well-functioning liver.

The neurological functioning of a transplant recipient may be compromised by a multitude of agents, including steroid therapy used in the treatment of acute rejection (Tarter, Switala, & VanThiel, 1994). The three primary ways in which delirium may present include

- Difficulty with memory and disorientation with little agitation
- Paranoid delusions, fear and hyperalertness with mild agitation
- Psychomotor agitation (Hackett & Cassem, 1987) (see Table 13.1)

Supportive care coupled with a psychiatric assessment and treatment (discussed later in this chapter) should be initiated.

Posttransplant delirium requires energetic intervention when agitation,

TABLE 13.1 Diagnostic Criteria for Delirium due to Multiple Etiologies

A. Disturbance of consciousness (i.e., reduced clarity of awareness of the environment) with reduced ability to focus, sustain, or shift attention

B. A change in cognition (such as memory deficit, disorientation, language disturbance) or the development of a perceptual disturbance that is not better accounted for by a preexisting, established, or evolving dementia

C. The disturbance develops over a short period of time (usually hours to days) and tends to fluctuate during the course of the day.

D. There is evidence from the history, physical examination, or laboratory findings that the delirium has more than one etiology (e.g., more than one etiological general medical condition, a general medical condition plus substance intoxication or medication side effect).

Reprinted with permission from the *Diagnostic and Statistical Manual of Mental Disorders* (4th ed.). Copyright © 1994 American Psychiatric Association.

mood lability, hallucinations, and delusions pose a threat to medical management.

Anxiety and Depression

The incidence of posttransplant anxiety and depression has been well documented (Chacko, Harper, Gotto, & Young, 1996; Jowsey, Bruce, & McGregor, 1994; Popkin, Callies, Colon, Lentz, & Sutherland, 1993; Squire et al., 1995). Patients without any prior history of anxiety and/or depression often will experience fear and vulnerability that challenge the best coping mechanisms. Virtually all of those patients with a pretransplant diagnosis of anxiety or depression will have an exacerbation of symptoms at some point during the transplant process (Paris, Muchmore, Pribil, Zuhdi, & Cooper, 1994).

Anxiety is the affective response to the tension or pressure produced by attitudes that conflict with one's social environment whereas fear is the affective response to an actual external danger (see Table 13.2). An anxious state ranges from unease to terror and panic. Anxiety is the persistent feeling of dread, apprehension, and impending disaster. It is often displaced by the patient from its true source (always unknown) to a more acceptable one.

Paris and colleagues have suggested that an unconscious fear of death among transplant patients produces numerous psychosocial challenges. Few, if any, patients will acknowledge their impending death, but the reality of this possibility will impact their communication and behavior with healthcare providers. The extent to which the patient addresses these challenges will have some impact on their compliance with the medical regimen (Paris, Brawner, Thompson, & Penido, 1997).

Depression is a mood disorder that produces impairment of physical functioning, social functioning, and perceived health; depression may also be associated with increased complaints of pain (Dubovsky & Buzan, 1999). At one extreme depression results in suicide, while at the other it produces dysthymia—a chronic, less severe, nonepisodic form of the disorder (see Table 13.3).

Though often mentioned synonymously, anxiety and depression should be considered as separate, though interrelated, disorders. The relationship between anxiety and depression is complex (Hackett & Cassem, 1987). The overlap makes the distinction between them difficult, but there are differences. Psychomotor retardation, persistent dysphoria, early morning awakening, a sense of hopelessness, and suicidal thoughts are more indicative of depression. Patients with an anxiety disorder have not lost interest in their usual activities, but rather have lost their ability to negotiate them.

TABLE 13.2 Diagnostic Criteria for Generalized Anxiety Disorder

A. Excessive anxiety and worry (apprehensive expectation), occurring more days than not for at least 6 months, about a number of events or activities (such as work or school performance).

B. The person finds it difficult to control the worry.

C. The anxiety and worry are associated with 3 (or more) of the following 6 symptoms (with at least some symptoms present for more days than not for the past 6 months. **Note:** Only one item is required in children.
   • Restlessness or feeling keyed up or on edge
   • Being easily fatigued
   • Difficulty concentrating or mind going blank
   • Irritability
   • Muscle tension
   • Sleep disturbance (difficulty falling or staying asleep, or restless unsatisfying sleep)

D. The focus of the anxiety and worry is not confined to features of an Axis 1 disorder, e.g., the anxiety or worry is not about having a panic attack (as in panic disorder), being embarrassed in public (as in social phobia), being contaminated (as in obsessive-compulsive disorder), being away from home or close relatives (as in separation anxiety disorder), gaining weight (as in anorexia nervosa), having multiple physical complaints (as in somatization disorder), or having a serious illness (as in hypochondriasis), and the anxiety and worry do not occur exclusively during posttraumatic stress disorder.

E. The anxiety, worry, or physical symptoms cause clinically significant distress or impairment in social, occupational, or other important areas of functioning.

F. The disturbance is not due to the direct physiological effects of a substance (e.g., a drug of abuse, a medication) or a general medical condition (e.g., hyperthyroidism) and does not occur exclusively during a mood disorder, a psychotic disorder, or a pervasive developmental disorder.

Reprinted with permission from the *Diagnostic and Statistical Manual of Mental Disorders* (4th ed.). Copyright © 1994 American Psychiatric Association.

TABLE 13.3 Criteria for Major Depressive Episode

A. Five (or more) of the following symptoms have been present during
    the same 2-week period and represent a change from previous func-
    tioning; at least one of the symptoms is either (1) depressed mood
    or (2) loss of interest or pleasure. **Note:** Do not include symptoms
    that are clearly due to a general medical condition, or mood-incon-
    gruent delusions or hallucinations.
    • Depressed mood most of the day, nearly every day, as indicated
       by either subjective report (e.g., feels sad or empty) or observa-
       tion made by others (e.g., appears tearful). **Note:** In children
       and adolescents, can be irritable mood.
    • Markedly diminished interest or pleasure in all, or almost all,
       activities most of the day, nearly every day (as indicated by either
       subjective account or observation made by others)
    • Significant weight loss when not dieting or weight gain (e.g., a
       change of more than 5% of body weight in a month), or
       decrease or increase in appetite nearly every day. **Note:** In chil-
       dren, consider failure to make expected weight gains.
    • Insomnia or hypersomnia nearly every day
    • Psychomotor agitation or retardation nearly every day (observ-
       able by others, not merely subjective feelings of restlessness or
       being slowed down)
    • Fatigue or loss of energy nearly every day
    • Feelings of worthlessness or excessive or inappropriate guilt
       (which may be delusional) nearly every day (not merely self-
       reproach or guilt about being sick)
    • Diminished ability to think or concentrate, or indecisiveness, nearly
       every day (either by subjective account or as observed by others)
    • Recurrent thoughts of death (not just fear of dying), recurrent
       suicidal ideation without a specific plan, or a suicide attempt or a
       specific plan for committing suicide

B. The symptoms do not meet criteria for a mixed episode.

C. The symptoms cause clinically significant distress or impairment in
    social, occupational, or other important areas of functioning.
    • The symptoms are not due to the direct physiological effects of a
       substance (e.g., a drug of abuse, a medication) or a general med-
       ical condition (e.g., hypothyroidism).

continued

TABLE 13.3 *(continued)*

- The symptoms are not better accounted for by bereavement, (i.e., after the loss of a loved one), the symptoms persist for longer than 2 months or are characterized by marked functional impairment, morbid preoccupation with worthlessness, suicidal ideation, psychotic symptoms, or psychomotor retardation.

Reprinted with permission from the *Diagnostic and Statistical Manual of Mental Disorders* (4th ed.). Copyright © 1994 American Psychiatric Association.

They are more likely to report hyperactivity, perceptual distortions, and impatience rather than hopelessness. Both disorders often have antecedents in major life events and their psychosocial stressors may be similar.

Adjustment Disorder

Several investigators have documented the incidence of adjustment disorder among transplant recipients (Dew, Roth, Thompson, Kormos, & Griffith, 1996; Dew et al., 1994).

An adjustment disorder is a stress-related phenomenon in which a stressor results in maladaptation and symptoms that are time-limited (usually less than 6 months) until the stressor is removed or a new state of adaptation has evolved (see Table 13.4). Unlike other psychological diagnoses, there is a known etiology that is central to the diagnosis. Although considered an imprecise term by many, its clinical benefit is that it serves as a diagnosis that can help explain previously unobserved behavior and one that can be modified with information from longer-term evaluation and treatment.

SIDE EFFECTS OF IMMUNOSUPPRESSANT MEDICATIONS

Corticosteroids have a number of significant side effects that may have psychological sequelae. These include facial erythema, increased sweating, dermatologoical petechiae and ecchymoses, weight gain, cushingoid features (adiposity of face, neck, and trunk), fatigue, muscle weakness, insomnia, and mental status changes (behavioral changes, aggression, mood swings, agitation). Similarly, calcineurin inhibitors can cause hirsutism, gum hyperplasia, and tremors (Sollinger & Pirsch, 1996). Although these side effects can adversely affect any transplant recipient's self-image, they are particularly problematic for adolescents.

Typically, the above side effects are most pronounced in the early post-

TABLE 13.4 Diagnostic Criteria for Adjustment Disorders

A. The development of emotional or behavioral symptoms in response
    to an identifiable stressor(s) occurring within 3 months of the onset
    of the stressor(s).

B. These symptoms or behaviors are clinically significant as evidenced
    by either of the following:
    • Marked distress that is in excess of what would be expected from
      exposure to the stressor
    • Significant impairment in social or occupational (academic)
      functioning

C. The stress-related disturbance does not meet the criteria for
    another specific Axis 1 disorder and is not merely an exacerbation
    of a preexisting Axis 1 or Axis 2 disorder.

D. The symptoms do not represent bereavement.

E. Once the stressor (or its consequences) has terminated, the symp-
    toms do not persist for more than an additional 6 months.
    Specify if
    • **Acute:** if the disturbance lasts less than 6 months
    • **Chronic:** if the disturbance lasts for 6 months or longer

Reprinted with permission from the *Diagnostic and Statistical Manual of Mental
Disorders* (4th ed.). Copyright © 1994 American Psychiatric Association.

transplant period when immunosuppressant doses are at their highest levels. Given the particularly adverse effects of corticosteroid therapy, a number of transplant centers have initiated a steroid-weaning program whereby
the corticosteroid dose is gradually tapered and eventually discontinued.
Some recipients, however, cannot tolerate a steroid-free regimen and must
remain on corticosteroid therapy indefinitely.

INTERVENTIONS

Psychotherapeutic Interventions

In transplant medicine, traditional psychotherapy is typically not the opti-
mum treatment option. Classical psychoanalysis requires a significant amount
of time and may induce additional anxiety and fear compared to other therapeutic interventions (e.g., cognitive therapy, behavioral therapy).

In the consultation-liaison psychiatric services, general hospital psychiatrists generally use various individualized psychotherapeutic techniques designed to enhance motivation for transplantation, maintain compliance after a transplant, support family relations, reduce feelings of guilt or anxiety, and alleviate distress. General psychotherapeutic techniques are effective in

- Promoting relaxation training, meditation, and self-hypnosis
- Alleviating guilt feelings
- Providing behavioral treatment for operative phobias and
- Enhancing interpersonal skills and coping strategies in patients with a history of personality disorder (Surman, 1998)

Table 13.5 lists psychotherapeutic interventions for psychiatric and/or psychosocial problems in transplantation.

Psychopharmacologic Interventions—General

Psychopharmacologic interventions for psychiatric and/or psychosocial problems in transplantation are typically based on the principles of consultation-liaison psychiatry in the general hospital setting. However, the metabolism of transplant candidates and recipients may differ significantly from that of other patients. General considerations include the following:

1. The bioavailability of medication may be affected by various factors including
   - The drug's volume of distribution
   - How much of the drug is bound or unbound to plasma proteins
   - How quickly the drug is metabolized into active or inactive metabolites
   - How quickly the drug is cleared
   - Any interactions with other drugs and their metabolic pathways
   - Variations in receptor sensitivity and density (DiMartini & Trzepacz, 1999)
2. First-pass metabolism can contribute a clinically significant but variable role in drug metabolism and may be affected by enzyme activity, plasma protein binding, and gastrointestinal motility.
3. Most psychotropic drugs are highly protein-bound, lipophilic, and metabolized in the liver.

Both hepatic and renal insufficiency can result in reduced levels of serum albumin, thereby increasing the unbound fraction of protein-bound drugs (the free and pharmacologically available fraction) and increasing the risk of side effects or toxicity due to increased drug availability (Levy,

TABLE 13.5 Psychotherapeutic Interventions for Psychiatric and/or Psychosocial Problems in Transplantation

Cognitive therapy
1. Shape or reframe patient reactions to postoperative events
2. Encourage strategies such as self-hypnosis for their relaxation effect.

Traditional therapy
1. Supportive psychotherapy for patients at risk for noncompliance
2. Individual therapy for those with psychiatric disorders
3. Family therapy
4. Group therapy

Behavioral therapy
1. Strategies for aiding patients with postoperative compliance
2. Treatment of anxiety states

1990). Reduced protein-binding during renal failure is most significant for drugs whose normal binding is high.

The cytochrome P-450 isoenzyme system is emerging as a clinically important feature of drug metabolism. For transplant recipients, the specific interactions of the CYP450 3A3/4 are most important due to the metabolism of immunosuppressive medications at this enzyme site, particularly cyclosporine, tacrolimus (FK506) and mycophenolate mofitil. Psychotropic medications that inhibit CYP450 3A3/4 system (e.g., in decreasing order: fluvoxamine, nefazodone, fluoxetine, sertraline, tricyclic antidepressants, paroxetine, and venlafaxine) can increase the serum levels of these drugs.

In patients with liver insufficiency, prudent treatment consists of starting at one half the normal dosage and gradually titrating the dose upward, while monitoring clinical response and side effects. Many patients can achieve clinical response at lower than usual therapeutic dosages. Because of the decreased protein binding associated with renal failure, it is suggested that the drug dosage be decreased by two thirds (Levy, 1990).

In severe heart failure, if there is evidence of passive congestion of the liver, follow the above guidelines for liver insufficiency.

Monoamine oxidase inhibiting (MAOI) antidepressants are felt to be too difficult to manage in transplant candidates/recipients due to possible unanticipated situations that would necessitate the use of anesthesia, narcotic analgesics, or pressor support. In these situations, the concomitant use of a MAOI would be dangerous. The use of reversible MAOIs has not been investigated in transplant recipients.

Psychopharmacologic interventions for psychiatric and/or psychosocial problems are summarized in Table 13.6.

PSYCHOPHARMACOLOGIC INTERVENTIONS—SPECIFIC

Liver Transplantation

Most psychotropic medications undergo hepatic metabolism, i.e., transformation into active or inactive metabolites. Many drugs undergo multistep biotransformation before elimination. The cytochrome P450 enzyme system is considered to be closely related to issues of drug metabolism and enzyme inhibition, competition, and induction.

Hepatic biotransformation of drugs occurs in two phases:

- Phase 1 enzymes are mostly affected by processes that involve the pericentral region: acute viral hepatitis, alcoholic hepatitis, and active cirrhosis (Leipzig, 1990).
- Phase 2 enzymes act on parent drugs (e.g., lorazepam) or metabolites generated from Phase I activity, to conjugate molecules to a more polar and usually inactive compound (Howden, Birnie, & Brodie, 1989).

In cirrhosis, glucuronidation (a conjugation pathway) is actually preserved (Pacifici et al., 1990), so that choosing medications that require only glucuronidation (e.g., oxazepam, lorazepam, morphine) or that do not require phase 1 biotransformation is advantageous. Haloperidol uses phase 1 enzymes (cytochrome P450 3A4 and 2D6) to become reduced-haloperidol that appears to be in equilibrium with haloperidol such that it can transform back to haloperidol, which is then metabolized via glucuronidation before excretion. Thus, it may have advantages when used in patients with cirrhosis.

For therapeutic dosages, the clearance of a drug at steady state can be characterized as being "high" or "low," depending on whether blood flow or enzyme saturation are the rate-limiting factors for hepatic metabolism. The hepatic metabolizing enzyme affinities determine whether drugs are enzyme or flow dependent.

Low-clearance drugs (e.g., diazepam, quinidine, phenytoin) have low hepatic enzyme affinity, saturate the enzymes, and are therefore metabolized more slowly than high-clearance drugs (e.g., beta-blockers, morphine, tricyclics, ketoconazole) that have a high hepatic enzyme affinity and faster metabolism.

TABLE 13.6 Preoperative Psychopharmacologic Interventions for Psychiatric and/or Psychosocial Problems in Organ Transplantation

Anxiolytics
1. Short-acting agents are preferable (lorazepam, oxazepam). Metabolites of long-acting agents may accumulate in patients with renal or hepatic failure.
2. Oxazepam is more readily metabolized by the liver, but dosing must be determined cautiously in patients with hepatic failure or obtundation may result.
3. Watch for excessive sedation and respiratory depression.

Antidepressants
1. Selective serotonin reuptake inhibitors and bupropion are well tolerated in patients with end-organ failure but should be initiated at a low dose.
2. Bupropion and methylphenidate are stimulating and therefore are preferable in patients prone to encephalopathy.
3. Tricyclics are helpful in patients with diabetic neuropathy and may be beneficial for those with insomnia. Start with a low dose, and monitor blood levels.
4. Treatment may be initiated for major or minor depression and should be continued for those on chronic maintenance.
5. Be alert to drug interactions secondary to suppression of the cytochrome p450 system by selective serotonin reuptake inhibitors (SSRIs) and its enhancement by bupropion.

Neuroleptics
1. Haloperidol is preferred in the management of delirium.
2. Maintenance therapy should be continued in those with psychotic disorders.

Mood stabilizers
1. Administer lithium carbonate at a low dose after dialysis in patients with bipolar illness who are receiving dialysis, and check the levels often at first. Be aware of increased toxicity with cyclosporine.
2. Substitute valproate for patients with lithium side effects and those who are lithium nonresponders. Be aware of cytochrome p450 enzyme stimulation and the potential effect on immunosuppressant regimens

Renal Transplantation

Most psychotropic agents are hepatically metabolized; therefore, renal drug clearance will not affect drug elimination unless the drug or its active metabolite is renally cleared (e.g., lithium) and there is renal function impairment or concomitant renal insufficiency (i.e., hepatorenal syndrome) (McLean & Morgan, 1991). Lithium, methylphenidate, and gabapentin are renally cleared; therefore, they can be problematic in renal failure. However, maintenance of stable lithium levels can be achieved even in patients with renal failure on dialysis because lithium is totally dialyzable and can be administered as a single dose after each dialysis. Because of decreased excretion during renal failure, it is generally recommended that dosing intervals be increased (Bennett et al., 1983; Levy, 1990).

In renal failure, both the accumulation of endogenous albumin binding inhibitors and uremia-induced impairment of drug binding affinities for albumin can cause increased free drug concentrations in the plasma, especially for acidic drugs with protein binding greater than 80% (i.e., many psychotropic agents) (Wilkinson, 1983).

Heart Transplantation

In congestive heart failure, drug metabolism and clearance may be decreased due to hypoperfusion of organs (including kidneys and liver) and reduced volume distribution of drugs due to third spacing into interstitial tissues (Shammas & Dickstein, 1988). Reduced blood flow to the liver can lower the metabolism of high clearance drugs. For example, even the short-acting benzodiazepine, midazolam, has reduced clearance in the presence of congestive heart failure (Patel et al., 1990).

Intramuscular injections should be avoided in patients with poor vascular perfusion. Acute hypoxia can also change blood flow dynamics, resulting in decreased drug metabolism as a result of reduced splanchnic blood flow to the liver and reduced renal blood flow (du Souich, McLean, Lalka, Erill, & Gibaldi, 1978).

Tricyclic antidepressants have an alpha-adrenergic blocking activity that can cause orthostatic hypotension. The negative inotropic effects of tricyclic antidepressants are not clinically significant except in severe cardiac failure when the ejection fraction is less than 20%.

Drugs with type 1A antiarrhythmic effects (quinidine-like effects) are contradicted in patients with cardiac conduction disease. After heart transplantation, clinically significant conduction disturbances could occur, unless the patient has a ventricular pacemaker (Kay et al., 1991).

Lung Transplantation

The lungs are known to have CYP450 isoenzymes that may contribute, in a minor way, to drug metabolism (Paine et al., 1996). Similar to platelets and brain tissue, serotonin transporter is expressed on human pulmonary membranes (Suhara et al., 1998). In pulmonary disease, the binding of some drugs to plasma proteins may be increased, thereby lengthening the time course of the drug effect, distribution, and hepatic and renal clearance (du Souich et al., 1978).

Acute hypoxia can reduce splanchnic blood flow to the liver, thereby decreasing drug metabolism, and can reduce renal blood flow (du Souich et al., 1978). Increased pulmonary vascular resistance can lead to decreased cardiac output (cor pulmonale), increased systemic venous pressures, and decreased perfusion of the liver and kidneys.

THE LONG-TERM ADAPTATION PHASE: RECIPIENT ISSUES

A number of psychosocial issues confront transplant recipients during the long-term adaptation phase. These include adherence to the medical regimen, return to work, physical rehabilitation, and psychological stressors.

ADHERENCE: ADULT RECIPIENTS

Most transplant programs expect patients to take their medications, attend clinic appointments, have all laboratory tests and other associated procedures done in a timely manner, follow a prescribed exercise program, abstain from alcohol, illicit drugs, or tobacco products, and in general, follow the prescribed medical regimens (Dew et al., 2000). Unfortunately, recipients often fail to meet these expectations. The causes of medical nonadherence are multifactorial.

Adherence to Medication, Dietary, and Follow-up Regimens

Twenty percent of heart recipients and 50% of kidney recipients have been found to be nonadherent with medications during a given 12-month period (Dew et al., 1996; House & Thompson, 1988; Paris, Muchmore, Pribil, Zuhdi, & Cooper, 1994). One recent study found that medication adherence among liver transplant recipients was directly related to financial factors (Paris, Dunham, Sebastian, Jacobs, & Nour, 1999). If medications were available, liver transplant recipients would take them. However, those patients who relied on public assistance or indigent drug programs were more likely to be noncompliant.

From 3% to 15% of heart transplant recipients fail to regularly keep follow-up appointments and/or have required blood work; 21% to 34% do not monitor vital signs regularly; 18% to 28% fail to follow dietary guidelines; 20% have morbid obesity (DeGeest, 1996; Dew et al., 1996; Paris et al., 1994).

The frequency of each medication dose is a primary factor that affects adherence (Cramer & Rosensheck, 1998). Medication adherence rates have been shown to decrease over time; therefore, there may be an important role for reeducation efforts by all health care providers (Cramer, Mattson, Prevey, Scheyer, & Ouellett, 1989).

Cultural factors may also influence overall adherence. The diagnosis and treatment of a particular ailment may have different meanings and implications for people from different cultural backgrounds. The extent to which a patient fully accepts and endorses a treatment regimen will be seen in the level of adherence. Each of these factors will have some impact on long-term morbidity and/or mortality, although their effects may not become apparent for many years.

Overall, it has been suggested that the best medical adherence rate any program could hope for is 75% to 80% (DeGeest, 1996).

Substance Abuse

Substance abuse has also been an important area of adherence research, particularly the incidence of alcohol abuse in liver transplant patients and smoking in heart patients (Dew et al., 2000). However, the identification of relapse rates for alcohol or tobacco is difficult because of the various criteria used to define, treat, and monitor usage. It has been reported that 11% to 48% of liver transplant recipients return to some level of alcohol consumption during the first year posttransplant; 5% to 10% resume drinking the following year. From 5% to 26% of heart recipients have smoked at least once posttransplant. Patient self-reports, when compared to random urine toxocologies, were unreliable 40% of the time (Paris et al, 2000; Sebastian et al., 2000).

There seems to be no significant differences in substance abuse among heart, lung, or liver transplant recipients. This suggests that an overall substance abuse assessment, treatment, and monitoring program would be appropriate for all types of transplant recipients. Table 13.7 summarizes major psychiatric and psychological factors associated with non-adherence.

TABLE 13.7 Psychiatric and Psychological Factors Associated with Nonadherence

Psychiatric factors
- Cognitive disorders such as delirium and dementia
- Mental retardation
- Schizophrenia
- Manic-depressive disorder
- Substance abuse disorder
- Personality disorder

Psychological factors
- Poor motivation for medical treatment
- Poor understanding of the significance of transplantation
- Strong belief system or inflexible attitude
- Willfulness or low self-efficacy
- Anxiety regarding the medical staff

ADHERENCE: PEDIATRIC RECIPIENTS

Medical adherence in pediatric transplant recipients is a unique challenge. Age of the recipient, strengths and weakness of the family system, financial resources, and community or extended family supports have all been shown to influence clinical outcomes (Rapoff, 1999). As a part of a family system, children are more vulnerable than adults. Pediatric adherence is complex and is associated with the child's developmental stage, the nature of family relationships and peer influences.

RETURN TO WORK

Transplantation survival rates have increased and the morbidity associated with long-term immunosuppressive therapy is decreasing (Cooper & Paris, 1993). The aim of transplantation should be to enable each recipient to return to an active lifestyle, including employment for recipients under retirement age. Unfortunately, this goal has not been achieved; fewer than 50% of recipients deemed medically able to work actually return to successful employment (Paris et al., 1999).

Prior to 1990, posttransplantation employment was considered to be feasible only for those who could return to a pretransplantation job. Multiple barriers were identified that precluded new posttransplantation employment, including

- Changes in priorities whereby patients value family and leisure activities over work
- Hiring discrimination based on medical history
- Restrictive cost or unavailability of workmen's compensation or medical insurance
- Poor local or regional economic conditions
- Limited education and/or work skills (Evans, 1986; Harvison et al., 1988; McBride et al., 1988; Meister, McAleer, Meister, Riley, & Copeland,1986; Niset, Coustry-Degre, & Degre, 1988; Samuelsson, Hunt, & Schroeder, 1984; Shapiro, 1990; Wallwork & Caine, 1985).

As a result, transplant programs frequently were liberal in their support of posttransplantation medical disability and were unlike to encourage patients to return to work.

In a series of studies conducted since 1990, when transplant centers began to focus on patient employment, 10% to 15% of recipients were able to secure new employment. Centers also reported a higher rate of patients returning to their previous employment (Paris et al., 1993; Paris, Tebow, Dahr, & Cooper, 1997).

The most difficult aspect of a patient's rehabilitation is the psychological component (Andrews et al., 1992; Shoemaker, Robin, & Robin, 1992). Before transplant recipients return to their former employment or before they can secure new posttransplantation employment, they must believe they are physically able to work (Grady, Jalowiec, Grusk, White-Williams, & Robinson, 1992; Paris, et al., 1999). Consistently, the patient's perception of physical disability is directly linked to posttransplantation employment status. The discrepancy between the 10% of transplant recipients who meet disability requirements (as determined by physician assessment) and the 40% of patients who perceive they have a work disability is problematic. Whether this reflects a real or imagined incapacity on the part of the transplant recipient is uncertain. As with other chronic illnesses, transplant recipients may not be totally disabled but may have specific physical limitations and complaints that preclude only certain types of work (Paris, et al., 1992).

Potential barriers to employment include the following:

- Depression, fear, or anxiety may limit the patient's capacity to function optimally in a vocational environment (Tarter, Edwards, & Van Thiel, 1994). With posttransplant depression and anxiety rates reported above 50%, psychological evaluation and treatment should be considered for patients whose health perceptions differ significantly from those of the physician (Maricle, Hosenpud, & Norman, 1989).

- Contrary to the fears of most employers, many of the numerous follow-up examinations can be done within the work or training program with minimal disruption. Potentially, the frequency of return visits to the transplant center could be reduced for those patients who are able to follow more detailed instructions and have a local health care provider who could perform part of the follow-up monitoring.
- A pretransplant history of substance abuse may be viewed as a barrier to posttransplant employment. However, having as few as 6 months sobriety or abstinence from alcohol or drugs may have a profound impact on a patient's posttransplant opportunity to obtain, and more importantly, sustain employment (Gish et al., 1993).
- Transplant recipients are typically instructed to avoid extremes of weather and physical exertion, exposure to physical irritants, industrial pollutants, or dust, and employment locations associated with the risk of recurrent infections (e.g., public information desks, cafeterias, and bars). Vocational rehabilitation programs are available for recipients who must learn a new skill in order to obtain employment.
- Posttransplant medication side effects may also pose some employment limitations. Jones, Taylor, and Dip (1990) found that recipients on steroid-free immunosuppressive regimens were more likely to be employed, presumably because they were in better physical condition. Tarter and colleagues (1994) reported that steroids, even in small doses, can exert subtle but detectable effects on cognitive functioning. Furthermore, physical appearance, most notably cushingoid features, obesity, acne, and hirsutism, may exacerbate negative self-appraisal, thereby contributing to social withdrawal.

Employment can offer structure and meaningful activity. Work can provide a sense of purpose that contributes to positive self-esteem, thus enhancing the patient's quality of life. However, unemployed transplant recipients who are experiencing relative satisfaction in their daily lifestyles and activities, along with sufficient financial security, will likely be reluctant to resume employment and disrupt this homeostasis.

PHYSICAL REHABILITATION

Clearly, the pretransplantation physical status of the patient may influence posttransplantation rehabilitation. For example, if a bedridden patient is physically weak at the time of transplantaton, posttransplant physical rehabilitation will be slow, and it is likely that social rehabilitation will be similarly prolonged (Cooper & Paris, 1993). Once transplantation has taken place and the organ is functioning satisfactorily, patients should begin a rapidly progressive physical rehabilitation program (Kempeneers et al., 1988; Noakes & Kempeneers, 1990).

A patient's progress will be limited largely by peripheral muscle strength. If this is depleted from pretransplant inactivity, then rehabilitation may be prolonged (Nicholas, Oleske, Robinson, Switala, & Tartar, 1994). For liver transplant recipients, a persisting encephalopathy, even of a low-grade subclinical severity, may impair concentration and psychomotor capacity and further delay rehabilitation (Tarter et al., 1986). Patients who recover well experience few limitations and are able to resume fairly normal daily activities. However, this positive outcome is often dependent on regular exercise, medication and dietary compliance, and an absence of psychological problems (Kavanagh, 1992).

PSYCHOLOGICAL STRESSORS

Numerous studies have examined the stressors that confront transplant recipients. The most common psychological stressors include fears regarding the following:

- Rejection of the transplanted organ
- Risk of infection
- Uncertainty about the future
- Cost and side effects of medications
- Rehospitalization for complications
- Changes in family responsibilities and spousal role reversal (Cupples, 1995).

Some recipients experience guilt over the fact that "someone had to die" in order for the transplant procedure to take place. The intrapsychic adaptive mechanism of denial may be used to cope with this guilt. For example, denial, directed at either the donated heart or the donor, may be used by heart transplant recipients. Graft denial may be reflected in comments such as "I try to forget about the new heart" or "I have no thoughts about my new heart." Donor denial may be expressed in statements such as "I have not asked where it [the heart] came from" and "I never think about the donor" (Mai, 1986, p. 1160).

PSYCHOSOCIAL ASPECTS OF LIVING DONATION

The success of renal allografts from living, unrelated donors has been found to be almost as good as that from human leukocyte antigen-identical siblings (Terasaki, Cecka, Gjertson, & Takemoto, 1995) and living donation has now expanded to include liver and lung transplantation. The critical shortage of donor organs is a compelling motivation for using living donors to increase the donor pool. Moreover, the development of new surgical techniques has helped to reduce the "costs" associated with living donation. For example, laparoscopic nephrectomy affords the donor a shorter length of stay, a faster recovery period, and reduced time away from work. Along with technological innovations, there has been an expansion in the criteria for suitable living donors.

Parents and siblings were originally considered as the only individuals suitable to donate organs. In recent years, however, friends, marital partners, adult children, and even anonymous individuals have been living donors. As the number of living donors increases, it is important to consider the psychosocial issues associated with living donation—from the perspective of both the donor and the recipient.

LIVING DONORS

The psychosocial dynamics that surround living donation are complex. Donation of a lung or liver lobe may be viewed as "life-saving" when a cadaveric organ is not available. Clearly, these are desperate situations and donors may feel internal or external pressure to donate to avoid the death of another human being. It is essential that transplant teams exercise great care in the identification of potential donors and provide counseling as needed.

Benefits of Living Donation

At present, there is little information on the psychosocial effects of living liver or lung transplant donation; however, the following benefits have been associated with kidney transplantation:

- It is generally accepted that the main psychological benefit to kidney donation is increased self-esteem for the donor (Spital, 1988).
- In a recent study, 90% of living donors indicated that they would make the same choice to donate again (Schrover, Streem, Boparai, Duriak, & Novik, 1997)

- For a family member, kidney donation may have further benefits such as freedom from supporting a dialysis patient, ability to travel more easily, and reduction of family and household responsibilities. If the recipient returns to work posttransplant, family income is increased.
- Living donation may offer an opportunity for the donor to make amends for past deeds or to assume a special place in the family or with the recipient. For example, the "black sheep" of the family may consider donation as a means of improving status within the family, the adult child may wish to try to atone for a troubled adolescence, or the adopted child may view donation as a vehicle for cementing their membership within the adoptive family.

Psychosocial Risks of Living Donation

Although living donation potentially confers many benefits, the following psychosocial risks have been identified:

- Although some living donors may be eligible for medical benefits during the period of hospitalization and postoperative recovery, many donors still incur financial loss due to absence from work. Donors who travel great distances to donate may not receive full compensation for their expenses and may have to depend on fundraising and financial support from friends, family and charitable organizations.
- After transplantation, the shift of attention from the donor to the recipient may increase the risk of donor depression (Kemph, Berman, & Coppolilo, 1969).
- Donors may be at increased risk of depression if the donated organ is rejected (Russell & Jacob, 1993).
- In a 12-year follow-up study of donors, investigators found that 15% of donors believed that donating had negatively affected their health; 23% thought that donation had hurt them financially (Schrover et al., 1997).
- Another study of nearly 600 living kidney donors found that 4% of donors experienced dissatisfaction and regretted that they had donated; 16% found the donation experience to be extremely or very stressful (Johnson et al., 1999).
- Living donors whose recipient died within 12 months of transplantation indicated that they would not donate again if it were possible (Johnson et al., 1999).

RECIPIENTS OF LIVING DONATION

For liver and lung transplant candidates, living donation is truly life-saving. For renal transplant patients, living donation provides a means of avoiding dialysis and its attendant psychosocial sequelae such as work disruption, role changes, financial hardship, anger, denial, and depression. For all organ recipients, living donation offers a means of dealing with problems proactively. The surgery is scheduled, thereby allowing a level of planning and organization of family, financial and work commitments denied to the recipients of cadaveric grafts whose lives are disrupted suddenly when they are called for transplant. Furthermore, the stress and uncertainty of waiting for a transplant is eliminated.

Adolescent Recipients

Adolescents may state very definitively whether they would consider the option of living donation and who would they accept as donors. For example, in a recent study of living donor lung transplant recipients, adolescent candidates expressed moral, social, and pragmatic concerns about potential donors (e.g., accepting an organ from a divorced parent; postlobectomy quality of life of the donor) (Markovitz, Doyle, Shaner, Schuller, & Sweet, 2001). Other psychosocial issues associated with living donation include the following:

- Adolescents may express concerns that the parent who donates will exert a "controlling presence" throughout the transplant process.
- Some adolescents have insisted their parents be the only donors, feeling that sharing the same genetic makeup, as well as spiritual and cultural beliefs, will enhance their chances of posttransplant survival.
- Both male and female adolescents have expressed fear about "owing" their donor.
- Most adolescents express reluctance about their mother donating because they want her to be with them during their surgery and initial recovery.
- Some adolescents may harbor distorted self-images and misperceptions of how their "self" will be altered posttransplant (i.e., a refusal to accept a donor from a "dead person" because they will "become like them").

Adult Recipients

The need for an organ from a living donor raises issues that may change family dynamics and equilibrium forever. Many patients are unable to ask family members to donate an organ; other family members often perform this task. Recipients often struggle to cope with the knowledge that another person underwent surgery, experienced pain and discomfort, and sacrificed part of their body in order to give them life or the chance of a better quality of life.

Although the notion of "gift giving" may be useful in conceptualizing living donation, the gift of an organ may be unique considering the invasiveness of such a procedure, its psychological consequences, and the fact that it cannot be returned.

Much is unknown about how living donation affects the relationships among recipients, their living donors, and other family members. One may speculate that the homeostasis of the family is altered by the event. Avenues for future research include

- Recipients' attitudes toward those family members who did not offer to donate or who proved unsuitable as donors
- Recipients' strategies for coping with feelings of indebtedness toward living donors
- The relationship between living donation and posttransplant compliance with treatment

More information on these and other aspects of living donation will be useful as the number of these donations increases in the future.

CONCLUSION

Transplant recipients, family members, and living donors are often confronted with a number of significant psychosocial issues. This chapter has examined the challenges faced by many transplant recipients in the early posttransplant phase. The major psychological disorders associated with transplantation have been discussed, as well as their respective psychotherapeutic and psychopharmacologic interventions. Recommendations regarding psychotropic medications have been provided. Three major psychosocial issues faced by recipients in the long-term adaptation phase have been discussed (adherence, return to work, and physical rehabilitation). The psychosocial aspects of living donation have been reviewed, both from the perspective of the living donor and the transplant recipient.

Although solid organ transplantation has become an accepted treatment modality for many end-stage diseases, many psychosocial issues are associated with this effective but oftentimes challenging therapeutic option. The interdisciplinary transplant team, in concert with the patient's primary health care providers, can help patients and families cope with these challenges and enjoy the longevity and quality of life that transplantation affords.

REFERENCES

American Psychiatric Association. (1994). *Diagnostic and statistical manual of mental disorders,* 4th ed. Washington, DC: Author.

Andrews, H., Barker, J., Pittman, J., Mars, L., Struening, E., & LaRocca, N. (1992). National trends in vocational rehabilitation: A comparison of individuals with physical disabilities and individuals with psychiatric disabilities. *Journal of Rehabilitation, 58,* 7–16.

Bennett, W. M., Aronoff, G. R., Morrison, G., Golper, T. A., Pulliam, J., Wolfson, M., & Singer, I. (1983). Drug prescribing in renal failure: Dosing guidelines for adults. *American Journal of Kidney Disease, 3*(3), 155–193.

Bright, J. M., Craven, J. L., & Kelly, P. J. (1990). Assessment and management of psychosocial stress in lung transplant candidates. *Health and Social Work, 15,* 125–132.

Cardin, S., & Clark, S. (1985). A nursing diagnosis approach to the patient awaiting cardiac transplantation. *Heart & Lung, 14,* 499–504.

Chacko, R., Harper, R., Gotto, J., & Young, J. (1996). Psychiatric aspects of heart transplantation: Preoperative evaluation and postoperative sequelae. *British Medical Journal, 292,* 311–313.

Cooper, D. K. C., & Paris, W. (1993). Rehabilitation and return to work after cardiac transplantation. In M. Bhannari, S. S. Agarwol, V. K. Kapoor, & P. K. Ghosh (Eds.), *Perspectives on organ transplantation* (pp. 137–140). New Delhi: B. I. Churchill Livingstone.

Cramer, J. A. & Rosenheck, R. (1998). Compliance with medication regimens for mental and physical disorders. *Psychiatric Services, 49,* 196–201.

Cramer, J. A., Mattson, R. H., Prevey, M .L., Scheyer, R. D., & Ouellette, V. L. (1989). How often is medication taken as prescribed? A novel assessment technique. *Journal of the American Medical Association, 261*(22), 3273–3277.

Craven, J. (1990). Psychiatric aspects of lung transplant. The Toronto Lung Transplant Group. *Canadian Journal of Psychiatry, 35*(9), 759–764.

Cupples, S. A. (1995). Stress and coping among transplant patients and their families. In M. T. Nolan & S. M. Augustine (Eds.), *Transplantation nursing: Acute and long-term management* (pp. 45–75). Norwalk, CT: Appleton & Lange.

Cupples, S. A., Nolan, M. T., Augustine, S. M., & Kynoch, D. (1998). Perceived stressors and coping strategies among heart transplant candidates. *Journal of Transplant Coordination, 8*(3), 179–187.

De Geest, S. (1996). Subclinical noncompliance with immunosuppressive therapy in heart transplant recipients: A Cluster analytic study. Doctoral dissertation, Catholic University of Leuven, Belgium.

De Groen, P., Aksamit, A., Rakela, J., Forbes, G., & Drom, R. (1987). Central nervous system toxicity after liver transplantation: The role of cyclosporine and cholesterol. *New England Journal of Medicine, 317,* 861–866.

Dew, M., Roth, L., Thompson, M., Kormos, R., & Griffith, B. (1996). Medical compliance and its predictors in the first year after heart transplantation. *Journal of Heart and Lung Transplantation, 15,* 631–645.

Dew, M., Simmons, R., Roth, L. H., Schulberg, H. C., Thompson, M. D., Armitage, J. M., & Griffith, B. P. (1994). Psychosocial predictors of vulnerability to distress in the year following heart transplantation. *Psychological Medicine, 24*(4), 929–945.

Dew, M., Switzer, G., DiMartini, A., Matukaitis, J., Fitzgerald, M., & Kormos, R. (2000). Psychosocial assessments and outcomes in organ transplantation. *Progress in Transplantation, 10,* 239–261.

DiMartini, A., & Trzepacz, P. T. (1999). Psychopharmacologic issues in organ transplantation. In M. Matsushita, & I. Fukunishi (Eds.), *Cutting-Edge Medicine and Liaison Psychiatry—Psychiatric Problems of Organ Transplantation, Cancer, HIV, and Genetic Counseling* (pp. 111–120). Amsterdam: Elsevier Science Publishers.

du Souich, P., McLean, A. J., Lalka, D., Erill, S., & Gibaldi, M. (1978). Pulmonary disease and drug kinetics. *Clinical Pharmacokinetics, 3,* 257–266.

Dubovsky, S., & Buzan, R. (1999). Mood disorders. In R Hales, S. Yudofsky, & J. Talbott (Eds.), *Textbook of Psychiatry,* (3rd ed., pp. 479–566). Washington, DC: American Psychiatric Press.

Evans, R. W. (1986). The economics of transplantation. *Circulation, 75,* 63–76.

Fricchione, G. (1989). Psychiatric aspects of renal transplantation. *Australian and New Zealand Journal of Psychiatry, 23,* 407–417.

Gish, R. G., Lee, A. H., Keeffe, E. B., Rome, H., Concepcion, W., & Esquivel, C. O. (1993). Liver transplantation for patients with alcoholism and end-stage liver disease. *American Journal of Gastroenterology, 88,* 1337–1342.

Gold, L. M., Kirkpatrick, B. S., Fricker, F. J., & Zitelli, B. J. (1986). Psychosocial issues in pediatric organ transplantation. *Pediatrics, 77,* 738–744.

Grady, K. L., Jalowiec, A., Grusk, B. B., White-Williams, C., & Robinson, J. A. (1992). Symptom distress in cardiac transplant candidates. *Heart & Lung, 21,* 434–439.

Hackett, T., & Cassem, N. (Eds.) (1987). *Handbook of General Hospital Psychiatry.* Littleton, MA: PSG Publishing Company, Inc.

Harvison, A., Jones, B. M., McBride, M., Taylor, F., Wright, F., Wright, O., & Chang, V. P. (1988). Rehabilitation after heart transplantation: The Australian experience. *Journal of Heart Transplantation, 7,* 337–341.

House, R., & Thompson, T. (1988). Psychiatric aspects of organ transplantation. *Journal of the American Medical Association, 160,* 535–539.

Howden, C. W., Birnie, G. G., & Brodie, M. J. (1989). Drug metabolism in liver disease. *Pharmacologic Therapy, 40,* 439–474.

Johnson, E. M., Anderson, J. K., Jacobs, C., Suh, G., Humar, A., Suhr, B. D., Kerr, S. R., & Matas, A. J. (1999). Long-term follow up of living kidney donors: Quality of life after donation. *Transplantation, 67,* 717–721.

Jones, B. M., Taylor, J., & Dip, S. W. (1990). Quality of life after heart transplantation in patients assigned to double or triple-drug therapy. *Journal of Heart Transplantation, 9,* 392–396.

Jowsey, S., Bruce, B., & McGregor, C. (1994). Decreased anxiety in lung transplant recipients. *American Journal of Psychiatry, 151,* 617.

Kavanagh, T. (1992). Physiological and psychological benefits of exercise rehabilitation after cardiac transplantation. In P. J. Walter (Ed.), *Quality of life after open heart surgery* (pp. 404–416). Dordrecht: Kluwer Academic.

Kay, J., Bienenfeld, D., Slomowitz, M., Burk, J., Zimmer, L., Nadolny, G., Maravel, N. T., & Geier, P. (1991). Use of tricyclic antidepressant in recipients of heart transplant. *Psychosomatics, 32*(2), 165–170.

Kempeneers, G. L. G., Myburgh, K. H., Wiggins, T., Adams, V., Van Zyl-Smit, R., & Noakes, T. D. (1988). The effect of an exercise training program on renal transplant recipients. *Transplantation Proceedings, 20,* 381.

Kemph, J. P., Berman, E. A., & Coppolilo, H. P. (1969). Kidney Transplant. *American Journal of Psychiatry, 125,* 39–44.

Leipzig, R. (1990). Psychopharmacology in patients with hepatic and gastrointestinal disease. *International Psychiatry in Medicine, 20,* 109–139.

Levy, N. B. (1990). Psychopharmacology in patients with renal disease. *International Psychiatry in Medicine, 20*(4), 325–334.

McBride, M., Taylor, F., Wright, O., Harvison, A., Jones, B., & Chang, V. (1988). Rehabilitation and employment following heart transplantation (Abstract). *Journal of Heart Transplantation, 7,* 46.

McLean, A. J., & Morgan, D. J. (1991). Clinical pharmacokinetics in patients with liver disease. *Clinical Pharmacokinetics, 21*(1), 42–69.

Mai, F. M. (1986). Graft and donor denial in heart transplant recipients. *American Journal of Psychiatry, 143,* 1159–1161.

Mai, R., Mckenzie, N., & Kostuk, W. (1986). Psychiatric aspects of cardiac transplantation: Preoperative evaluation and postoperative sequelae. *British Medical Journal, 292,* 311–313.

Maricle, R. A., Hosenpud, J. D., & Norman, D. J. (1989). Depression in patients being evaluated for heart transplantation. *General Hospital Psychiatry, 11,* 418–424.

Markovitz, M. S., Doyle, A., Shaner, M. A., & Sweet, S. C., (2001). Pediatric living donor lung transplantation: Psychosocial considerations. (Abstract). *Journal of Heart and Lung Transplantation, 20*(2), 245.

Medical Economics Company (2000). *Physicians' Desk Reference.* 54th ed. Montvale, NJ: Medical Economics Company, Inc.

Meister, N. D., McAleer, M. J., Meister, J. S., Riley, J. E., & Copeland, J. G. (1986). Returning to work after heart transplantation. *Journal of Heart Transplantation, 5,* 154–161.

Muirhead, J., Meyerowitz, B. E., Leedham, B., Eastburn, T. E., Merrill, W. H., & Frist, W. H. (1992). Quality of life and coping in patients awaiting heart transplantation. *Journal of Heart and Lung Transplantation, 11*(2, Pt. 1), 265–271.

Nicholas, J. J., Oleske, D., Robinson, L. R., Switala, J. A., & Tarter, R. (1994). The quality of life after orthotopic liver transplantation: An analysis of 166 cases. *Archives of Physical Medicine Rehabilitation, 75,* 431–435.

Niset, G., Coustry-Degre, I. C., & Degre, S. (1988). Psychosocial and physical rehabilitation after heart transplantation: 1–year follow-up. *Cardiology, 75,* 311–317.

Noakes, T. D., & Kempeneers, G. L. G. (1990). Exercise rehabilitation. In D. K. C. Cooper & D. Novitzky (Eds.), *Transplantation and replacement of thoracic organs* (pp. 233–240). London: Kluwer Academic.

Pacifici, C. M., Viani, A., Franchi, M., Santerini, S., Temellini., A., Giuliani, L., & Carrai, M. (1990). Conjugation pathways in liver disease. *British Journal of Clinical Pharmacology, 30*(3), 427–435.

Paine, M. F., Shen, D. D., Kunze, K. L., Perkins, J. D., Marsh, C. L., McVicar, J. P., Barr, D. M., Gillies, B. S., & Thummel, K. E. (1996). First-pass metabolism of midazolam by the human intestine. *Clinical Pharmacology and Therapeutics, 60*(1), 14–24.

Paris, W., Brawner, N., Thompson, S., & Penido, M. (1997). Psychosocial issues in heart transplantation: A review for transplant coordinators. *Journal of Transplant Coordination, 7*, 88–92.

Paris, W., Dunham, S., Sebastian, A., Jacobs, C., & Nour, B. (1999). Medication nonadherence and its relation to financial barriers. *Journal of Transplant Coordination, 9*, 149–152.

Paris, W., Muchmore, J., Pribil, A., Zuhdi, N., & Cooper, D. K. C. (1994). Study of the relative incidences of psychosocial factors before and after heart transplantation and the influence of posttransplantation psychosocial factors on heart transplantation outcome. *Journal of Heart and Lung Transplantation, 13*, 424–430.

Paris, W., Paradis, I., Nelson, D., Kessinger, S., Tripp, J., Wood, J., Smith, C., Vanhooser, D., & Chaffin, J. (2000). Patient self-report vs toxicology to confirm abstinence from tobacco products, alcohol, or illicit drugs (Abstract). *Journal of Heart and Lung Transplantation, 19*(12), 59–60.

Paris, W., Tebow, S., Dahr, A. S., & Cooper, D. K. C. (1997). Returning to work after heart transplantation-a replication study. *Research on Social Work Practice, 7*, 370–377.

Paris, W., Woodbury, A., Thompson, S. Levick, M., Nothegger, S., Arbuckle, P., Hutkin-Slade, L., & Cooper, D. K. (1992). Social rehabilitation and return to work posttransplant: A multicenter survey. *Transplantation, 53*, 433–438.

Paris, W., Woodbury, A., Thompson, S., Levick, M., Nothegger, S., Arbuckle, P., Hutkin-Slade, L., & Cooper, D. K. (1993). Returning to work after heart transplantation. *Journal of Heart and Lung Transplantation, 12*, 46–54.

Patel, I. H., Soni, P. P., Fukuda, E. K., Smith, D. F., Leier, C. V., & Boudoulas, H. (1990). The pharmacokinetics of midazolam in patients with congestive heart failure. *British Journal of Clinical Pharmacology, 29*(5), 565–569.

Popkin, M. K., Callies, A. L., Colon, E. A., Lentz, R. D., & Sutherland, D. E. (1993). Psychiatric diagnosis and the surgical outcome of pancreas transplantation in patients with type I diabetes mellitus. *Psychosomatics, 34*(3), 251–258.

Rapoff, M. A. (1999). *Adherence to pediatric medical regimens.* New York: Kluwer Academic/Plenum Publishers.

Russell, S., & Jacob, R. G. (1993). Living related organ donation: The donor's dilemma. *Patient Education and Counseling, 21*(1–2), 89–99.

Samuelsson, R. G., Hunt, S. A., & Schroeder, J. S. (1984). Functional and social rehabilitation of heart transplant recipients under age thirty. *Scandinavian Journal of Thoracic and Cardiovascular Surgery, 18*, 97–103.

Schrover, L. R., Streem, S. B., Bopari, N., Duriak, K., & Novick, A. C. (1997). The psychosocial impact of donating a kidney: Long term follow-up from a urology based centre. *The Journal of Urology, 157*, 1596–1601.

Sebastian, A., Carlson, J., Smith, C., Pennington, S., Emmett, C., McMillon, G., Lancaster, M., Sigle, G., Duffy, J., Wright, H., Gurake, A., Jazzar, A., Nour, B., McFadden, R., Guillory, N., & Paris, W. (2000). Liver transplant candidate self-report vs toxicology to confirm abstinence from alcohol, or illicit drugs (Abstract). *Liver Transplantation, 19,* 59–60.

Shammas, F. V., & Dickstein, K. (1988). Clinical pharmacokinetics in heart failure: An updated review. *Clinical Pharmacokinetics, 15,* 94–113.

Shapiro, P. A. (1990). Life after heart transplantation. *Progress in Cardiovascular Disease, 32,* 405–418.

Shoemaker, R. J., Robin, S. S., & Robin, H. S. (1992). Reaction to disability through organization policy: Early return to work policy. *Journal of Rehabilitation, 58,* 18–24.

Sollinger, H., & Pirsch, J. (1996). *Transplantation Drug Pocket Reference Guide,* 2nd ed. Austin, TX: Landes.

Spital, A. (1988). Living kidney donation: Still worth the risk. *Transplantation Proceedings, 20*(5), 1051–1058.

Squire, H., Ries, A., Kaplan, R., Prewitt, L. M., Smith, C. M., Kriett, J. M., & Jamieson, S. W. (1995). Quality of well-being predicts survival in lung transplantation candidates. *American Journal of Respiratory and Critical Care Medicine, 152*(6, Pt. 1), 2032–2036.

Suhara, T., Sudo, Y., Yoshida, K., Okubo, Y., Fukuda, H., Obata, T., Yoshikawa, K., Suzuki, K., & Sasaki, Y., (1998). Lung as reservoir for antidepressants in pharmacokinetic drug interactions. *Lancet, 351*(9099), 332–335.

Surman, O. S. (1998) Approach to the patient undergoing organ transplantation. In T. A. Stern, J. B. Herman, & P. L. Slavin (Eds.), *The MGH guide to psychiatry in primary care* (pp. 401–408). New York: McGraw-Hill.

Tarter, R., Edwards, K., & Van Thiel, D. (1986). Hepatic encephalopathy. In G. Goldstein & R. Tarter (Eds.), *Advances in clinical neuropsychology* (pp. 243–263). New York: Plenum Press.

Tarter, R., Switala, J., & Van Thiel, D. (1994). Psychosocial factors in organ transplantation in adults. In D. Cook & P. Davis (Eds.), *Anesthetic Principles of Organ Transplantation* (pp. 302–340). New York; Raven Press.

Terasake, P. I., Cecka, I. M., Gjertson, D. W., & Takemoto, S. (1995), High survival rates of kidney transplant from spousal and living unrelated donors. *New England Journal of Medicine, 333,* 333–336.

Wallwork, J., & Caine, N. (1985). A comparison of the quality of life of cardiac transplant patients before and after surgery. *Quality of Life and Cardiovascular Care, 2,* 317–33

Wilkinson, G. R. (1983). Plasma and tissue binding considerations in drug disposition. *Drug Metabolism Reviews, 14*(3), 427–465.

14

Pregnancy and Transplantation

Lisa A. Coscia, Carolyn H. McGrory,
Lydia Z. Philips, John M. Davison,
Michael J. Moritz, and Vincent T. Armenti

The first known pregnancy after transplantation occurred in 1958 in a recipient who had received a kidney from her identical twin sister (Murray, Reid, Harrison, & Merrill, 1963). Since then, thousands of pregnancies have been reported in female solid organ recipients via case report, single-center, and registry experiences. When recipients have stable and adequate graft function, pregnancy is generally well tolerated. Each type of organ transplant has its own particular issues and problems. Graft function can deteriorate unexpectedly and irreversibly, even in recipients with previously stable function. No specific pattern of birth defects has been noted among the offspring, although there is a high incidence of prematurity and low birthweight. The overall consensus, therefore, is that pregnancy can be safe in this population, although continued surveillance is needed, especially in light of newer immunosuppressants.

To study posttransplant pregnancies, the National Transplantation Pregnancy Registry (NTPR) at Thomas Jefferson University in Philadelphia, PA began collecting data in 1991 from female transplant recipients who have had pregnancies and male transplant recipients who have fathered pregnancies. Data are collected via questionnaires, telephone interviews, and hospital records. To date, 1,436 recipients have reported 2,140 pregnancies, with 2,185 outcomes, including twins and triplets.

PRE-PREGNANCY ISSUES

RETURN OF FERTILITY

Sexual dysfunction, menstrual abnormalities and amenorrhea are often present in the setting of chronic organ failure. Return of fertility can occur soon after a successful transplant. Normal menstrual cycles and ovulation often quickly resume and conception has occurred shortly after transplant. Recipients in the childbearing years should be given information about appropriate contraception. Pregnancy issues should be reviewed with couples both before and shortly after the transplant procedure, and reiterated at routine follow-up visits. Female recipients may not realize they are now fertile and in need of birth control. There are no grounds for routine sterilization.

BIRTH CONTROL

Oral Contraceptives

Oral contraceptives can cause or aggravate hypertension and thromboembolism, and may also produce subtle changes in the immune system. Interactions with immunosuppressive agents have also been reported, so immunosuppressive drug levels should be monitored. These factors do not necessarily contraindicate their use, but careful surveillance is needed. In particular, liver transplant recipients may be susceptible to cholestatic drug reactions.

Intrauterine Devices

An intrauterine contraceptive device (IUD) may aggravate menstrual problems, which in turn may obscure signs and symptoms of abnormalities of early pregnancy. Increased long-term risks of pelvic infection in an immunosuppressed recipient with an IUD make this method worrisome. Insertion or replacement of an IUD causes bacteremia in at least 1 in every 10 women; therefore, antibiotic coverage at this time should be considered in transplant recipients.

The efficacy of the IUD may be reduced by immunosuppressive and anti-inflammatory agents, possibly due to modification of the leukocyte response. As many women request this method, careful counseling and follow-up are essential.

Barrier Devices

In transplant recipients, male and female condoms are often the contraceptive of choice as they prevent conception and provide protection from sexually transmitted diseases. Other barrier devices include diaphragms and spermacidal creams, foams, tablets, or jellies.

Long-Acting Contraceptives

Long-acting contraceptives such as medroxyprogesterone (Depo-Provera) and levonorgestrel (Norplant), incur the same concerns and side effects as oral contraceptives. However, in the right situation, and with careful monitoring, there is a place for their usage.

PRECONCEPTION GUIDELINES

It is generally thought that with stable graft function, pregnancy does not adversely affect graft function, and the chances for a successful pregnancy and maternal long-term graft survival are good (Davison, 1994). Davison and colleagues' case report of a pregnancy in a renal transplant recipient first presented management guidelines for women before conception, during pregnancy, and at delivery (Davison, Lind, & Uldall, 1976). Current prepregnancy guidelines for female renal transplant recipients are adapted from this case report. These guidelines, which may also be suitable for recipients of other organs, include the following:

- Recipients are advised to wait 1 to 2 years after transplantation before becoming pregnant.
- Immunosuppressive medications should be at maintenance levels. Recommendations regarding newer immunosuppressive medications are evolving.
- Recipients should have good, stable graft function with no recent rejection episodes.
- Medical conditions such as hypertension or diabetes should be well controlled.
- Stature should be compatible with good obstetric outcome.
- There should be no evidence of urinary obstruction on ultrasound.

These guidelines can be utilized for developing a risk assessment profile, but are not exclusive of additional factors that may include abnormal laboratory values, graft dysfunction, or infections such as cytomegalovirus

(CMV) or hepatitis. Data from the NTPR would suggest that female liver transplant recipients with evidence of worsening graft function related to hepatitis are at risk for further deterioration of graft function during pregnancy. Although the numbers are small, female lung transplant recipients may be at an increased risk for serious consequences related to rejection during pregnancy and the postpartum period; however successful cases have been reported to the NTPR. In addition, depending upon the original disease, transplant recipients may wish to consider genetic counseling.

PERIPARTUM ISSUES

In Vitro Fertilization

There have been a few cases of successful in vitro fertilization reported to the NTPR and in the literature, but the experience is limited. (Lockwood et al., 1999).

Peripartum Management of Maternal Comorbid Conditions

Hypertension

Hypertension should be well controlled before conception, and control should be emphasized during prepregnancy counseling.

Certain antihypertensive medications should not be used during pregnancy such as angiotensin-converting enzyme (ACE) inhibitors, due to possible harmful effects on the fetus and neonate including: renal function abnormalities, oligohydramnios, pulmonary hypoplasia, and long-lasting neonatal anuria (Hanssens, Keirse, Vankelecom, & Van Assche, 1991). The use of ACE inhibitors during the second and third trimesters has been associated with injury and even death in the developing fetus (category D third trimester) (*Physicians' Desk Reference,* 2001). Appropriate prepregnancy changes should be made to the antihypertensive regimen.

Close monitoring of the recipient's blood pressure and proteinuria during pregnancy is advisable in this high-risk population, as hypertensive recipients are more likely to develop preeclampsia (Lindheimer, Grunfeld, & Davison, 2000).

Hypertension during pregnancy is common among female recipients reported to the registry.

Diabetes

Diabetes should be under good control prior to conception with close monitoring during pregnancy. Data from the NTPR comparing pregnancies in diabetic kidney recipients to pancreas–kidney recipients indicated that pancreas–kidney recipients were euglycemic and did not require insulin. In this study, the infants born to kidney transplant only diabetic recipients requiring insulin had a higher incidence of newborn complications (Armenti et al., 1997).

Preeclampsia

Preeclampsia complicates 7% to 10% of pregnancies in the general population. Transplant recipients are at an increased risk for preeclampsia with an occurrence rate of 23–38% in female kidney transplant recipients reported to the NTPR. Serum uric acid levels and 24-hour urinary protein excretion may be increased above normal values in renal transplant recipients; therefore, these "markers" of preeclampsia may be misleading (Davison, 1994).

The incidence of preeclampsia reported to the NTPR among pancreas–kidney recipients is 48%. Liver transplant recipients taking cyclosporine microemulsion (Neoral) report a higher rate of preeclampsia (24%) than those taking tacrolimus (Prograf) (5%) (Armenti et al., 2000).

The management of preeclampsia is palliative and may include bed rest and treatment of hypertension. Delivery is the only definitive treatment (Barron, 2000).

Rejection Surveillance and Treatment

Appropriate laboratory values and studies should be monitored during pregnancy to assess graft function. Any change in values warrants further investigation to determine the presence of rejection. In most cases, biopsies may be safely performed. In heart transplant recipients, endomyocardial biopsy guided by echocardiography rather than fluoroscopy may be preferred to prevent radiation exposure to the fetus (Wagoner et al., 1994). Corticosteroids are often used safely for the initial treatment of rejection. Muromonab-CD3 (OKT3) or antilymphocyte globulins have also been used during pregnancy, with no reported malformation pattern in the newborn; however, data are limited (Armenti, Moritz, Jarrell, & Davison, 2000). There are three cases that have been reported to the NTPR of OKT3 use during pregnancy resulting in a livebirth. One kidney recipient was treated in the first trimester, and two recipients (one liver and one pancreas–kidney) were treated in the second trimester.

INFECTION

Infections should be treated with appropriate antibiotics that are deemed safe for use during pregnancy and that do not interact with the patient's immunosuppressants. Registry data indicate that urinary tract infections are the most common type of infections in female kidney transplant recipients. These infections are rarely life-threatening (Armenti, Moritz, & Davison, 1998).

Cytomegalovirus (CMV)

The incidence of CMV infection in the nontransplant recipient population is approximately 0.2% to 2.2% of livebirths. The incidence in the transplant population is unknown. Immunosuppressive therapy predisposes transplant recipients to CMV infection; therefore, recipients should be closely monitored for CMV infection during pregnancy

CMV infection can be difficult to detect; therefore, screening should take place at the onset of the pregnancy and at each trimester (Lindheimer et al., 2000). Positive serology with anti-CMV antibodies denotes prior exposure and low probability of reactivation. Accurate diagnosis of active CMV infection can be obtained from one of three assays performed on blood: (1) shell vial assay for CMV early antigens, (2) CMV antigenemia assay, and (3) PCR for CMV genome.

At least four cases of CMV infection in kidney transplant recipients have been reported to the NTPR. One of these pregnancies resulted in a stillbirth; another in a miscarriage. The other two pregnancies resulted in liveborn infants; one infant required treatment for a CMV-related infection. These mothers were not treated with ganciclovir during the pregnancies.

At least five cases of CMV infection complicating pregnancy have been reported to the NTPR in female liver transplant recipients. Two cases had documented ganciclovir treatment. Both cases resulted in liveborn infants. One infant had no complications; the other infant had pyloric stenosis and bronchopulmonary dysplasia. There is a case report of a liver recipient who received Cytovene (oral ganciclovir) for CMV prophylaxis early in pregnancy; the pregnancy resulted in a 30-week livebirth with no structural malformations (Pescovitz, 1999).

Sequelae of CMV infection in utero or in the newborn include:

- Thrombocytopenia
- Prolonged neonatal jaundice
- Growth retardation
- Microencephaly
- Neurological deficits

Hepatitis

Transplant recipients who develop hepatitis B within 2 months of conception or who are chronically infected may transmit hepatitis B to their offspring. For their offspring, hepatitis B immune globulin (HBIG) and hepatitis B virus vaccine must be given within a few hours of birth. When given within 48 hours, these agents are 90% effective in preventing chronic hepatitis B in infants.

The rate of transmission of hepatitis C infection from mother to child in nontransplant patients is approximately 5% (Conte, Fraquell, Prati, Colucci, & Minola, 2000). There has been no systematic reporting of vertical transmission of hepatitis C to offspring in transplant recipients.

Toxoplasmosis

It is recommended that transplant recipients undergo screening for toxoplasmosis at the beginning of the pregnancy and at each trimester (Lindheimer et al., 2000). The greatest fetal danger from toxoplasmosis occurs when the mother acquires a primary case during the first trimester of pregnancy. However, concerns about other trimesters also exist; infection transmission is more likely to occur when the mother acquires the infection during the third trimester. Pregnancy termination may have to be considered if toxoplasmosis is diagnosed early in pregnancy (Peddler and Orr, 2000).

IMMUNOSUPPRESSION DURING PREGNANCY

The commonly used immunosuppressive drugs and their respective Federal Drug Administration pregnancy categories are listed in Table 14.1. General principles regarding immunosuppression therapy include the following:

- If a recipient is on a stable immunosuppressive regimen, it is generally recommended that the woman remain on that regimen during pregnancy, regardless of each agent's pregnancy category. There is appropriate reluctance to modify the regimen due to the potential adverse effect on graft function.
- There is a low incidence of rejection episodes during pregnancy; therefore, it is recommended that immunosuppression during pregnancy should, at the very least, be continued at maintenance levels.
- Typically, drug levels during pregnancy decrease concomitantly with the increased volume of distribution, altered gut absorption, fetal

TABLE 14.1 Pregnancy Safety Information for Immunosuppressive Drugs Used in Transplantation

	FDA pregnancy category
Corticosteroids (prednisone, methylprednisolone, etc.)	B
Cyclosporine (Sandimmune, Neoral)	C
Tacrolimus, FK506 (Prograf)	C
Sirolimus, rapamycin (Rapamune)	C
Azathioprine (Imuran)	D
Mycophenolate mofetil (CellCept)	C
Antithymocyte globulin (ATGAM, ATG)	C
Antithymocyte globulin (Thymoglobulin)	C
Muromonab-CD3 (orthoclone OKT3)	C
Basiliximab (Simulect)	B
Daclizumab (Zenapax)	C

FDA categories A: controlled studies, no risk
B: no evidence of risk in humans
C: risks cannot be ruled out
D: Evidence of risk
Adapted from *Graft 2000, vol. 3,* 12–16.

drug metabolism, and other metabolic alterations. Drug doses and levels must be reassessed after delivery. Some practitioners have chosen to maintain constant doses of immunosuppression throughout pregnancy while others have adjusted doses depending on measured drug levels.

- Of the newer immunosuppressive drugs, mycophenolate mofetil (CellCept), a category C agent, has generated greater concern because animal reproductive studies appear to show a potential for fetal malformations. The NTPR has received reports of exposure to mycophenolate mofetil in eleven pregnancies in female kidney transplant recipients. Among the seven offspring of these pregnancies, there were 2 infants with structural malformations. In 29 pregnancies fathered by male transplant recipients taking mycophenolate mofetil at the time of conception, there were no major complications among 29 live-born children (Armenti et al., 2000).

COLLABORATION WITH THE HIGH-RISK OBSTETRICAL TEAM

Pregnancies among transplant recipients should always be regarded as high-risk cases, and multidisciplinary teamwork is essential to ensure a good outcome for mother and child. Management requires attention to serial assessment of organ function, blood pressure control, and diagnosis and treatment of rejection, infection and pre-eclampsia. Meticulous serial fetal surveillance is essential. It is also essential to carefully review the mother's emotional attitude and the overall support she receives from her partner and family.

INTRAPARTUM PERIOD

METHOD OF DELIVERY

General

- Unless there are specific indications for induction of labor, spontaneous onset of labor can be awaited. Cesarean section is only necessary for purely obstetric reasons.
- The reported cesarean section incidences range from 25% to 57% in the NTPR database. This is certainly much higher than the general population and may reflect a "fear of the unknown," rather than certainty that vaginal delivery would be hazardous (see Tables 14.2–14.4).
- Pelvic problems should be recognized during pregnancy so that delivery by cesarean section, when necessary, can be planned
- Pain relief during delivery is provided as for healthy women.

Renal Transplant Recipients

- Vaginal delivery does not cause mechanical injury to the kidney allograft, nor does the allograft obstruct the birth canal.
- For cesarean section, a lower uterine segment approach is usually feasible, but previous surgery may make this difficult. For pelvic grafts (kidney, pancreas), care must be taken that the graft, its blood supply, and ureter (or duodenal segment) are not damaged or compromised.
- Renal transplant recipients may have pelvic osteodystrophy related to previous renal failure and dialysis or prolonged steroid therapy. If there is any question of cephalopelvic disproportion or kidney compression, at 36 weeks gestation an ultrasound may be performed.

TABLE 14.2 NTPR Female Kidney Recipients—CsA (304 Recipients, 456 Pregnancies), Neoral (56 Recipients, 68 Pregnancies), Tacrolimus (19 Recipients, 23 Pregnancies)

	CsA	*Neoral*	*tacrolimus*
Maternal factors			
Mean transplant to conception interval	3.1 years	4.7 years	2.4 years
Hypertension during pregnancy	62%	70%	48%
Diabetes during pregnancy	12%	9%	17%
Graft dysfunction during pregnancy	11%	0%	9%
Infection during pregnancy	22%	29%	32%
Rejection episode during pregnancy	4%	3%	17%
Preeclampsia	27%	23%	38%
Creatinine (mean) mg/dL Before pregnancy	1.4	1.3	1.4
During pregnancy	1.4	1.4	1.9
After pregnancy	1.6	1.5	1.8
Graft loss within 2 years of delivery	8%	1.8%	10.5%
Outcomes (*n*)*	(465)	(71)	(24)
Therapeutic abortions	8%	1.4%	0%
Spontaneous abortions	13%	17%	29%
Ectopic	0.70%	0%	0%
Stillborn	3%	1.4%	0%
Live births	75%	80%	71%

continued

TABLE 14.2 *(continued)*

	CsA	*Neoral*	*tacrolimus*
Live births (*n*)	(350)	(57)	(17)
Gestational age (mean)	35.9 weeks	35.8 weeks	33.0 weeks
Premature (< 37 weeks)	52%	51%	63%
Birthweight (mean)	2485 g	2449 g	2151 g
Low birthweight (< 2,500 g)	46%	54%	63%
Cesarean-section	51%	48%	44%
Newborn complications	40%	49%	53%
Neonatal deaths (within 30 days of birth)	1%	0%	6%

CsA = Sandimmune brand cyclosporine.
Neoral = Neoral brand cyclosporine.
Tacrolimus = Prograf (FK506).
* Includes twins, triplets.
Adapted from *Clinical Transplants, 1999.*

Antibiotic Prophylaxis and Pulse Steroids

All surgical procedures with risk of bacteremia should be covered by pro-phylactic antibiotics. Current practice is to augment steroids to cover the stress of delivery; however, the necessity of this is questionable. (Bromberg et al., 1995)

OUTCOMES

PREGNANCY

Ectopic Pregnancy

There may be an increased risk of ectopic pregnancy in this population, especially in kidney recipients, because of previous pelvic surgery and/or sequelae of peritoneal dialysis.

Ectopic pregnancy may also be difficult to diagnose in both kidney and pancreas–kidney recipients as the symptoms may be mistaken for a trans-plant-related problem (Davison, 1994).

TABLE 14.3 NTPR Pregnancy Outcomes in Female Recipients of Other Organs

	Pancreas–Kidney (27)	Heart (24)	Lung (10)
Maternal factors			
Hypertension during pregnancy	82%	47%	64%
Diabetes during pregnancy	0%	2%	18%
Infection during pregnancy	58%	14%	18%
Rejection episode during pregnancy	9%	24%	36%
Preeclampsia	48%	10%	0%
Graft loss within 2 years of delivery	19%	0%	30%
Outcomes (n)[1]	(37)	(43)	(11)
Therapeutic abortions	8%	12%	36%
Spontaneous abortion	8%	21%	9%
Ectopic	3%	2%	0%
Stillbirth	0%	0%	0%
Live births	81%	65%	55%
Live births (n)	(30)	(28)	(6)
Gestational age (mean)	34 weeks	37 weeks	34 weeks
Premature (< 37 weeks)	80%	43%	67%
Birthweight (mean)	2,075 g	2,703 g	2,149 g
Low birthweight (< 2,500 g)	67%	36%	67%

continued

TABLE 14.3 *(continued)*

	Pancreas– Kidney (27)	Heart (24)	Lung (10)
Cesarean-section	57%	29%	50%
Newborn complications	57%	29%	83%
Neonatal deaths (within 30 days of birth)	3%[2]	0%	0%
Immunosuppression during pregnancy[3]			
CsA, aza, prednisone	51%	70%	55%
CsA, prednisone	17%	14%	9%
Neoral, aza, prednisone	17%	7%	9%
Neoral, prednisone	3%	0%	0%
tacro, aza, prednisone	6%	5%	18%
tacro, aza	3%	0%	0%
tacro, prednisone	0%	2%	0%
tacro alone	0%	2%	9%

[1] Includes twins.
[2] One neonatal death due to sepsis.
[3] CsA—Sandimmune, aza—azathioprine, tacro—tacrolimus.
Adapted from *Clinical Transplants, 1999.*

Therapeutic Abortion

The incidence of therapeutic abortion has decreased over time. This decrease may be due to greater familiarity with transplant pregnancies and/or improvement in management (Davison, 1994).

Spontaneous Abortion

The incidence of spontaneous abortion reported to the registry varies between 9% and 29%, depending on the organ transplanted (Tables

TABLE 14.4 NTPR Pregnancy Outcomes in Neoral or Tacrolimus-based Female Liver Recipients

	Neoral *(n = 14)*	*tacrolimus* *(n = 15)*
Maternal factors		
Hypertension during pregnancy	50%	24%
Diabetes during pregnancy	0%	14%
Graft dysfunction during pregnancy	6%	24%
Infection during pregnancy	29%	10%
Rejection episode during pregnancy	6%	14%
Preeclampsia	24%	5%
Graft loss within 2 years of delivery	8%	0%
Outcomes (n)	(18)	(21)
Therapeutic abortions	0%	0%
Spontaneous abortion	28%	19%
Ectopic	0%	0%
Stillbirth	0%	5%
Live births	72%	76%
Live births (n)	(13)	(16)
Gestational age (mean)	37 weeks	37 weeks
Premature (< 37 weeks)	46%	31%
Birthweight (mean)	2,565 g	3,069 g
Low birthweight (< 2500 g)	42%	19%
Cesarean-section	25%	31%
Newborn complications	23%	38%
Neonatal deaths (within 30 days of birth)	0%	0%

Adapted from *Clinical Transplants, 1999.*

14.2–14.4). They may not represent the true incidence in the transplant population, as a registry does not capture every pregnancy.

Stillbirth

In developed countries, the stillbirth rate has been reported at 7 to 12 per 1,000 births (Beischer, Mackay, & Colditz, 1997). Some stillbirths have been reported among transplant recipients; however, because the registry is voluntary and not inclusive of all births, the true incidence of stillbirths is not known (see Tables 14.2–14.4).

Live Births

- The majority of pregnancies result in a healthy live birth, although many babies are born preterm and may also be small for gestational age.
- Low birth weight is common among offspring of all types of female organ transplant recipients.
- Low birth weight has been reported to occur in 32% to 67% of live births, depending on the organ transplanted and the immunosuppressive regimen.
- Preterm birth is defined as gestational age of less than 37 weeks. Mean preterm gestational age ranges from 34 weeks in lung and pancreas–kidney transplant recipients to 37 weeks in heart transplant recipients.
- Although the majority of infants reported to the NTPR have birth weights appropriate for gestational age, there are some reports of intrauterine growth retardation.

Multiple Births

Although multiple births are not common, both twin and triplet births have been reported to the NTPR.

NEONATAL MORBIDITY AND MORTALITY

Morbidity—Infection

There have been few infections reported in infants born to female transplant recipients. Infections were generally not life-threatening and responded to appropriate antibiotics.

Mortality

Very few neonatal deaths have been reported to the NTPR (see Tables 1–3). The most common cause of death in these infants was severe prematurity. A few interesting cases are presented below.

- There were two neonatal deaths reported in the group of female kidney transplant recipients receiving cyclosporine (Sandimmune). Neither woman reported rejection or preeclampsia during pregnancy. In the first case, the mother noted decreased fetal movement at 29 weeks gestation and a cesarean section was performed. An 800 g infant was delivered with multiple complications including respiratory distress syndrome, patent ductus arteriosus, renal failure and asphyxia and died after 3 days. In the second case, premature rupture of the membranes occurred at 26 weeks and a 921 g infant was delivered. The neonate died at 13 days of life with an atrial septal defect, hyaline membrane disease, sepsis, and adrenal insufficiency.
- In a third case, a neonate was born to a pancreas–kidney recipient whose pregnancy occurred 1.4 years posttransplant with a prepregnancy creatinine of 1.2 mg/dL. Immunosuppression during pregnancy included cyclosporine (Sandimmune), azathioprine (Imuran), and prednisone. At 26 weeks gestation, a cesarean section was performed due to worsening preeclampsia. A 624 g infant was delivered. A maternal kidney biopsy performed at the time of cesarean section demonstrated an acute cellular rejection, for which the mother was subsequently treated. The neonate appeared to progress and was weaned from ventilatory support, but died of sepsis at 14 days of age.
- In a fourth case previously reported by Vyas and colleagues (1999), a kidney transplant recipient conceived twins at 2.9 years posttransplant, with a prepregnancy creatinine of 2.3 mg/dL. Her immunosuppression regimen included tacrolimus (Prograf), prednisone, and azathioprine (Imuran). Azathioprine was discontinued at 10 weeks gestation. No rejection episodes were reported during pregnancy. At 32 weeks gestation, an emergency cesarean section was performed for fetal distress and pregnancy-induced hypertension. The twins had birth weights of 1,055 g (twin A) and 1,445 g (twin B). At 12 hours of life, twin A required ventilatory support, continued to decline, and subsequently died at 3 days of age. Autopsy indicated thrombotic cardiomyopathy and extensive pulmonary hemorrhage as the causes of death. Twin B survived after a prolonged hospitalization. At last follow-up, ventilator-induced asthma-like symptoms were reported, although expected to resolve.

These few reports illustrate the high-risk nature of pregnancy in transplant recipients.

POSTPARTUM PERIOD ISSUES

BREAST-FEEDING

The current opinion is that women taking immunosuppressive medications should not breast-feed. However, given the lack of long-term studies of the effects of the relatively high in utero exposure to immunosuppressive agents, some clinicians believe that the documented benefits of breast-feeding outweigh the theoretical risks of relatively low drug exposure via breast milk. Prednisolone and prednisone are believed to be safe for breast-feeding mothers to take, as less than 0.1% of an infant's therapeutic dose is received by the nursing baby (Davison, 1994; Ito, 2000). Experience with breast-feeding while on azathioprine-based regimens is limited, but there were no adverse events reported in eight cases (Grekas, Vasiliou, & Lazarides, 1984; Nyberg, Haljamae, Frisenette-Fich, Wennergren, & Kjellmer, 1998).

For the calcineurin inhibitors (cyclosporine and tacrolimus [Prograf]), the two areas of concern are immunosuppression and neonatal nephrotoxicity (Armenti, Herrine, Radomski, & Moritz, 2000). There have been a small number of women, both in the literature and reported to the NTPR, who have chosen to breast-feed with no adverse effects reported in the infants (Nyberg et al., 1998). To adequately counsel recipients on this subject, further study is warranted, as there has been no long-term follow-up of these children.

BIRTH CONTROL

Postpartum counseling should include education for the resumption of contraception.

SUBSEQUENT BIRTHS

When additional pregnancies are considered, the general prepregnancy guidelines noted above are again appropriate. Ehrich and colleagues (1996), in a study of first and subsequent pregnancies among 102 female kidney transplant recipients, found that the two groups were similar with respect to mean gestational age (36 weeks), birth weight (2,490 g first pregnancy, 2,587 g subsequent pregnancy), neonatal mortality (4%), and incidence of congenital abnormalities (5% first pregnancy, 3% subsequent pregnancies). These investigators concluded that a subsequent pregnancy does not appear to be deleterious to the graft or infant. Data in the NTPR also support this conclusion for recipients with stable graft function.

REJECTION SURVEILLANCE

Those recipients who have had rejection episodes during pregnancy are more likely to have postpartum rejection and should be very closely monitored during this period. In a recent NTPR study of 10 liver transplant recipients (11 pregnancies) with biopsy-proven acute rejection during pregnancy, 5 (45%) women had a rejection episode within 3 months postpartum (Armenti et al., 2000).

IMMUNOSUPPRESSION POSTPARTUM

Recipients require frequent monitoring to restabilize doses of immunosuppressive medications that may have changed during pregnancy. Healthcare professionals should be alert to the possibility that recipients may have altered or stopped their immunosuppression regimens during and/or after the pregnancy. The NTPR has received reports of recipients with postpartum depression who have discontinued their immunosuppression agents. In a few cases, this has resulted in maternal death. Postpartum depression may have greater risks and may tend to be overlooked in this population. The high-risk nature of these pregnancies justifies continued close surveillance, not only during the pregnancy, but in the immediate postpartum period as well.

CHILDHOOD OUTCOMES

Overall, with few exceptions, the majority of children of transplant recipients are consistently reported as healthy and developing well. There have been no malformation patterns noted in their offspring. In an NTPR report of an ongoing study of 175 offspring born to 133 recipients taking cyclosporine (Sandimmune), only 3 children (1.7%) had major disabilities (Stanley et al., 1999). It will be important to continue to study these children to determine if age-related developmental delays or other problems with fertility or immune function develop later in life.

OUTCOMES OF PREGNANCIES FATHERED BY MALE RECIPIENTS

The NTPR has reported that male transplant recipients have fathered pregnancies with outcomes, complication rates and malformations that appear to be similar to those of the general population (Ahlswede, Ahlswede, Jarrell, Moritz, & Armenti, 1994). In 1999, the NTPR reported on 29 fathered pregnancies with mycophenolate mofetil exposure; there were no malformations reported among the 29 children (Armenti et al, 2000). Overall, the outcomes of pregnancies fathered by male transplant recipients appear to be excellent, but continued study is needed.

ACKNOWLEDGMENTS

The authors are indebted to the recipients, physicians, and transplant coordinators who have contributed their time and information to the registry. For further information, please call the NTPR at (215) 955-2840, fax (215) 923-1420, or e-mail NTPR.Registry@mail.tju.edu.

The NTPR is supported by grants from Novartis Pharmaceuticals Corp., Fujisawa Healthcare, Inc. Roche Laboratories Inc., and Wyeth-Ayerst Pharmaceuticals, Inc.

REFERENCES

Ahlswede, K. M., Ahlswede, B. A., Jarrell, B. E., Moritz, M. J., & Armenti, V. T. (1994). *National Transplantation Pregnancy Registry: Outcomes of pregnancies fathered by male transplant recipients*. In D. R. Mattison and A. F. Olson (Eds.), *Male mediated developmental toxicity* (pp. 335–338). New York: Plenum Press.

Armenti, V. T., McGrory, C. H., Cater, J., Radomski, J. S., Jarrell, B. E., & Moritz, M. J. (1997). The National Transplantation Pregnancy Registry: Comparison between pregnancy outcomes in diabetic cyclosporine-treated female kidney recipients and CyA-treated female pancreas-kidney recipients. *Transplantation Proceedings, 29,* 669–670.

Armenti, V. T., Moritz, M. J., & Davison, J. M. (1998). Medical management of the pregnant transplant recipient. *Advances in Renal Replacement Therapy, 5*(1), 14–23.

Armenti, V. T., Wilson, G. A., Radomski, J. S., Moritz, M. J., McGrory, C. H., & Coscia, L. A. (2000). *Report from the National Transplantation Pregnancy Registry (NTPR): Outcomes of pregnancy after transplantation.* In J. M. Cecka and P. I. Tarasaki (Eds.), *Clinical transplants 1999,* p. 111–119. Los Angeles, CA: UCLA Tissue Typing Laboratory.

Armenti, V. T., Moritz, M. J., Jarrell, B. E., & Davison, J. M. (2000). Pregnancy after transplantation. *Transplantation Reviews, 14*(3), 145–157.

Armenti, V. T., Herrine, S. K., Radomski, J. S., & Moritz, M. J. (2000). Pregnancy after liver transplantation. *Liver Transplantation, 6*(6), 671–685.

Barron, W. M. (2000). Hypertension. In W. M. Barron and M. D. Lindheimer (Eds.), *Medical disorders during pregnancy* (3rd ed., pp. 39–70). St. Louis: Mosby.

Bromberg, J. S., Baliga, P., Cofer, J. B., Rajagopalan, P. R., & Friedman, R. J. (1995). Stress steroids are not required for patients receiving a renal allograft and undergoing operation. *Journal of the American College Surgeons, 180,* 532–536.

Beischer, N. A., Mackay, E. V., & Colditz, P. (1997). Perinatal mortality. In N. A. Beischer, E. V. Mackay, and P. Colditz (Eds), *Obstetrics and the Newborn* (pp. 141–150). London: W. B. Sanders.

Case, A. M., Weissman, A., Sermer, M., & Greenalatl, E. Successful twin pregnancy in a dual-transplant couple resulting from in vitro fertilization and intracyto-plasmic sperm injection: Case Report. *Human Reproduction, (2000), 15*(3), 626–628.

Conte, D., Fraquell, M., Prati, D., Colucci, A., & Minola, E. (2000). Prevalence and clinical course of chronic hepatitis C virus (HCV) infection and rate of vertical transmission in a cohort of 15,250 pregnant women. *Hepatology, 31,* 751–755.

Davison, J. M. (1994). Pregnancy in renal allograft recipients: problems, prognosis and practicalities. In J. M. Davision and M. D. Lindheimer (Eds.), *Bailliere's clinical obstetrics and gynaecology* (pp. 501–525). London: Bailliere Tindall.

Davison, J. M., Lind, T., & Uldall, P. R. (1976). Planned pregnancy in a renal transplant recipient. *British Journal of Obstetrics and Gynaecology, 83,* 518–527.

Ehrich, J. H. H., Loirat, C., Davison, J. M., Rizzoni, G., Wittkop, B., Selwood, N. H., & Mallick, N. P. (1996). Repeated successful pregnancies after kidney transplantation in 102 women (Report by the EDTA Registry). *Nephrology Dialysis Transplantation, 11,* 1314–1317.

Grekas, D. M., Vasiliou, S. S., & Lazarides, A. N. (1984). Immunosuppressive therapy and breast-feeding after renal transplantation. *Nephron, 37,* 68.

Hanssens, M., Keirse, M. J. N. C., Vankelecom, F., & Van Assche, F. A. (1991). Fetal and neonatal effects of treatment with angiotensin-converting enzyme inhibitors in pregnancy. *Obstetrics and Gynecology, 78,* 128–135.

Ito, S. (2000). Drug therapy for breast-feeding women. *New England Journal of Medicine, 343,* 118–126.

Lindheimer, M. D., Grunfeld, J. P., & Davison, J. M. (2000). Renal disorders. In W. M. Barron and M. D. Lindheimer (Eds.), *Medical disorders during pregnancy* (3rd ed., pp. 39–70). St. Louis: Mosby.

Lockwood, G. M., Redger, W. L., & Barlow, S. H. (1995). Successful pregnancy outcome in a renal transplant patient following in vitro fertilization. *Human Reproduction, 10*(6), 1528–1530.

Murray, J. E., Reid, D. E., Harrison, J. H., & Merrill, J. P. (1963). Successful pregnancies after human renal transplantation. *New England Journal of Medicine, 269,* 341–343.

Nyberg, G., Haljamae, U., Frisenette-Fich, C., Wennergren, M., & Kjellmer, I. (1998). Breast-feeding during treatment with cyclosporine. *Transplantation, 65,* 253–255.

Peddler, S. J., & Orr, K. E. (2000). Bacterial, fungal and parasitic infections. In W. M. Barron & M. D. Lindheimer (Eds.), *Medical disorders during pregnancy* (3rd ed., pp, 411–465). St. Louis: Mosby.

Pescovitz, M. D. (1999). Absence of teratogenicity of oral ganciclovir used during early pregnancy in a liver transplant recipient. *Transplantation, 67,* 758–759.

Physicians' desk reference. (2001). Montvale, NJ: Medical Economics.

Stanley, C. W., Gottlieb, R., Zager, R., Eisenberg, J., Richmond, R., Moritz, M. J., & Armenti, V. T. (1999). Developmental well-being in offspring of women receiving cyclosporine post-renal transplant. *Transplantation Proceedings, 31,* 241–242.

Vyas, S., Kumar, A., Piecuch, S., Hidalgo, G., Singh, A., Anderson, V., Markell, M.S., & Baqi, N. (1999). Outcome of twin pregnancy in a renal transplant recipient treated with tacrolimus. *Transplantation, 67*(3), 490–492.

Wagoner, L. E., Taylor, D. O., Olsen, S. L., Price, G. D., Rasmussen, L. G., Larsen, C. B., Scott, J. R., & Renlund, D. G. (1994). Immunosuppressive therapy, management, and outcome of heart transplant recipients during pregnancy. *Journal of Heart and Lung Transplantation, 12*(6), 993–999.

Appendix

Review of Transplant Immunology for Community Health Care Providers

Linda Ohler

PRE-TRANSPLANT IMMUNOLOGY

Most transplant candidates must be evaluated from an immunologic perspective to determine compatibility with potential donors and to determine if there are any reactive antibodies. This practice varies among transplant centers and is often dependent on the organ being transplanted. Because of the costs associated with immunologic testing, it is usually reserved until after the patient is accepted as a candidate for transplantation. Important testing of the immune system for solid organ transplantation includes

- Panel of reactive antibodies (PRA)
- HLA tissue typing
- Cross-matching
  - Retrospective cross-matching
  - Prospective cross-matching

PANEL OF REACTIVE ANTIBODIES (PRA)

This test is done on most candidates accepted for solid organ transplantation. Results are reported in percentages with the normal value being

0%. Elevations in antibody levels indicate the presence of preformed cyto-toxic antibodies that are likely to be reactive with donor lymphocytes. Factors that may contribute or cause a rise in this value include a history of:

- Blood transfusions
- Pregnancies
- Previous transplants
- Connective tissue disease
- Mechanical assist devices used as a bridge to cardiac transplantation

It has been recommended that candidates have repeated PRA levels on a weekly or monthly basis if the level is greater than 10%. Most transplant programs recommend prospective cross-matching when a candidate for transplantation demonstrates a PRA > 10% to 15% (Smith, Danskine, Laylor, Rose, & Yacoub, 1993). This, again, varies from center to center and with the organ being transplanted.

FREQUENCY OF PRA TESTING

- Most renal transplant candidates send PRA samples to the transplant center monthly.
- Candidates with a PRA > 10% to 15% may also have monthly speci-mens sent to the transplant center.
- Cardiac transplant candidates who are being supported with mechan-ical assist devices often have a weekly PRA specimen to check PRA and to be available for prospective crossmatching.

ROLE OF THE HEALTH CARE PROVIDER IN THE COMMUNITY

Send PRA specimens (5–10 mL red top tube) to the transplant center.

- Most transplant centers provide transplant candidates with the spec-imen tube for the blood sample and a mailing container.
- Frequency of specimens to be mailed is determined on an individ-ual basis and is communicated to referring/community physicians and dialysis centers.

CROSS-MATCHING TRANSPLANT CANDIDATES AND DONORS

Alloreactive antibodies in transplant candidates have been studied for their impact on long term outcomes of the graft including acute, chronic, and hyperacute rejection (Zachary & Hart, 1997; Leech et al., 1996; Zachary, Griffin, Lucas, Hart, & Leffell, 1995; Lazda, 1994; Gammie et al., 1997). Cross-match testing was established in transplantation once clinicians recognized that a positive cross-match was associated with hyperacute rejections. Federal regulations now require cross-match tests for donor-reactive alloantibodies on all patients. Testing is done either prospectively or retrospectively

Prospective cross-matching is done prior to the actual transplant. In this way, it can be determined that levels of cytotoxic antibodies are or are not directed towards donor lymphocytes. Prospective cross-matching is performed

- Most commonly in renal transplantation
- In candidates demonstrating an elevation in PRA

Retrospective cross-matching is done after the transplant is performed. This is a common practice in heart, lung, liver, and islet cell transplantation when the patient has a PRA level < 10%.

RISKS OF ALLOANTIBODIES

The presence of alloantibodies in candidates for transplantation presents certain risks for transplantation:

- The transplant may be delayed by months or even years (Glotz et al., 1993)
- Graft survival is affected (Smith et al., 1993; Leech et al., 1996; Kerman et al., 1996)

TREATMENT OF ALLOANTIBODIES

Suppression of HLA specific alloantibodies has been attempted with varying degrees of success prior to transplantation (Glotz et al., 1996; Shweitzer et al., 2000; Massad et al., 1997). Current treatment interventions to decrease alloantibodies include single or combination therapies of the following:

- Plasmapheresis
- IVIg
- Cyclophosphamide
- Mycophenolate mofetil
- Calcineurin inhibitors
- Steroids

Decisions about treatment interventions are often made after discussions with the immunologist. Determinations are based on the types of alloantibodies present. For instance, IgG antibodies present a greater challenge than IgM antibodies. In candidates for cardiac transplantation, a highly sensitized patient may undergo treatment with plasmapheresis, cyclophosphamide and IVIg while awaiting a suitable donor heart. Because the PRA level may fluctuate between treatments, some transplant programs have performed plasmapheresis during the actual transplant with subsequent treatments post transplantation (Tsau et al., 1998).

REJECTION AFTER TRANSPLANTATION

There are several types of rejection possible after solid organ transplantation.

1. Hyperacute rejection usually occurs within minutes to a few days posttransplantation. This form of rejection is rare now that cross-match testing for preformed antibodies is done.
2. Acute rejection occurs most frequently in the first 6 months after transplantation and is treated with steroids. If acute rejections episodes persist or do not respond to steroid therapy, monoclonal or polyclonal antibody therapies are used.
3. Acute rejections are mediated by lymphocyte infiltrations in the transplanted organ.
4. Chronic rejection occurs over time and often involves the intimal layers of vessels causing ischemia in the transplanted organ.
5. Humoral rejection is also called vascular rejection. This form of rejection is much more difficult to detect and to treat. Special immunofluorescence stains on tissue from the biopsy of the transplanted organ may suggest the presence of humoral rejection. Treatment includes plasmapheresis, cyclophosphamide, and IVIg. However, the effectiveness of these treatment interventions has had varying reports of success (Montgomery et al., 2000; Grauhan et al., 2001)

EACH ORGAN TRANSPLANTED HAS METHODS
FOR DETECTING REJECTION

1. The endomyocardial biopsy has been the gold standard for cardiac transplantation and is performed on a center specific protocol.
2. Renal transplant biopsies are done when there are elevations in serum creatinine. Some transplant centers are tracking beta-2 microglobulins as a precursor to a rise in serum creatinine.
3. Liver rejection may be determined by elevations in laboratory testing including bilirubin, AST, ALT, GGT, alkaline phosphatase, and INR. Ultrasound of the liver may be used to evaluate the biliary ducts. A liver biopsy may be indicated to confirm rejection.
4. Lung rejection is often difficult to differentiate from infection. A decrease in spirometry may be an indicator of lung rejection or infection. Lung biopsies can be performed with bronchoscopy but may ultimately require the open lung route to truly determine rejection.
5. Islet cell and pancreas rejection continue to challenge clinicians in terms of developing standardized, proven diagnostic criteria. Currently, changes in blood glucose levels are followed closely. Pancreas recipients are observed for rises in serum amylase and lipase levels. Islet cell function is, at this time, determined through C-peptide tracking with arginine stimulation testing.

ROLE OF THE PRIMARY CARE OR COMMUNITY HEALTH CARE PROVIDERS

Many transplant recipients are followed by primary care physicians and nurses in their home communities. Working closely with the recipient's transplant center facilitates the care of the patient and increases the chances for improving outcomes. Referring recipients back to the transplant center with symptoms of rejection or infection improve the likelihood of positive outcomes. Early recognition of potential problems and communication with the transplant center allows for early interventions. It is not uncommon for a patient to require follow-up treatments for rejection or infection in the community. The following treatments have been provided in the community through collaborative efforts between primary physicians, emergency room personnel, home health nurses, and the transplant center staff:

- Antirejection treatment with intravenous steroids
- Intravenous antibiotic therapy

- Antiviral therapies such as intravenous immunoglobulins and ganciclovir
- Tissue biopsies (with tissue being sent to the transplant center for histopathology)
- Laboratory testing

A positive outcome for transplant recipients frequently depends on effective communication between the transplant center and community physicians.

REFERENCES

Gammie, J. S., Pham, S. M., Colson, Y. L., Kawai, A., Keenan, R. J., Weyant, R. J., & Griffith, B. P. (1997). Influence of panel-reactive antibody on survival and rejection after lung transplantation. *Journal of Heart and Lung Transplantation, 16*(4), 408–415.

Glotz, D., Haymann, J. P., Sansonetti, N., Francois, A., Menoyo-Calonge, V., Bariety, J., & Druet, P. (1993). Suppression of HLA-specific alloantibodies by high dose intravenous immunoglobulins (IVIg). *Transplantation, 56*(2), 335–337.

Grauhan, O., Knosalla, C., Ewert, R., Hummel, M., Loebe, M., Weng, Y., & Hetzer, R. (2001). Plasmapheresis and cyclophosphamide in the treatment of humoral rejection after heart transplantation. *Journal of Heart and Lung Transplantation, 20*(3), 316–321.

Kerman, R. H., Susskind, B., Buelow, R., Regan, J., Pouletty, P., Williams, J., Gerolami, K., Kerman, D., Katz, S. M., VanBuren, C. T., & Kahan, B. D. (1996). Correlation of Elisa—detected IgG and IgA anti-HLA antibodies in pre-transplant sera with renal allograft rejection. *Transplantation, 62*(2), 201–205.

Lazda, V. A. (1994). Identification of patients at risk for inferior renal allograft outcome by a strongly positive B cell flow cytometry cross-match. *Transplantation, 57*(6), 964–969.

Leech, S. H., Mather, P. J., Eisen, H. J., Pina, I. L., Margulies, K. B., Bove, A., & Jeevanandam, V. (1996). Donor-specific HLA antibodies after transplantation are associated with deterioration in cardiac function. *Clinical Transplantation, 10*, 639–645.

Massad, M. G., Cook, D. J., Schmitt, S. K., Smedira, N. G., McCarthy, J. F., Vargo, R. L., & McCarthy, P. M. (1997). Factors influencing HLA sensitization in implantable LVAD recipients. *Annals of Thoracic Surgery, 64*(4), 1120–1125.

Montgomery, R. A., Zachary, A. A., Racusen, L. C., Leffell, M. S., King, K. E., Burdick, J., Maley, W. R., & Ratner, L. E. (2000). Plasmapheresis and intravenous immune globulin provides effective rescue therapy for refractory humoral rejection and allows kidneys to be successfully transplanted into cross-match positive recipients. *Transplantation, 70*(6), 887–895.

Schweitzer, E. J., Wilson, J. S., Fernandez-Vina, M., Fox, M., Gutierrez, M., Wiland, A., Hunter, J., Farney, A., Philosophe, B., Colanna, J., Jarrell, B. E., & Bartlett,

S. T. (2000). A high panel-reactive antibody rescue protocol for cross-match positive live donor kidney transplants. *Transplantation, 70*(10), 1531–1536.

Smith, J. D., Danskine, A. J., Laylor, R. M., Rose, M. L., & Yacoub, M. H. (1993). The effect of panel reactive antibodies and the donor specific cross-match on graft survival after heart and heart-lung transplantation. *Transplant Immunology, 1*(1), 60–65.

Tsau, P. H., Arabia, F. A., Toporoff, B., Paramesh, V., Sethi, G. K., & Copeland, J. G. (1998). Positive panel reactive antibody titers in patients bridged to transplantation with a mechanical assist device: Risk factors and treatment. *American Society of Artificial Internal Organs (ASAIO) Journal, 44*(5), 634–637.

Zachary, A., Griffin, J., Lucas, D. P., Hart, J., & Leffell, M. S. (1995). Evaluation of HLA antibodies with the PRA-STAT test. *Transplantation, 60*(12), 1600–1606.

Zachary, A., & Hart, J. (1997). Relevance of antibody screening and cross-matching in solid organ transplantation. In M. S. Leffel, A. D. Donnenberg, & N. R. Rose (Eds.), *Handbook of human immunology*. Boca Raton and New York: CRC Press.

Index